Advances in Glaucoma Management and Intraocular Pressure Physiology

Advances in Glaucoma Management and Intraocular Pressure Physiology

Guest Editor
Kevin Gillmann

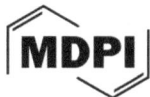

Basel • Beijing • Wuhan • Barcelona • Belgrade • Novi Sad • Cluj • Manchester

Guest Editor
Kevin Gillmann
Genève Ophtalmologie
Geneva
Switzerland

Editorial Office
MDPI AG
Grosspeteranlage 5
4052 Basel, Switzerland

This is a reprint of the Special Issue, published open access by the journal *Journal of Clinical Medicine* (ISSN 2077-0383), freely accessible at: https://www.mdpi.com/journal/jcm/special_issues/U0751L8G0M.

For citation purposes, cite each article independently as indicated on the article page online and as indicated below:

Lastname, A.A.; Lastname, B.B. Article Title. *Journal Name* **Year**, *Volume Number*, Page Range.

ISBN 978-3-7258-3375-7 (Hbk)
ISBN 978-3-7258-3376-4 (PDF)
https://doi.org/10.3390/books978-3-7258-3376-4

Cover image courtesy of Kevin Gillmann

© 2025 by the authors. Articles in this book are Open Access and distributed under the Creative Commons Attribution (CC BY) license. The book as a whole is distributed by MDPI under the terms and conditions of the Creative Commons Attribution-NonCommercial-NoDerivs (CC BY-NC-ND) license (https://creativecommons.org/licenses/by-nc-nd/4.0/).

Contents

About the Editor vii

Preface ix

Murray Johnstone, Chen Xin, Elizabeth Martin and Ruikang Wang
Trabecular Meshwork Movement Controls Distal Valves and Chambers: New Glaucoma Medical and Surgical Targets
Reprinted from: *J. Clin. Med.* **2023**, *12*, 6599, https://doi.org/10.3390/jcm12206599 1

Philip Keye, Daniel Böhringer, Alexandra Anton, Thomas Reinhard and Jan Lübke
Comparison between Intraocular Pressure Profiles over 24 and 48 h in the Management of Glaucoma
Reprinted from: *J. Clin. Med.* **2023**, *12*, 2247, https://doi.org/10.3390/jcm12062247 32

Kangyi Yang, Zhiqiao Liang, Kun Lv, Yao Ma, Xianru Hou and Huijuan Wu
Anterior Segment Parameter Changes after Cataract Surgery in Open-Angle and Angle-Closure Eyes: A Prospective Study
Reprinted from: *J. Clin. Med.* **2022**, *12*, 327, https://doi.org/10.3390/jcm12010327 38

Seung Hyen Lee, Tae-Woo Kim, Eun Ji Lee and Hyunkyung Kil
Association between Optic Nerve Sheath Diameter and Lamina Cribrosa Morphology in Normal-Tension Glaucoma
Reprinted from: *J. Clin. Med.* **2023**, *12*, 360, https://doi.org/10.3390/jcm12010360 50

Peter Wostyn
Could Young Cerebrospinal Fluid Combat Glaucoma? Comment on Lee et al. Association between Optic Nerve Sheath Diameter and Lamina Cribrosa Morphology in Normal-Tension Glaucoma. *J. Clin. Med.* 2023, *12*, 360
Reprinted from: *J. Clin. Med.* **2023**, *12*, 3285, https://doi.org/10.3390/jcm12093285 60

Seung Hyen Lee, Tae-Woo Kim, Eun Ji Lee and Hyunkyung Kil
Reply to Wostyn, P. Could Young Cerebrospinal Fluid Combat Glaucoma? Comment on "Lee et al. Association between Optic Nerve Sheath Diameter and Lamina Cribrosa Morphology in Normal-Tension Glaucoma. *J. Clin. Med.* 2023, *12*, 360"
Reprinted from: *J. Clin. Med.* **2023**, *12*, 3784, https://doi.org/10.3390/jcm12113784 63

Yosuke Ueno, Yusuke Haruna, Mami Tomita, Atsushi Sakai, Shogo Ogawa and Shigeru Honda
The Effectiveness of Pattern Scanning Laser Trabeculoplasty as an Additional Treatment for the Patients of Open-Angle Glaucoma Receiving Full Ocular Hypotensive Medications
Reprinted from: *J. Clin. Med.* **2024**, *13*, 3266, https://doi.org/10.3390/jcm13113266 65

Brenda Nana Wandji, Noélie Bacq and Adèle Ehongo
Efficacy and Safety of Rho Kinase Inhibitors vs. Beta-Blockers in Primary Open-Angle Glaucoma: A Systematic Review with Meta-Analysis
Reprinted from: *J. Clin. Med.* **2024**, *13*, 1747, https://doi.org/10.3390/jcm13061747 72

Yu Mizuno, Kaori Komatsu, Kana Tokumo, Naoki Okada, Hiromitsu Onoe, Hideaki Okumichi, et al.
Safety and Efficacy of the Rho-Kinase Inhibitor (Ripasudil) in Bleb Needling after Trabeculectomy: A Prospective Multicenter Study
Reprinted from: *J. Clin. Med.* **2023**, *13*, 75, https://doi.org/10.3390/jcm13010075 85

Yusuke Orii, Eriko Kunikane, Yutaka Yamada, Masakazu Morioka, Kentaro Iwasaki, Shogo Arimura, et al.
Ocular Distribution of Brimonidine and Brinzolamide after Topical Instillation of a 0.1% Brimonidine Tartrate and 1% Brinzolamide Fixed-Combination Ophthalmic Suspension: An Interventional Study
Reprinted from: *J. Clin. Med.* **2023**, *12*, 4175, https://doi.org/10.3390/jcm12134175 98

Qëndresë Daka, Maja Sustar Habjan, Andrej Meglič, Darko Perovšek, Makedonka Atanasovska Velkovska and Barbara Cvenkel
Retinal Ganglion Cell Function and Perfusion following Intraocular Pressure Reduction with Preservative-Free Latanoprost in Patients with Glaucoma and Ocular Hypertension
Reprinted from: *J. Clin. Med.* **2024**, *13*, 1226, https://doi.org/10.3390/jcm13051226 110

Qëndresë Daka, Nina Špegel, Makedonka Atanasovska Velkovska, Tjaša Steblovnik, Miriam Kolko, Burim Neziri and Barbara Cvenkel
Exploring the Relationship between Anti-VEGF Therapy and Glaucoma: Implications for Management Strategies
Reprinted from: *J. Clin. Med.* **2023**, *12*, 4674, https://doi.org/10.3390/jcm12144674 122

Ioannis Halkiadakis, Kalliroi Konstantopoulou, Vasilios Tzimis, Nikolaos Papadopoulos, Klio Chatzistefanou and Nikolaos N. Markomichelakis
Update on Diagnosis and Treatment of Uveitic Glaucoma
Reprinted from: *J. Clin. Med.* **2024**, *13*, 1185, https://doi.org/10.3390/jcm13051185 132

Charlotte L. L. I. van Meerwijk, Astrid B. Edema, Laurentius J. van Rijn, Leonoor I. Los and Nomdo M. Jansonius
Goniotomy for Non-Infectious Uveitic Glaucoma in Children
Reprinted from: *J. Clin. Med.* **2023**, *12*, 2200, https://doi.org/10.3390/jcm12062200 152

Hyun Jee Kim, Mi Sun Sung and Sang Woo Park
Factors Associated with Visual Acuity in Advanced Glaucoma
Reprinted from: *J. Clin. Med.* **2023**, *12*, 3076, https://doi.org/10.3390/jcm12093076 161

About the Editor

Kevin Gillmann

Dr. Kevin Gillmann is an ophthalmologist, glaucoma specialist, and researcher with a career spanning multiple countries. After training at world-leading institutions such as Moorfields Eye Hospital and Stanford University, he currently serves as Medical Director of Genève Ophtalmologie in Switzerland.

Dr. Gillmann holds qualifications from renowned institutions, including the universities of Newcastle (MBBS), Lausanne (MD), Kingston (PhD), and Harvard (PgCert). Recognized among the top 0.5% global experts in glaucoma by ExpertScape, he is dedicated to advancing care and research in the field.

A prolific contributor to the scientific community, Dr. Gillmann has authored over 50 peer-reviewed articles and edited the *Elsevier* textbook "The Science of Glaucoma Management". His work focuses on minimally invasive glaucoma surgery (MIGS), intraocular pressure physiology, neuroprotection, and personalized medicine, with groundbreaking studies featured in journals such as Nature's *Eye* and the *British Journal of Ophthalmology*. As Chief Medical Officer of PeriVision, he further contributes to advancing glaucoma care through the development of novel visual field technologies. His contributions have been recognized with awards and funding from organizations such as the BrightFocus Foundation and the Swiss Glaucoma Research Foundation.

Dr. Gillmann is also a passionate educator. He has taught at the University of Liverpool and the University of London, where he lectures on quality improvement in healthcare services and was awarded a prize for academic excellence. Beyond ophthalmology, he explores the intersections of hospital design and patient care through architectural research. An architect by training, he holds a Master of Architecture (MArch) from Paris and an MBA from the University of London. His multidisciplinary expertise underscores his holistic approach to healthcare, blending clinical proficiency with innovative strategies to improve system design and patient experience.

Preface

We are pleased to present the reprint of *"Advances in Glaucoma Management and Intraocular Pressure Physiology"*, a collection of cutting-edge research addressing some of the most pressing questions and unmet needs in glaucoma care. This Special Issue was developed to advance our understanding of glaucoma pathophysiology, particularly intraocular pressure (IOP) dynamics, and to foster innovative approaches to treatment and management.

The articles in this reprint cover a range of topics, from novel insights into aqueous outflow physiology to pressure-independent neuroprotective therapies and new IOP measurement strategies. Featured studies explore Schlemm's canal physiology, the efficacy of newer therapeutics like Rho-kinase inhibitors, the role of pattern scanning laser trabeculoplasty, and the relationship between cerebrospinal fluid dynamics and glaucoma progression. Additionally, unique perspectives on pediatric and uveitic glaucoma management, as well as advances in imaging and diagnostics, are highlighted.

We extend our gratitude to the authors for their invaluable contributions, the reviewers for their insightful feedback, and the editorial team of the *Journal of Clinical Medicine* for their unwavering support. We hope this Special Issue serves as a valuable resource for clinicians, researchers, and educators striving to enhance the care and quality of life of those affected by glaucoma.

Kevin Gillmann
Guest Editor

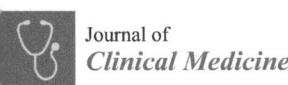

Review

Trabecular Meshwork Movement Controls Distal Valves and Chambers: New Glaucoma Medical and Surgical Targets

Murray Johnstone [1,*], Chen Xin [2,3], Elizabeth Martin [4] and Ruikang Wang [1,5]

1. Department of Ophthalmology, University of Washington, Seattle, WA 98195, USA; wangrk@u.washington.edu
2. Beijing Tongren Eye Center, Beijing Institute of Ophthalmology, Beijing 100730, China; xinchen0322@ccmu.edu.cn
3. Beijing Tongren Hospital, Capital Medical University, Beijing 100730, China
4. Department of Ophthalmology, Indiana University School of Medicine, Indianapolis, IN 46202, USA; martin.elizabethann@gmail.com
5. Department of Bioengineering, University of Washington, Seattle, WA 98195, USA
* Correspondence: murrayj2@uw.edu

Abstract: Herein, we provide evidence that human regulation of aqueous outflow is by a pump-conduit system similar to that of the lymphatics. Direct observation documents pulsatile aqueous flow into Schlemm's canal and from the canal into collector channels, intrascleral channels, aqueous veins, and episcleral veins. Pulsatile flow in vessels requires a driving force, a chamber with mobile walls and valves. We demonstrate that the trabecular meshwork acts as a deformable, mobile wall of a chamber: Schlemm's canal. A tight linkage between the driving force of intraocular pressure and meshwork deformation causes tissue responses in milliseconds. The link provides a sensory-motor baroreceptor-like function, providing maintenance of a homeostatic setpoint. The ocular pulse causes meshwork motion oscillations around the setpoint. We document valves entering and exiting the canal using real-time direct observation with a microscope and multiple additional modalities. Our laboratory-based high-resolution SD-OCT platform quantifies valve lumen opening and closing within milliseconds synchronously with meshwork motion; meshwork tissue stiffens, and movement slows in glaucoma tissue. Our novel PhS-OCT system measures nanometer-level motion synchronous with the ocular pulse in human subjects. Movement decreases in glaucoma patients. Our model is robust because it anchors laboratory studies to direct observation of physical reality in humans with glaucoma.

Keywords: aqueous valves; aqueous outflow pump; intraocular pressure; aqueous outflow; pulsatile flow; tissue biomechanics; trabecular meshwork; Schlemm's canal valves; intraocular pressure regulation; MIGS

1. Introduction

1.1. A New Model of Aqueous Outflow Regulation

This article reviews evidence that the aqueous outflow and vascular systems use similar physiologic mechanisms to control pressure and flow. We describe pulsatile aqueous outflow in normals that is absent in humans with glaucoma [1–3]. (Video 1) shows pulsatile aqueous outflow [4]. Figure 1 demonstrates pump-like behavior that controls intraocular pressure (IOP) by regulating the pulsatile stroke volume of aqueous discharge (Figure 1). (Video 2) shows stroke volume regulation of IOP [4]. Table 1 describes the contents of videos documenting aqueous flow and motion, which are dynamic behaviors not easily captured in text and static figures.

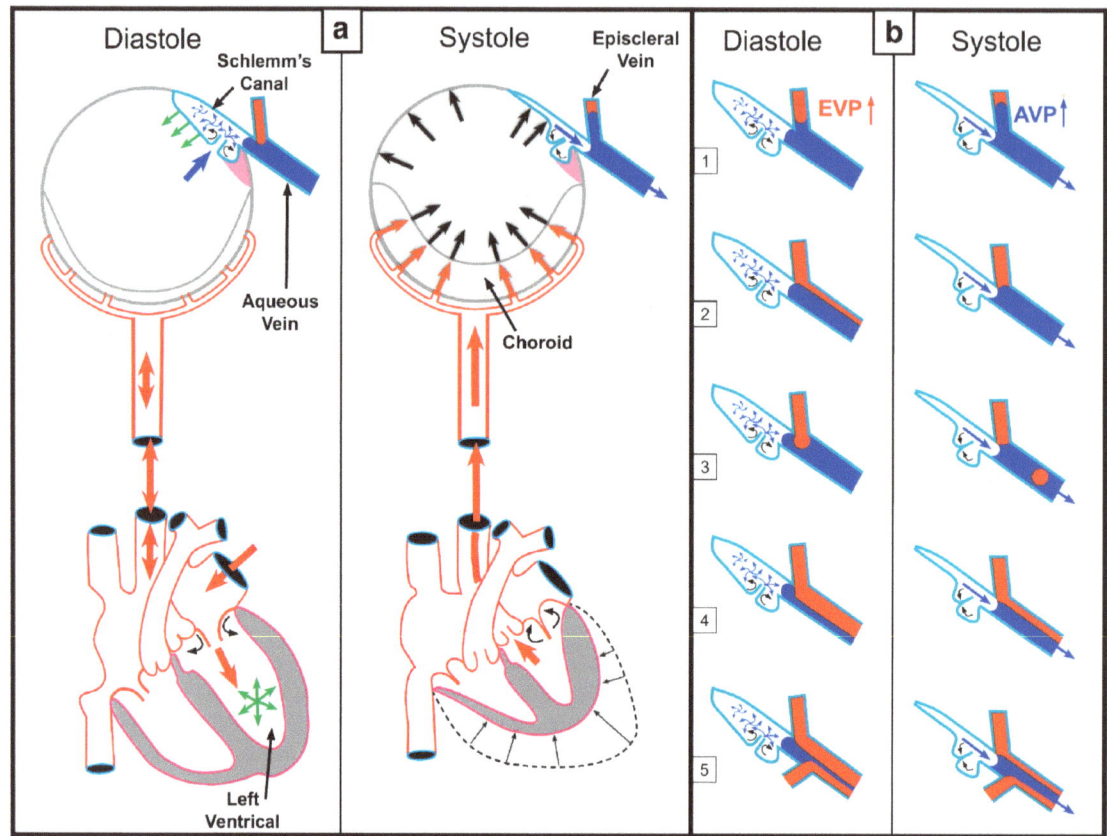

Figure 1. Cardiac-induced pulsatile aqueous outflow mechanisms. Cardiac source of (**a**) pulsatile aqueous outflow and (**b**) resultant pulsatile flow into the aqueous veins. The cardiac cycle results in pulsatile blood flow into the choroid, causing a rise in IOP. The IOP increase causes the TM to move outward, compressing SC. The oscillatory Schlemm's canal (SC) compression causes a pulse wave of aqueous to enter the episcleral veins. (**b**) 1–5 represent different manifestations of pulsatile flow observed in diastole and systole. (EVP) episcleral vein pressure, (AVP) aqueous vein pressure [4].

Table 1. Videos and descriptions. Click either item number or thumbnails for links to videos (SC) Schlemm's canal, (IOP) intraocular pressure, (SIVs) Schlemm's canal inlet valves, (AC) anterior chamber, (CC) collector channel, (HR-OCT) high-resolution OCT, (ISCC) intrascleral collector channel (SOV) SC outlet valve.

#	What the Videos Demonstrate: Pulsatile Flow and Outflow Tissue Motion	Links
1	• Aqueous exiting SC enters aqueous veins in pulsatile waves. • Propagating aqueous waves cyclically enter episcleral veins.	
2	• Increase in IOP increases pulse stroke volume, discharging more aqueous. • Increases aqueous discharge, then reduces IOP to setpoint. A feedback loop.	
3	• SC inlet valve (SIV) lumen is a direct AC to CC aqueous conduit. • Perfused tracers are in the TM, SIV, and CC.	

Table 1. *Cont.*

#	What the Videos Demonstrate: Pulsatile Flow and Outflow Tissue Motion	Links
4	• Synchronous pressure-dependent TM and distal outflow channel motion. • Fresh tissue and HR-OCT. HR-OCT is at 05:27 in the video.	
5	• SC inlet valve relationships and elasticity shown in an operating room @ 00:53. • Pulsatile aqueous flow from the anterior chamber into SC @ 02:19.	
6	• Pulse waves directed at a limbal segment cause TM distention and recoil. • The TM rapidly distends into SC storing elastic energy. Recoil follows.	
7	• Ciliary muscle tension in the radial limbal section opens SC and CC. • Tension causes TM lamellae elongation, rotation toward AC, and then recoil.	
8	• TM motion is synchronous with SC, CC, and ISCC (SOV) volume changes. • In a glaucoma eye, TM motion slowed and was limited by SC wall adhesions	
9	• TM position is tightly linked to IOP changes with baroreceptor-like behavior. • TM movement opens distal valves to control aqueous discharge.	

IOP control results from pressure-dependent tissue motion that regulates the aqueous outflow pathway dimensions that regulate stroke volume. The force of IOP determines the trabecular meshwork (TM) setpoint position between the anterior chamber and Schlemm's canal (SC) (Figure 2).

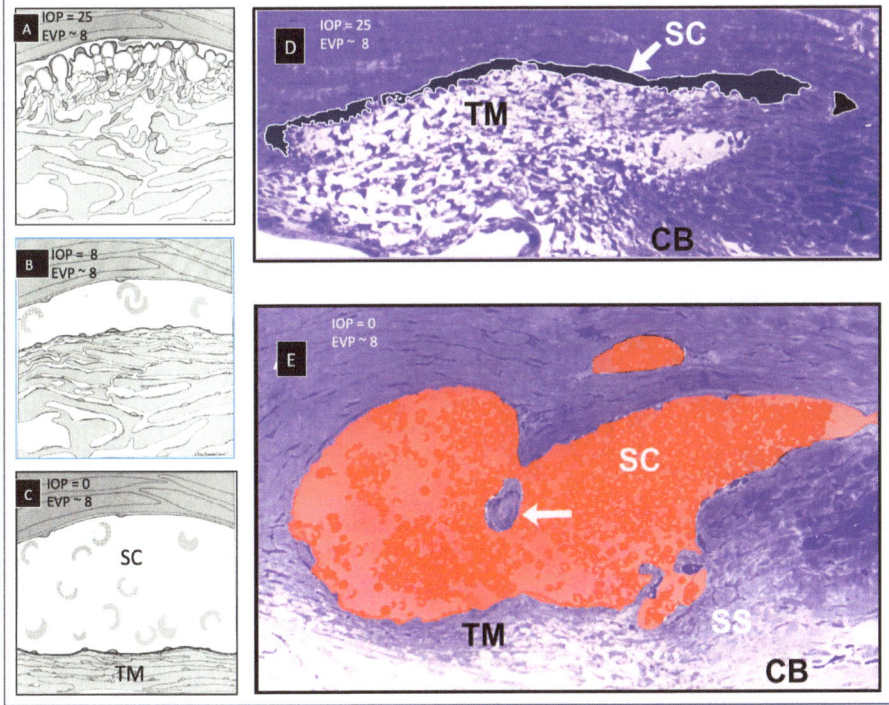

Figure 2. Pressure-dependent configuration of the TM, scleral spur, and ciliary body. Images (**A–C**) depict the tissue configuration IOP and EVP in a primate eye fixed in vivo (**D**) IOP of 25 mm Hg. (**E**) Fellow eye IOP of 0 mm Hg. (**A**) Cellular connections between the TM, juxtacanalicular cells,

and SC endothelium provide tethering of the SC inner wall that prevents SC collapse. The white arrow in (**E**) indicates an SIV suspended in the canal. (TM) trabecular meshwork, (SS) scleral spur, (CB) ciliary body, (IOP) intraocular pressure, (EVP) episcleral venous pressure, (SIV) Schlemm's canal inlet valve [4].

The ocular pulse causes the TM to undergo continuously oscillating deformation centered around the TM setpoint position (Figure 2) [5]. Section 1 TM deformation causes cyclic volume changes in SC that cause pulsatile aqueous flow from SC into the aqueous veins (Figure 3) (Section 5).

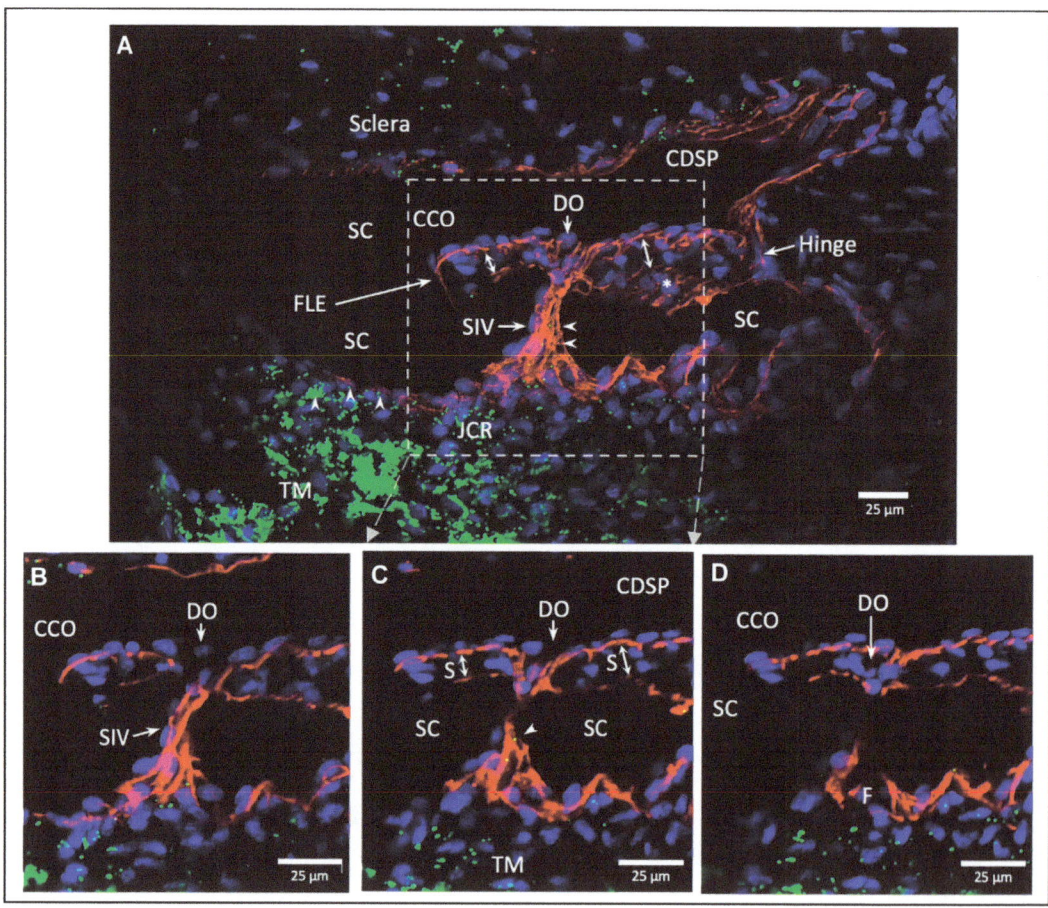

Figure 3. An SIV conduit connects the juxtacanalicular region to a collector channel ostia. Schlemm's canal inner wall narrows to form an SIV (double arrows) with a continuous lumen that spans SC. The SIV passes directly through a septum to a distal opening at a collector channel ostia. The septum has an unattached edge, appearing as a flap-like extension hinging at its scleral attachment providing mobility as a SC outlet valve. (**B**–**D**) boxed area in (**A**). Merged confocal CD31 (red), DAPI (blue), and 1 μm fluorescent microsphere (green) channels. (TM) trabecular meshwork, (F) funnel shaped region, (SC) Schlemm's canal, (SIV) SC inlet valve, (S) septum, (CC) collector channel, (CCO) collector channel ostia, (FLE) flap-like extension, (CDSP) circumferential deep scleral plexus, (JCR) juxtacanalicular region, (DO) distal opening (indented arrowheads); green fluorescent microspheres in the juxtacanalicular region, and the SIV lumen. See (Video 3) detailing TM/SIV/CC/CDSP relationships [6].

SC outlet valves (SOVs) at collector channel (CC) entrances control the flow of aqueous from SC. SIVs connect TM and SOVs [6] (Video 3). The connections ensure that the transmission of IOP-dependent TM motion is tightly linked to outlet valve opening and closing [7] (Video 4) [4]. The linkage provides the distal outflow system with a direct role in IOP control (Figures 3 and 4) (Sections 6 and 7). Evidence in humans demonstrates that the system fails in glaucoma because of abnormal TM lamellae tissue motion responses to IOP [8–11] (Figure 5) (Sections 3 and 8–10).

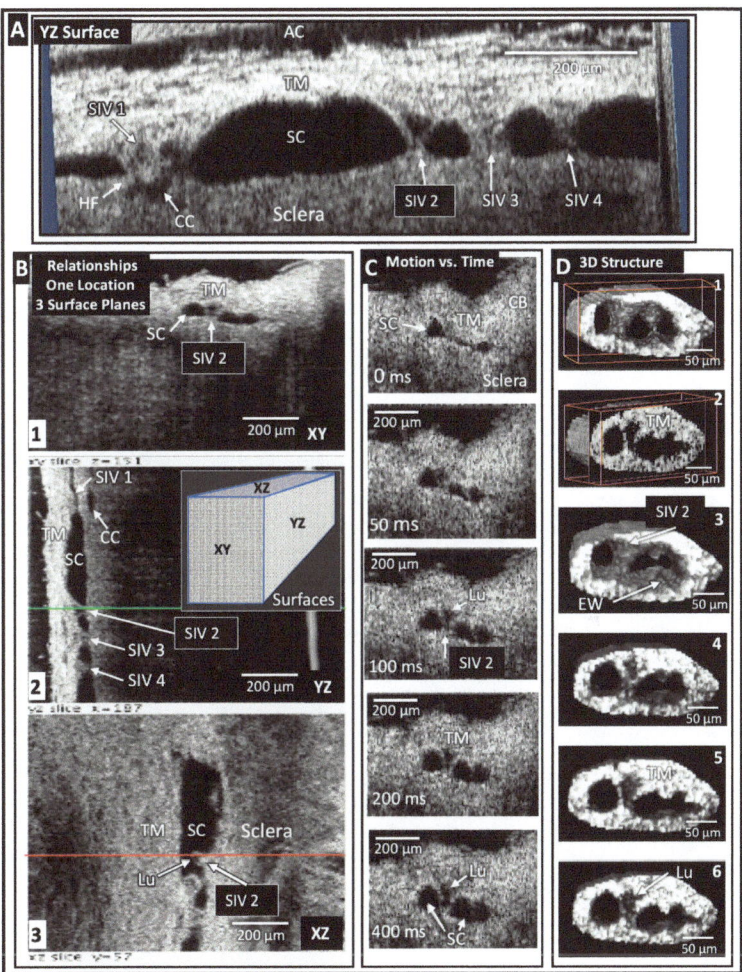

Figure 4. Schlemm's canal inlet valve-like structure (SIV) 3D relationships and motion. Images (XYZ) are from 3D OCT volumes captured at 30 mm Hg SC pressure. (**A**) Four SIV crossing SC. The three surface planes in (**B1–B3**) clarify SIV relationships at SIV1; a hinged flap is visible at a CC entrance. (**B**) The SIV2 appearance in each plane at one location is seen in XY, YZ (green line), and XZ (red line). (**C**) Motion capture—OCT 2D imaging while SC pressure changed from 0 to 30 mm Hg. Most SIV2 lumen volume changes occurred in <200 ms. (**D**) A mask provided 3D images of SC surface appearance (**D1**) and internal structure at increased depths (**D2–D6**). (C) The funnel-shaped deformation of the TM and SIV lumen (Lu) exiting from the TM is consistent with the strain induced by pressure-dependent stresses. (SC) Schlemm's canal, (SIVs) Schlemm's canal inlet valves, (TM) trabecular meshwork, (EW) external wall of SC, (HF) hinged flap [12].

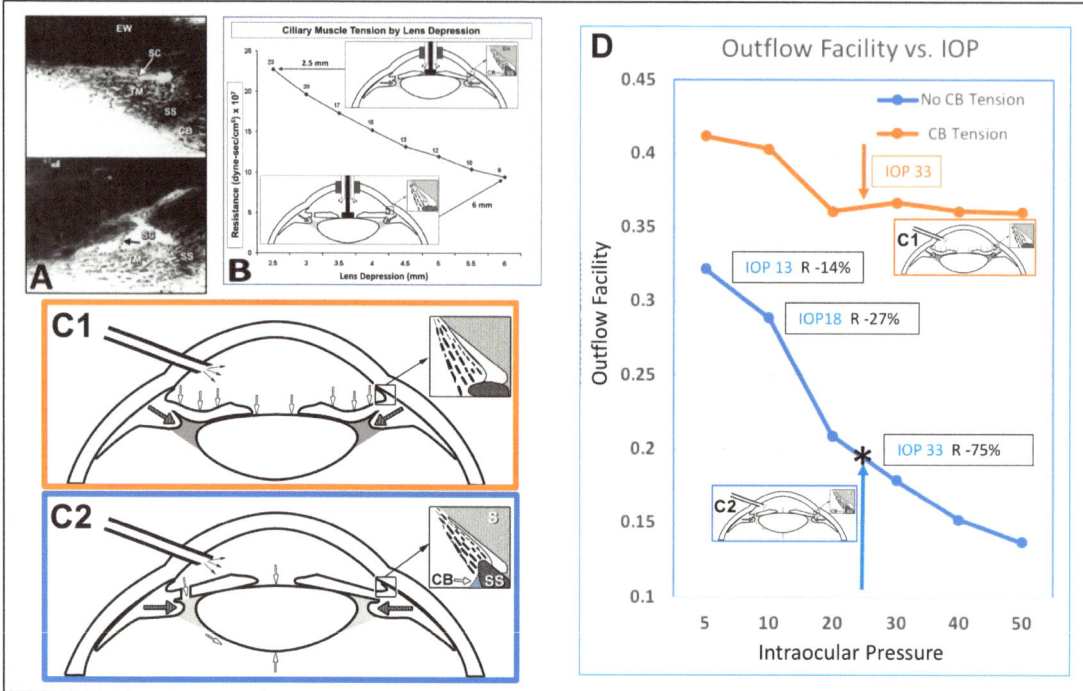

Figure 5. Ciliary muscle tension, intraocular pressure (IOP), and TM removal: impact on outflow facility. (**A–C**) depict experiments to induce ciliary muscle tension that prevents SC collapse. (**D**) illustrates the profound effects of IOP elevation on resistance and SC collapse in the absence of ciliary muscle tension. Grant's 1958 [13] and 1963 [14] experiments were performed at an effective IOP of 33 mm Hg without ciliary muscle tension. The * indicates the effective IOP of 33 mm Hg in vivo that would result from the ex vivo IOP of 25 mm Hg pressure because of absent 8 mm Hg episcleral venous pressure, leading to the resultant high resistance. Subsequent studies performed at physiologic pressures of 13 and 18 mm Hg found that the TM accounted for 14–27% of the resistance. The addition of ciliary muscle tension to prevent SC collapse resulted in a much-improved facility that was not reduced by increasing pressure levels. (**C1**) depicts the ball valve effect of chamber deepening with resultant CB, SS, and TM tension; (**C2**) iridectomy eliminates chamber deepening and tension. (Note that 25 mm Hg IOP requires an 8 mm Hg upward adjustment for EVP correction.) (IOP) intraocular pressure, (SC) Schlemm's canal, (EW) external wall of SC, (TM) trabecular meshwork, (SS) scleral spur, (CB) ciliary body, (EVP) episcleral venous pressure, (black arrow in (**A**)) SC inlet valve [4] Grant 1958 https://doi.org/10.1001/archopht.1958.00940080541001, Grant 1963 https://doi.org/10.1001/archopht.1963.00960040789022.

1.2. Pressure-Dependent Configuration of the TM, Scleral Spur, and Ciliary Body

Although we use a multiplicity of laboratory techniques to validate the model, this article's proposals are grounded in objective evidence, including direct observation of pulsatile flow throughout the outflow system in vivo in humans [1–3] (Video 5) [4] (Video 1) (Video 2) (Section 2). Knowledge of pulsatile flow is coupled with direct dissecting microscope observations of a mobile pressure-dependent TM [4] (Video 6). TM motion results in SC dimension changes synchronous with the opening and closing of pressure-dependent valves [7,15] (Video 7) [4].

1.3. Optical Coherence Tomography (OCT) Validation of Dynamic Outflow System Motion

Crucial evidence validating our model comes from optical coherence tomography (OCT) studies (Figure 4). The studies validate predictions from prior studies and introduce previously unrecognized synchrony of TM and distal system motion (Figure 4). Development of our high-resolution OCT platform permitted quantifying TM and motion at millisecond resolution in the laboratory (Figure 4). Clinical evidence and our laboratory model predicted human pulsatile outflow system motion. However, the technologies were inadequate to test the hypothesis. To solve the problem, Wang's lab developed phase-based OCT (PhS-OCT) capable of nanometer resolution. His lab's critical studies established pulse-dependent TM motion in humans and decreased motion in glaucoma, validating the dynamic model's predictions [16].

We then developed a high-resolution OCT platform that permitted capturing unprecedented detail comparable to that obtained using scanning electron microscopy (SEM) [7]. Unlike SEM, our OCT system permitted imaging of fine structural details with millisecond resolution (Video 4). OCT characterized pressure-dependent relationships among the TM, structures within SC, and collector channel entrances. Prior studies of pressure-dependent behavior involved steady-state measurements in fixed tissue that prevented the resolution of time-dependent motion. Our platform permitted millisecond-level resolution of both the proximal and distal outflow structures' movement [7].

The platform revealed synchronous motion of the TM and hinged flaps at CC entrances. The synchrony resulted from connections provided by the SIV spanning SC. Subsequent OCT studies developed an approach to characterize TM elastance/stiffness using quantitative steady-state and instantaneous TM motion studies. Glaucomatous tissue exhibited increased stiffness compared with normals and apposition and adhesion between SC walls [4]. (Video 8) shows OCT motion and stiffness in glaucoma. The OCT evidence of TM and distal valve motion led to the development of dynamic animation modeling of the unified tissue motion of the entire outflow system [7,15]. (Video 9) shows the unified motion of the entire outflow system [6].

1.4. The Passive Flow-Filter Model

Current textbooks and research papers regularly present a passive flow-filter model of IOP control as a definitive explanation for aqueous outflow regulation without acknowledging model limitations or rival hypotheses. The approach suggests that theory includes all relevant alternatives and that there are no viable rival hypotheses, which leads to foreclosure of further discussion. Consequently, it is difficult for research scientists and clinicians to gain awareness of the rapidly accumulating body of evidence challenging the passive model. This paper's length reflects the need to introduce readers to unfamiliar evidence, conclusions, and the resulting concepts of a rival hypothesis.

Those engaged in clinical research and surgery may benefit from reassessing their reliance on the traditional belief system for the following reasons. (1) Minimally invasive glaucoma surgery (MIGS) documents that TM removal does not reduce IOP to episcleral venous pressure (EVP) levels as the model requires. (2) Grant's evidence demonstrates that control of IOP is not within the TM but instead results from relationships between SC walls.

Evidence from passive flow studies points to further theory weaknesses. (1) Pores occur as a reproducible titratable artifact, and all pores may be artifactual [17–20]. No current technologies can prove or disprove their presence, leaving them in the realm of conjecture rather than theory [21]. (2) Hydraulic conductivity is orders of magnitude beyond what passive flow theory can explain, requiring a different explanation for aqueous passage into SC [18,22]. Inadequate extracellular matrix is present in the juxtacanalicular region to explain resistance, suggesting that the passive flow-filter model's fundamental thesis is unsupported [23–25].

The passive flow-filters theory's dependence then rests on an ad hoc funneling idea proffered to sustain the model's framework. However, the concept was not formulated based on empirical data demonstrating funneling behavior and remains unsupported by meaningful objective evidence. No current technology can prove or falsify funneling behavior, leaving funneling in the realm of speculation and best described as a conjecture rather than a theory [21]. Review articles by authorities [23–25] point out that funneling conjecture is now the sole means of retaining support for the passive flow theory of resistance control.

2. Noninvasive Aqueous Angiography: Stealth Paradigm Transformation

Slitlamp development introduced a technology that permitted the most crucial breakthrough discovery of the 20th century: direct observation of aqueous flow from SC to the episcleral veins. Our current concepts of aqueous outflow and its abnormality in glaucoma rely on Ascher's discovery of the aqueous veins [1–3]. Scientists actively disputed the idea of aqueous circulation before his discovery. By studying readily available videos, we can easily verify pulsatile flow in the aqueous veins. For example, see the aqueous vein pulsations in (Video 1) and (Video 2).

Evidence was insufficient to support the theory of aqueous circulation before Ascher's discovery. The concept of angle-closure glaucoma was disputed; open-angle glaucoma was an enigma. Reports by Asher and others removed the controversies, opening the way for the widespread use of peripheral iridectomy, and identifying circulation and its blockage at the level of the outflow system [1–3] provided the rationale for outflow drugs and MIGS surgery, which are the subjects of this report.

Pulsatile flow has been recognized as a salient feature since the aqueous veins were first identified. DeVries noninvasively explored the undisturbed distribution of aqueous veins. Aqueous outflow in humans is highly asymmetric and concentrated in the inferior hemisphere (87%), particularly the inferior nasal quadrant (56%), a distribution well documented in his exhaustive report [26].

Aqueous vein patterns are likely stable for a lifetime [3], with two or three typically visible, four and, at most, five are present only occasionally [3,26]. Stepanik's videography measured the velocity and volume of pulsatile flow in the aqueous veins under noninvasive physiologic conditions. His quantitative study demonstrated that two aqueous veins could carry all aqueous outflow [27,28].

2.1. Pulsatile Flow into Aqueous Veins Requires Specific Structural Outflow System Features

The arterial, venous, and lymphatic systems all have continuous, pulsatile flow as components of vascular circulatory loops. The aqueous outflow system is one such circulation. An arterial arm of the loop delivers aqueous from the heart to the eye, then returns it to the venous system and the heart. Pulsatile mechanisms in the systemic veins and lymphatic vessels return fluid to the heart [29]. Pulsatile flow requirements for the vasculature are three-fold: (1) compressible chambers, (2) valves, and (3) an energy source. Sections between venous and lymphatic system valves act as mini ventricles or chambers [29].

Initial lymphatics and small veins rely on energy from the cardiac system to alter tissue turgor, causing chamber compression during systole and relaxation during diastole. Valves prevent backflow. Pulsatile flow in the outflow system imposes equivalent requirements to permit pulsatile flow. Requirements are compressible chambers, valves, and a chamber wall that can respond to the cardiac pulse. As noted in the following sections, pulsatile aqueous flow is well-characterized in humans [1–3]. Structural features and functional behavior within the outflow system also explain and predict pulsatile flow behavior [7].

2.2. Pulsatile Flow in Aqueous Veins, Intrascleral Channels, Collector Channels, and SC

In response to cardiac-dependent changes in choroidal volume, the anterior chamber experiences continuous pulsatile alterations in pressure [30]. Pressure oscillations force the TM outward in systole, followed by recoil in diastole. SC volume oscillates as a result.

SC inlet valve-like structures (SIVs) are regularly distributed around the circumference of SC in human eyes. The SIVs have a funnel-like proximal origin from SC inner wall endothelium, and their lumen communicates with the juxtacanalicular space. The SIVs develop a cylindrical shape and attach to SC's external wall at CC entrances [6].

In response to the ocular pulse, waves of aqueous propagate from funnel-shaped origins at SC's inner wall into a cylindrical region, culminating in aqueous ejection from the distal end. The ejected aqueous creates swirling eddies in SC as it mixes with blood. A recurring pattern over thirty cardiac cycles demonstrates that aqueous entry to SC is synchronous with the ocular pulse [5]. Objective evidence using direct observation is visible in readily available peer-reviewed video material [4], for example, (Video 5) shows pulsatile aqueous flow into SC (start the video at 2:19 min to see SC pulsatile flow).

A generalizable pattern is apparent in the propagating wave of clear aqueous. A specific configuration outlines funnel-shaped and cylindrical areas in each cycle as aqueous moves through a clearly defined constraining structure. The shape configuration changes rapidly as aqueous passes through the conduits, demonstrating that their constraining walls are highly compliant. Real-time pulsatile aqueous entry into SC in humans provides a benchmark for assessing the validity of the dynamic model. Blood-stained aqueous moving outward in CC and intrascleral channels in synchrony with the cardiac pulse provides confirmatory evidence of pulsatile flow in the outflow system [5]. To summarize, pulse waves of aqueous progress through the TM into SC and then into CC, intrascleral channels, aqueous veins, and, finally, episcleral veins.

2.3. IOP Oscillations and Pressure Transients

The AC pressure and volume continually oscillate due to cardiac-dependent changes in choroidal volume. Eye movements and blinking cause the IOP to undergo multiple transients above baseline each minute. In healthy people, dynamic contour tonometry demonstrates an ocular pulse amplitude of 3 mm Hg ranging from 0.0 to 7.2 mm Hg [31].

Blinking and eye movements cause recurring instantaneous IOP spikes reaching 20–30 mm Hg. Eye movements are frequent in daily activities, with approximately 170,000 daily saccades. Monkey eye telemetry demonstrates that the eye experiences transient IOP spikes 2.5 mm Hg above baseline about 5000 times per hour [32]. These oscillatory and transient pressure spikes are the source of pulsatile aqueous outflow from SC.

2.4. Clinical Studies Confirm Rapid Trabecular Meshwork Motion in Humans

TM motion effects can be directly observed by watching rapid blood reflux into SC [33–35]. Episcleral vein compression with the flange of a goniolens causes a reversal of pressure gradients with EVP > IOP. The TM moves toward the AC within seconds as blood refluxes into SC in response to the pressure gradient reversal. Pressure gradient reversal in living primate eyes followed by histology studies confirms clinical findings [36]. In vivo studies demonstrate that blood widely dilates SC. SC dilation results from the complete collapse of the inner portion of the TM tissues with associated outward movement of all the trabecular lamellae. The directly observable blood reflux and SC dilation in humans can be coupled with comparable evidence in living primates that experience pressure reversal. In each case, the TM rapidly deforms in response to the pressure changes. TM motion associated with SC filling slows and eventually stops as glaucoma progresses. The finding is well documented in multiple quantitative clinical studies [33–35,37,38].

3. Outflow Abnormalities in Glaucoma—Directly Verifiable Clinical Evidence

Initial aqueous vein studies identified pulsatile flow as a salient feature [1–3]. Soon after the initial studies, Ascher and others published evidence that pulsatile flow slows and eventually stops as glaucoma worsens [3].

3.1. The Aqueous Influx and Compensation Maximum Outflow Tests for Glaucoma

Aqueous vein pulsatile flow increases in normal subjects when EVP rises. We can clinically observe the pulsatile flow increase when pressure on a distal episcleral vein causes pressure in the more proximal vein to rise. An increased stroke volume per pulse causes aqueous influx into adjacent previously blood-filled ESVs. The pulsatile aqueous influx reflects the TM's ability to alter its stiffness/elastance in response to changing the pressure differential across its surface. A more vigorous distention and recoil then occur with each ocular pulse wave. In glaucoma, the outflow system loses the ability to increase pulsatile flow in response to increasing EVP [1,3], a behavior consistent with the loss of elastance of the TM.

When IOP increases in a compensation maximum test, the stroke volume of pulsatile aqueous flow also increases in normal subjects. In contrast, pulsatile flow decreases and eventually stops when IOP increases in glaucoma patients [39,40]. Clinicians use an ophthalmodynamometer that presses on the eye to increase IOP. The instrument provides a quantitative assessment of the induced pressure. The test assesses the ability of the TM to withstand increased IOP distending forces above its homeostatic setpoint. The TM loses its ability to withstand distending forces in glaucoma, resulting in an initial decrease and an eventual absence of pulsatile aqueous outflow as glaucoma worsens [39,40].

3.2. Miotic Responses Identify a Mechanistic Cause of the IOP Increase in Glaucoma

Pulsatile aqueous outflow slows and then stops in advanced glaucoma. Miotics reduce IOP in glaucoma patients, a response preceded by increased pulsatile aqueous outflow. As the duration of mitotic action ends, pulsatile flow stops. Recurrent elevation of IOP follows [1,3]. Ciliary muscle contractile responses increase in response to miotics [41]. Contractile responses of the muscle cause increased tension on the scleral spur and TM lamellae. The TM tissues move away from the SC external wall, and the TM lamellae experience increased tension-induced stress (Figure 5). The increase in TM lamellae stress alters their elastance, restoring their ability to distend and recoil within their homeostatic response range [5].

The ciliary body's role in controlling aqueous outflow has robust experimental support (Section 8). In the absence of ciliary muscle tone, increasing IOP results in IOP elevation and SC collapse in ex vivo eyes. The introduction of ciliary body tension allows the tissue to respond with stable resistance over an extensive range of pressures [9]. Ciliary muscle tension and outflow resistance are tightly linked. Laboratory studies support the conclusion that ciliary muscle tension is a crucial parameter of aqueous outflow regulation in both normal and glaucoma eyes [8–11,41,42].

4. TM—Mobile Wall of a Compressible Chamber Called SC

4.1. TM Structural Organization and Composition That Determines Function

Trabecular lamellae typically originate at Schwalbe's line, quickly branching into three lamellae. The lamellae course posteriorly, and then further branch to form a series of 8–14 parallel beams or sheets, each about 5–12 μm in thickness (Figure 2). The branching results in a fan-shaped appearance of the TM with the base of the fan at Schwalbe's line (Figure 2). The trabecular sheets are generally circumferentially arranged, with the sheets parallel to one another and the limbal circumference [43].

The trabecular lamellae of the corneoscleral TM extend from Schwalbe's line posteriorly in a meridional fashion. Their posterior anchoring distributes about equally between the scleral spur and the ciliary muscle tendons. Lamellae near the AC are considerably thicker than the ones close to SC (Figure 3). The composition of the corneoscleral trabecular lamellae is similar to that of other organ systems with marked elasticity and compliance such as the lung, blood vessel walls, and tendons.

4.2. TM Composition Determines TM Lamellae Energy Storage and Release

The trabecular lamellae's organization and distribution of elastin and collagen are like that of a tendon. Pulsatile changes in IOP are forces that cause oscillatory TM tissue loading. The composition can explain the observed reversible TM deformation. TM lamellae endothelial cells have a rich endowment of cytoplasmic organelles responsible for protein synthesis and secretion. TM lamellae experience about 30 million oscillations per year. Constantly optimizing elastin and collagen fiber properties is essential for maintaining homeostasis in such a dynamic environment. Cytoskeletal elements in the trabecular endothelial cells and their cytoplasmic processes are microfilaments (F-actin), intermediate filaments (vimentin), and microtubules (alpha-tubulin) [43].

4.3. TM Lamellae, Juxtacanalicular Cells, and SC Inner Wall Connect by Cell Processes

Trabecular lamellae endothelial cells project many cytoplasmic processes into the intertrabecular spaces. Processes of adjacent lamellae join, creating cellular connections. TM lamellae cytoplasmic processes from the TM lamellae also project into the juxtacanalicular space, attaching to juxtacanalicular cell processes. The relationships result in the TM lamellae being tethered to the SC inner wall endothelium. The TM lamellae move outward as IOP increases because the numerous processes tether them to the JCT and SC endothelium [20,36,44–47] (Figure 2). The inner wall endothelium initially moves outward, but the TM lamellae process connections limit the SC inner wall distention into the SC lumen.

4.4. Immediate Responses to Pressure Changes Result from Continuous Tensile Forces

SC endothelium experiences continuous pressure-dependent baseline, oscillatory, and transient stresses at physiologic pressures, as illustrated using in vivo fixation studies [20,36,44–46]. The tensile stresses at SC inner wall endothelium transmit to the TM lamellae through the numerous tethering cytoplasmic processes. The force of IOP exerts continuous uniformly distributed tensile forces on SC endothelial cells, juxtacanalicular cells, and endothelial cells covering the trabecular lamellae.

4.5. Tensile Stress Status and Changes—An Information-Dense Sensory System

The IOP-induced force creates tension on SC's inner wall endothelium. The stresses are transmitted to the entire TM complex through cellular process connections. The uniformly distributed tension provides TM cells with information that permits instantaneous, simultaneous sensing of pressure and changes in pressure. The pressure-dependent sensory input enables TM cells to maintain optimized elastance through mechanotransduction mechanisms. Cardiovascular system walls elsewhere experience comparable pressure-dependent sensory input and responses [29].

TM biomechanical properties determine SC dimensions. Control of TM biomechanical properties determines how far the TM distends into the canal. In unfixed ex vivo eyes, experimentally induced pulsatile motion is directly observable. Pulse-dependent TM distension causes SC progressive collapse. After the pulse wave stops, the TM recoils to the baseline configuration. Direct observation of the pulsatile TM behavior is visible using videography. Scale bars on the images permit the capture and quantitation of TM motion speed and amplitude in this living tissue [4], for example, see (Video 6) of TM motion and SC collapse.

4.6. New OCT Technology Permits TM Elastance Determination

TM biomechanics quantitative studies have been significantly advanced by recently developed high-resolution spectral domain OCT (SD-OCT) capture of movement in ex vivo TM tissues. Using these technologies, we explored a new TM biomechanical parameter, elastance. Elastance is a measure that quantifies the ability of a tissue surrounding a volume to store and release energy [48]. The TM is the deforming tissue that determines the volume of SC. In this setting, the TM is the tissue storing and releasing energy as it responds to IOP changes by deforming. Stiffness is an alternative term for elastance. Our studies permitted us to generate TM elastance curves. The curves characterize the TM tissues' stiffness and ability to respond to pressure changes. They explore both the dynamic volume changes and response speeds. TM distension and recoil are very rapid, occurring within about 250 milliseconds [7,12].

Another technique, PhS-OCT, provides motion sensitivity at the nanometer level with a 1000 nm dynamic range [7,48]. Recent ex vivo experimental platforms and algorithm developments demonstrated measurement feasibility. Subsequently, PhS-OCT was translated into a clinical imaging system that identifies TM pulsatile flow in vivo in humans and motion changes in glaucoma. Diurnal IOP fluctuation is an elusive but essential parameter in glaucoma management. PhS-OCT can assist in assessing IOP control by identifying the propensity for diurnal changes [16,47].

5. SC Inlet Valves (SIVs): Discovery and Operating Room Documentation

SIVs were discovered during experiments that identified SC as a dynamically compressible chamber [36] (Figure 2). A study on the SIVs or informed commentary about their presence, absence, or behavior is not feasible without the dilation of SC. The SIV course is circumferentially in SC. At normal pressures, the distended TM tissues obscure the presence of SIVs, their origins at the level of the TM, and their insertion at CC entrances along the SC external wall.

Initial awareness that the outflow system could function as a pump resulted from three discoveries: (1) pressure-dependent TM motion permits SC to behave as a compressible chamber, (2) an SIV has a pressure-dependent lumen, and (3) an SIV acts as a conduit that allows aqueous passage directly from the juxtacanalicular space into SC.

5.1. Multiple Imaging Modalities Confirm SIV Presence and Function

Operating room unroofing of SC provides directly observable evidence of SIV structural features, function as conduits carrying aqueous, and tensile nature of the connections with the inner and outer wall of SC [5]. (Video 5): surgical stretching and disruption of SIV by Stegmann (starting at 1:10) provides evidence. The SIVs undergo structural failure in response to experimentally induced axial stresses, leading to rupture and aqueous gushing from the disrupted lumen [5]. Direct observation of aqueous flow from the AC through the SIV to SC is made possible using operating room gonioscopy (see (Video 5) for evidence of pulsatile aqueous flow into SC starting at 2:19).

5.2. SIV Structure and Motion Responses: Clinical and Laboratory Correlation

Many modalities demonstrate the SIV structure, the effects of ciliary muscle tension and pulse-induced motion. They also show that pressure-dependent TM motion creates stress on the SIV that induces movement of the SC outlet valves (SOVs). Modalities that characterize the SIV structure are the dissecting and brightfield, phase contrast, differential interference contrast [4], and confocal microscope [6]. Additional modalities that characterize features and relationships include standard and blockface scanning electron microscopy (SEM) [5,36,49] and spectral domain OCT (SD-OCT) [7,12,49].

5.3. Protocols to Study SIV

Protocols to assess SIV motion include in vivo fixation at controlled steady-state pressures [5,15,36], controlled ciliary muscle tension, and direct pulsatile infusions at the dissecting microscope [4]. In vivo imaging protocols include high-resolution OCT while perfusing at steady-state pressures and during experimentally induced pulsatile motion. The findings reveal axial and radial SIV lumen dimension changes [4]. (Video 4) of linked TM/CC motion PhS-OCT demonstrates that IOP-dependent TM motion changes must induce SIV configuration changes because the SIVs connect to both the TM and SC external wall (Section 4.3).

The SIV endothelial walls and the lumen can be traced from their funnel-shaped origin at the SC inner wall to their outer wall attachments. The technique involves SC lumen viscoelastic dilation, clarification, IHC labeling, tracers, and confocal microscopy. These combined approaches establish the constituent properties of the walls and lumen of the SC inlet valves [6] (Figures 3, 6 and 7). Labeling studies reveal that SIV walls are those of a vascular endothelium continuous with SC inner wall cells. Microspheres perfused into the AC can be traced as they pass from the juxtacanalicular space of the TM into the SIV lumen followed by passage into CC entrances and circumferential vascular channels (CVCs) [6].

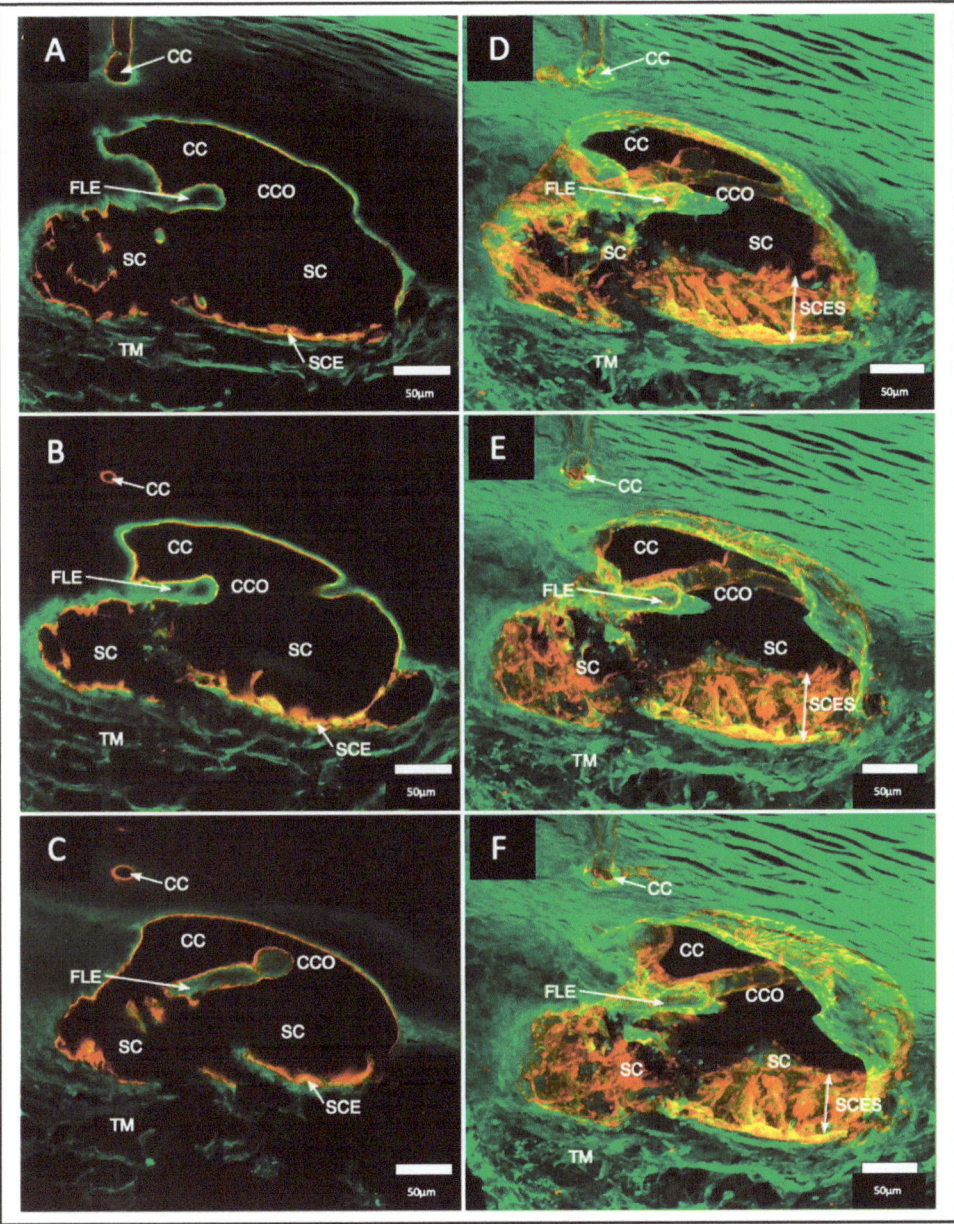

Figure 6. Confocal stack projections display Schlemm's canal flap-like collagenous extensions at collector channels. (**A–C**) are 2D and (**D–F**) are 3D projections of a 129 μm stack of merged CD31 (red) and Col type 1 (green) images. Viscodilation of Schlemm's canal (SC), clarification, and deep stack projections characterize the organization and relationships between tissues surrounding collector channels (CCs) and their ostia (CCO). 2D images show Schlemm's canal endothelium (SCE) and Schlemm's canal inner wall endothelial surface (SCES) is visible in the 3D stack projection. Flap-like collagenous extensions (FLEs) from the sclera wall protrude into SC. The unanchored distal end of the FLE provides a hinged configuration. (TM) trabecular meshwork [6].

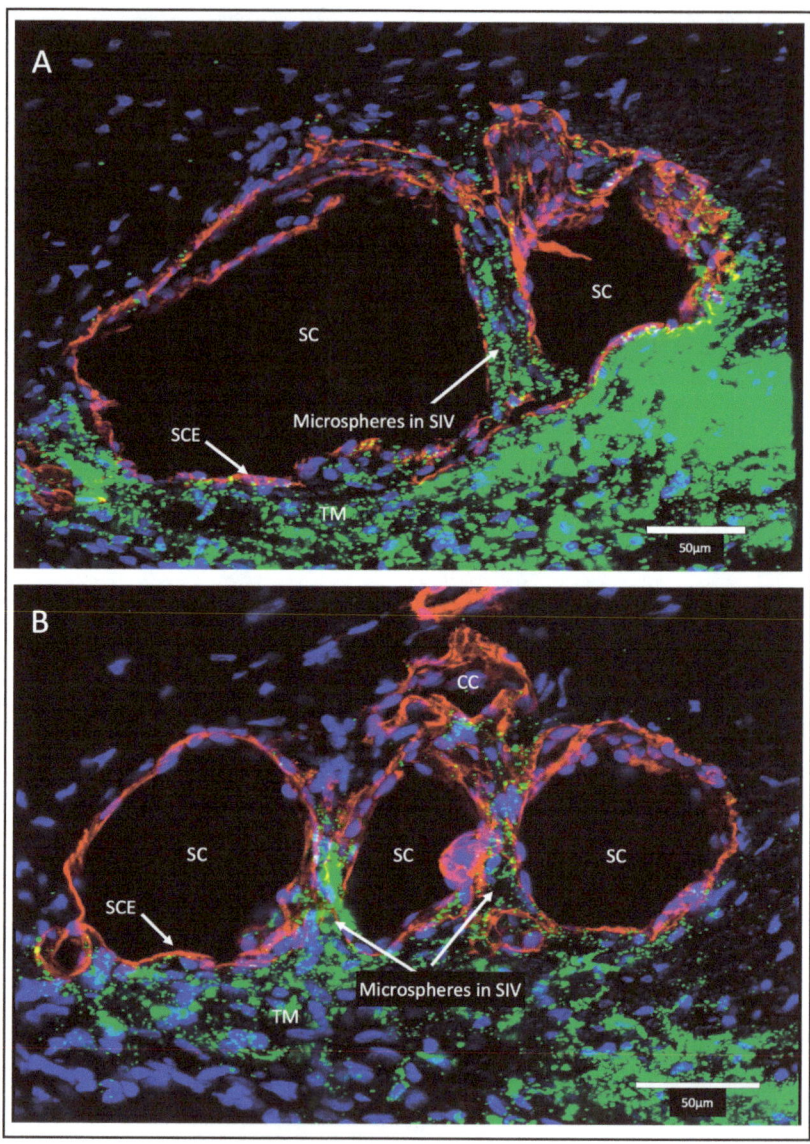

Figure 7. Schlemm's canal inner wall valve-like structures. Tracer studies (**A**,**B**) merged CD31 (red) DAPI (blue), and 500 nm fluorescent microsphere (green) channels. The stack size is 40 µm in (**A**) and 43 µm in (**B**). Schlemm's canal (SC) inner wall endothelium forms a valve-like structure (SIV). The SIVs arise from the SC inner wall endothelium (SCE) that forms the outer wall of the trabecular meshwork (TM). The funnel-shaped configuration extends into SC to form a cylindrical conduit attaching to the SC external wall at collector channels (CCs). The TM fills with fluorescent microspheres. The microspheres also fill the juxtacanalicular region, the SIV, and their connections with intrascleral channels (ISCs) [6].

Perfusion of nucleated avian red cells into the AC results in their passage through the entire length of the SIV lumen, as revealed with light and TEM [5]. In vivo reduction of

IOP below EVP results in blood filling the SC lumen. At the same time, primate red cells pass through the entire SIV length, reaching the JCS level. No red blood cells or plasma pass directly across the distended endothelium of the SC inner wall [5,15].

6. Schlemm's Canal Outlet Valve (SOV) Structure and Function

6.1. Circumferential Channels Parallel to SC in Humans: The Definitive Study

Ramirez et al. deserve credit for the discovery, clear articulation of anatomy, and embryogenesis of what they describe as "an outer collector that runs parallel to SC" [50]. Our later reports, unaware of the Ramirez group's discovery, used the terms circumferential deep scleral plexus, circumferential vascular channel, and intrascleral collector channel for the "outer collectors". The group's landmark discovery compares with that of Ashton's vascular casting studies [51], which established pathways from SC to the episcleral vessels. The "outer collector" clinical importance is comparable to that of the TM in understanding pressure control mechanisms and identifying surgical treatment targets.

The Ramirez group studied the embryology of distal "outer collector" pathways in 60 eyes. They explored five gestation intervals beginning at 24 weeks and compared them with the appearance after birth at two months, eight years, and adulthood. At 24 weeks, the anlage of "outer collectors" was present; at 36 weeks, it was clearly defined, and at two months after birth, its circumferential connections continued to develop. At eight years, the structures compared with those of adult. The structures were circumferential extensions of collector channels that arose from the SC ectomesenchyma. The episcleral plexus developed separately.

In seven randomly selected adult eyes, the mean number of CC connecting to the "outer collectors" was 39 (± 6.24). Circumferential "outer collectors" were divided into sectors but were continuous for as much as $120°$. Numerous ramifications from the external wall of the "outer collectors" formed intrascleral channels entering the episcleral veins. The report's description of the circumferential channels appears identical to that in our group's studies. Our later independent studies were performed without awareness of the Ramirez detailed report. However, our studies confirmed the earlier work using microscopy by manipulating fresh tissue, light microscopy, SEM, micro-vascular casting, and high-resolution OCT.

6.2. SOV Structural Features Assessed Using Multiple Approaches

IOP regulation includes distal resistance regulation as an essential factor. However, structural relationships and behavior that can control distal resistance are unclear [52]. Below, we describe evidence of distal resistance-controlling structures and their functional behavior. Studies include capturing the effects of direct manipulation while imaging with a microscope [4], histology [5,49], SC viscoelastic dilation, and examination of three thousand individual SEM preparations involving images at 12,000 locations and magnifications [7,49]. Studies also include microvascular casting [4,49] (Figure 5), tissue clarification [6], confocal microscopy [6], and IHC [6].

6.3. Septa, Hinged Flaps at CCs, and a Second Compressible Chamber

Septa oriented parallel to the external wall of SC separated SC from a second compressible chamber (Figure 6). Regularly recurring septa are found along the external wall of SC. At CC entrances, they appear as hinged flaps (Figures 3 and 6). A circumferentially oriented deep scleral plexus of channels (CDSP) extends around much of the outer wall periphery of SC, and the lumen communicates directly with CCs, SIVs, and the juxtacanalicular region (Figure 7).

The CDSP are partitioned from SC by thin septa and are also referred to as circumferential vascular channels (CVCs) [4–7,12,49]. Septa are thin and highly mobile. The properties of the septa result in high mobility, permitting pressure-dependent compression of the CDSP/CVC.

The septa mobility results in the CDSP acting as a second compressible chamber, distal but adjacent to SC (Figure 8). CC entrances are typically perpendicular to the circumference of SC and course only a short distance before entering the CVC. When sections are cut in an oblique plane, SEM captures the entirety of the relationships, including a short CC entrance, circumferential intrascleral path of the CVC, and radial intrascleral channels exiting the CVC that pass to the episcleral veins. Precise positioning is required because the relationships disappear with the slightest movement in any XYZ plane or rotation around the XYZ axis.

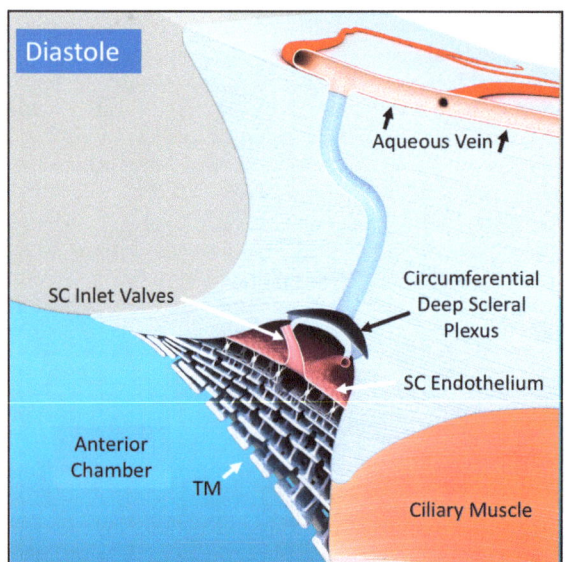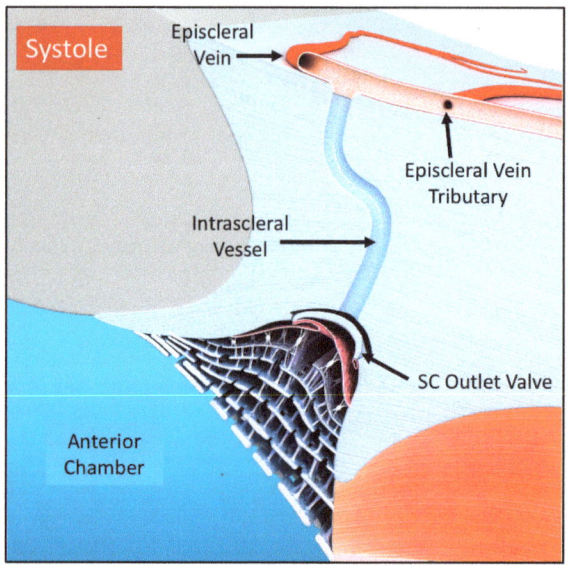

Figure 8. Aqueous pump model incorporating valves and compressible chambers. From the resting state in diastole, systole induces an intraocular pressure (IOP) rise, causing an ocular pulse wave in the anterior chamber (AC). The trabecular meshwork (TM) distends as IOP rises. TM distention causes Schlemm's canal (SC) to narrow, reducing its volume while forcing fluid through the collector channel (CC) outlet valve entrances which are initially in an open configuration, followed by septa movement outward, forcing aqueous out of the CDSP. TM recoil during the following diastole causing CC entrances to open into the circumferentially oriented deep scleral plexus (CDSP). Aqueous flows into the intertrabecular spaces, into SC through the conduits of the SC inlet valves, and into CDSP. The cycle then repeats. The proposed anatomic relationships and pressure-dependent sequences are provisional and warrant further study [4].

Only recently has the consistent presence and likely functional significance of a second compressible chamber adjacent to SC come into focus. A study identified and quantified relationships with SEM using limbal segments from human and primate eyes. About half the segments had CVC that coursed parallel to SC. In the segments, the mean length of SC was 1130 ± 586 µm, and CDSP/CVC was 565 ± 486 µm. The CDSP/CVC length is also a measure of the septa length that separates the two chambers. The mean scleral septa diameter was 23 ± 11 µm, and the thin diameter relative to length explained the septa mobility. SD-OCT and confocal microscopy 3D volume analysis using serial imaging 3D reconstructions, associated projections, and SD-OCT further confirmed CDSP/CVC characteristics [6,12].

6.4. SOV Structural Features Assessed Using Microvascular Casting Approaches

The technique injects microvascular casting material into SC. Tissue clarification follows, allowing imaging deep into the tissue, which is ideal for exploring distal sclera relationships (Figure 9). A clarification technique, new to ophthalmology, uses benzyl alcohol/benzyl benzoate (BABB) that rapidly clears the scleral tissues in the distal outflow pathway (Figure 7) [6].

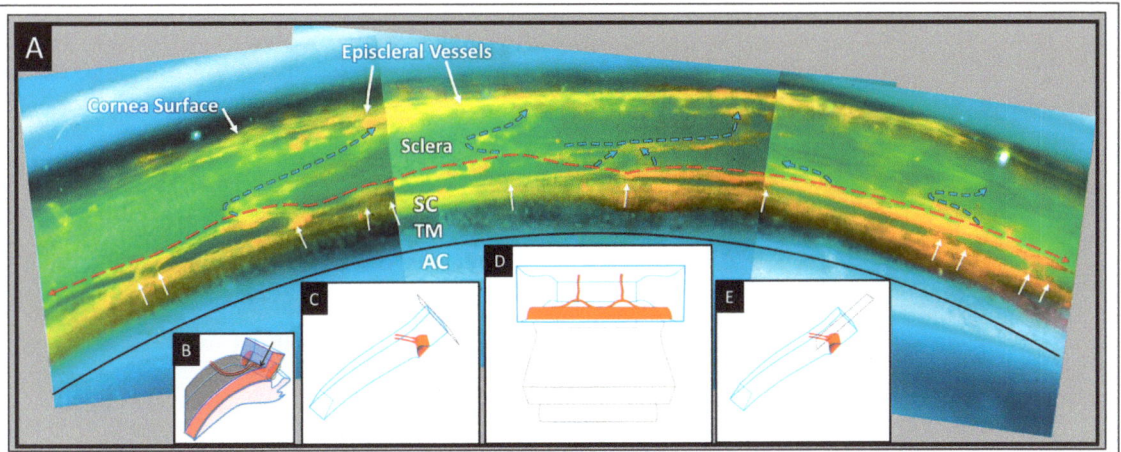

Figure 9. Circumferentially oriented deep scleral plexus visualization. A microvascular cast of the outflow system following tissue clarification. (**A**) The transparent TM is between the black curved line and SC. Collector channels arise from the outer wall of SC (white arrows) and connect to a circumferentially oriented deep scleral plexus (CDSP) (thin dashed red line). The CDSP forms a relatively continuous communicating ring adjacent and parallel to SC. Intrascleral vessels exit the CDSP and pass through the sclera (blue arrows) to the eye's surface, where episcleral and aqueous veins are visible. Between SC and CDSP are long, thin, collagenous septa, which are transparent and seen as a void between SC and the CDSP. The CDSP provides a compressible valve-like conduit/chamber because it opens and closes with pressure-dependent septa movement. (**B**–**E**) illustrate the need to visualize the CC/CDSP connections through the cornea surface to capture their uniform perpendicular plane of exit from SC. (AC) anterior chamber, (TM) trabecular meshwork, (SC) Schlemm's canal [4].

We found that cutting specimens at the corneoscleral interface was necessary to define the CC exit sites clearly. Visualization through the corneoscleral interface permitted us to visualize the CC perpendicular to where they exit the SC lumen (Figure 9). The protocol enables grasping global relationships involving SC, CC, septa, and CDSP/CVC. The ensemble provides the structural framework for understanding how SOV can function as outlet valves [4,6,49].

6.5. SOV Structure and Related Motion Motion—OCT Imaging Approaches

High-resolution SD-OCT imaging permits tracing TM, SC, SIV, CC, septa, and CDSP/CVC configuration changes. The experimental platform enables examination under steady-state conditions at different pressures. Experimentally controlled changing of pressure gradients while imaging permits quantifying motion in real-time with millisecond resolution in NH primates and human eyes [7,12]. The related new technology (PhS-OCT) provides millisecond motion resolution in glaucoma patients and identifies motion differences compared with normals [16,48].

The discovery of a collapsible chamber distal to SC was unexpected, and the evidence was initially discounted. However, regular organization, occurrence, and behavior are consistent with an essential role in controlling IOP. Multiple segments that all function to control flow, like miniventricles in series, are a feature of the lymphatics. The complex circular torus of SC may have used a similar evolutionary solution using an in-parallel approach adapted to the peculiar needs of a torus.

7. Outflow Regulation by an Aqueous Pump

7.1. First Mechanism: A Baroreceptor—IOP-induced Stretch—A Sensory System

The outflow system controls the return of aqueous to the heart. As a vascular circulatory loop, the outflow system functions by four homeostatic mechanisms identical to other vessel loops [29] (Figure 10). First, the TM is tensionally integrated and prestressed by IOP under physiologic conditions, as demonstrated with in vivo fixation (Figure 3) [15,20,36,44,46,53–55]. Continuous IOP-induced prestress links the TM configuration and IOP. Because of the prestress, the TM responds to small changes in IOP with profound shape changes. Optimized elastance causes TM deformation to track IOP with high fidelity. The close coupling of configuration and pressure permits the TM to function like other systemic baroreceptors, such as those of the aortic arch that sense stress-induced tissue deformation resulting from changes in volume that are tightly linked to pressure [29

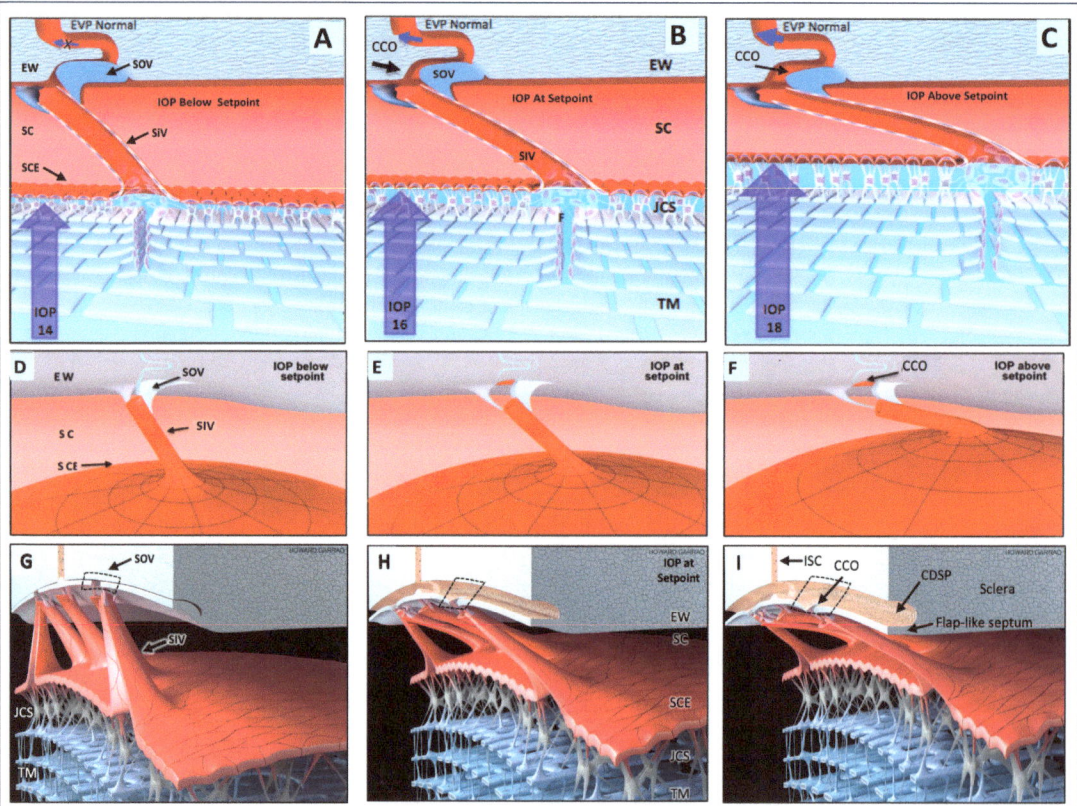

Figure 10. Depiction of the pressure-dependent relationships between trabecular meshwork Schlemm's canal, and valve-like structures. Images (**A,D,G**) depict the outflow system configuration at an intraocular pressure (IOP) below a homeostatic setpoint, images (**B,E,H**) are at the setpoint and images (**C,F,I**) are above the setpoint. In this provisional model, aqueous passes through the trabecular meshwork to the juxtacanalicular region and then flows through Schlemm's canal inlet valves into the SC lumen at collector channel ostia present at the external wall of SC. An SC outlet valve consists of a mobile flap-like septum between SC and a circumferentially oriented deep intrascleral

vascular plexus. The circumferential plexus serves as a closable conduit or chamber controlling aqueous flow. Blue arrows with increasing size indicate increased flow. See (Video 9) for animation of dynamic tissue motion and aqueous flow sequence. (TM) trabecular meshwork, (SC) Schlemm's canal, (SCE) Schlemm's canal inner wall endothelium, (SIV) SC inlet valve, (JCS) juxtacanalicular space, (EW) SC external wall, (CDSP) deep intrascleral vascular plexus, (IOP) intraocular pressure, (SOV) SC outlet valve, (CCO) channel entrances ostia, (ISC) intrascleral channel. See (Video 2) showing outflow feedback relationships that can control IOP [6].

7.2. Second Mechanism: SIV Link IOP-Induced TM Motion to SC Outlet Valves

Coupling the TM to SOV through SIV connections provides a second regulatory mechanism (Figures 3, 4, 7 and 8). The SIV connections between the TM and SOV hinged flaps at CCs are obliquely arranged [7]. Increasing pressure-induced outward movement of the TM results when IOP increases and permits fine adjustments of SOV dimensions through tensional integration and continuous IOP-induced prestress.

An increase in SOV lumen size can increase aqueous flow and reduce IOP. When IOP decreases, the TM moves toward the AC, permitting restoration of the setpoint. TM inward movement reduces tension on the obliquely arranged SIV. The reduced tension results in reduced flow IOP return to the homeostatic setpoint. A conduit-like behavior can be achieved close to the setpoint with the valves remaining slightly open. At the setpoint, visible pulsatile flow in the aqueous veins may be minimal or absent. When IOP rises significantly above the setpoint, the pulsatile flow becomes manifest [40]. See Video 2 showing stroke volume regulation of IOP.

7.3. Third Mechanism: Stroke Volume Regulation As an Innate Physical Feedback Loop

A third IOP regulatory mechanism is the control of stroke volume. The ocular pulse increases as IOP rises, thus increasing TM oscillatory amplitude. The increased TM amplitude increases SC volume, resulting in increased pulsatile aqueous discharge from SC to the aqueous veins [4]. See (Video 2) showing stroke volume regulation of IOP.

The pressure-dependent TM motion responses provide a physical, sensory error detection mechanism to identify pressure elevation. The physical TM motor responses act as a feedback mechanism. An increase in IOP causes increased stroke volume, restoring pressure to its homeostatic setpoint. When IOP is below the setpoint, TM cyclic decreases, the per pulse stroke volume decreases, total aqueous flow decreases, and IOP rises, returning to its homeostatic setpoint [4].

7.4. Fourth Mechanism: Pulsewave-Dependent Shear Stress in TM and Distal Pathways

In 2004, Johnstone first recognized evidence leading to the conclusion that shear stress is present in the entire outflow system and that NO and endothelin are major aqueous outflow regulatory factors [5]. The evidence and reasoning follow. In the human outflow system, rapid pulsatile flow into SC, the CCs, intrascleral channels, and the aqueous veins was directly observable, providing reality-based evidence of its presence (Section 2.2). Cyclic pulsatile aqueous flow from the TM into SIV progressed into SC. Pulsatile aqueous ejected into SC. Pulsatility was maintained as aqueous entered CCs and intrascleral channels. The speed of the cyclic pulsatile outflow system motion was synchronous with the cardiac pulse.

The cardiac pulse induces shear stress signals in the endothelium of vessel walls throughout the vascular system. Aqueous outflow system pathways have a comparable vascular endothelium and experience the same pulse speed. Outflow system structures can be expected to use identical mechanisms [29]. Initial evidence in human subjects led to the conclusion that shear stress-dependent nitric oxide signaling must be present in the outflow system in humans. Laboratory studies began seven years later with extensive follow-up studies validating the initial clinical evidence and conclusions, including evidence of effects on distal outflow [56–65].

8. Ciliary Body: Central Role in the Regulation of Aqueous Outflow

8.1. The Role of Ciliary Muscles in Preventing SC Collapse and TM Stiffness/Elastance

Ciliary body properties are central to IOP control. The ciliary body and the TM are anatomically and functionally inseparable units. The ciliary body regulates TM distention into SC by continually maintaining tension, preventing persistent SC collapse. Ciliary body tension moves the TM toward the AC then the SC lumen size increases, the spaces between TM lamellae enlarge, and the TM elastance/stiffness increases [8,10,11,41,41,66–74].

The tensional stress from SC enlargement increases SIV tension on CC hinged flaps, increasing CC and CDSP lumen dimensions. The improved vector forces enlarge outflow pathways, reducing outflow pathway resistance and improving responsiveness to IOP setpoint deviations as well as oscillatory and pulse transients. Increasing ciliary body tension favors outflow pathway enlargement, and stroke volume increases. Enhancing the dual pump/conduit function can thus reduce IOP.

8.2. Ciliary Body Attachments and Geometric Relations That Permit Regulation

The scleral spur is an anterior extension of the sclera that encompasses the posterior portion of SC, resulting in a mobile hinged region. The vector forces associated with scleral spur movement cause it to move inward and posteriorly with ciliary muscle tension. Thus, the ciliary muscle induces stress on the TM lamellae through direct ciliary muscle connections and scleral spur connections. The tension causes rotation of the TM inward, enlarging the SC area. The stress-induced tension also increases interspaces between trabecular lamellae and causes elongation. The ciliary muscle's geometric position and contractile state determine the TM lamellae's anatomic position and mechanical properties essential to flow regulation (Figure 2). The importance is illustrated by evidence that clinical disinsertion of the ciliary muscle results in severe angle recession glaucoma [41,75]. For example, see (Video 7) showing the effects of ciliary body tension on TM.

Phenomenological ground truth is easily determined using direct observation. Ciliary muscle tension results in the TM moving away from the external wall of SC and toward the AC. Lamellae move posteriorly, but their attachment to Schwalbe's line is maintained resulting in TM lamellae elongation. The elongation increases tensional stress and increases the stored potential energy (Figure 2). Evidence of the lamellae storage of potential energy is evident when ciliary muscle tension is released. The TM lamellae immediately shorten, and the TM complex moves toward the outer wall of SC.

8.3. TM Elastance/Stiffness Curve of the TM Controlled by the Ciliary Muscle

Stiffness/elastance of biological tissues is not a static property but is instead tightly linked to instantaneous tissue loading forces. As ciliary muscle tension increases, the TM lamellae move up the elastance curve, reflecting increased stiffness [48]. An elastance curve defines the tissue's ability to distend and recoil, and in the case of the TM, it involves measuring stiffness under varying loads. For homeostasis, a narrow range of elastance/stiffness must be maintained.

If the TM lamellae are abnormally compliant or stiff, they cannot move appropriately in response to IOP changes. The ciliary muscle is a primary determinant of TM elastance. For example, see the (Video 7) showing TM-ciliary muscle elastance. Optimized TM elastance governs the degree of pressure-dependent TM distention into SC and responses to oscillatory forces such as eye movement/blinking-related transients and associated pulsatile behavior [48].

8.4. Opposing Forces of IOP and Ciliary Muscle Tension Control TM Position

Two opposing forces govern the TM's position in the 3D space between the AC and SC. The compressive forces are (1) IOP, (2) superimposed transient pulses, and (3) oscillatory forces. These forces impinge on SC endothelium, which deforms in response and moves toward the SC lumen. Opposing forces involving tension are (1) the TM lamellae elastance as a tethering force limiting SC endothelial distention, (2) the anterior–posterior geometric position of the ciliary muscle, and (3) the contractile properties of the ciliary muscle. The combined tensile forces continually oppose the compressive forces, providing a homeostatic equilibrium position of the TM.

The TM may be likened to a stringed instrument constantly adjusting its properties to remain in tune. When optimally tuned, its position in 3D space provides an ideal relationship between the inner and outer walls of the SC. At the same time, the optimized elastance permits the TM to dance to the tune of the ocular pulse. Accurate tonal responses to the IOP, IOP transients, and oscillations are necessarily lost with too little or too much tension.

The seamless anatomic connections between TM lamellae and ciliary muscle ensure that vector forces act synchronously. This inextricable linkage requires synchronous dual regulation to maintain optimized SC dimensions, TM elastance, and IOP control. The relationships and elastance/stiffness requirements are necessary to maintain a highly regulated ciliary muscle contractile state. Age-related changes in position and contractile state are thought to alter the ciliary muscle's ability to participate in the control of IOP [74,76,77].

8.5. Ciliary Muscle Control of Distal Pathway Resistance

When ciliary muscle tension increases, SC enlarges, and SIV elongation increases. The SIV elongation transmits increased stress from the TM to septa that function as hinged flaps at CC entrances. The integrated structural CB-TM-SIV-SOV relationships allow the ciliary muscle to alter CC entrance dimensions (Figure 2).

The crystalline lens attachment to the ciliary muscle causes stresses that pull the ciliary muscle anteriorly with progressing age [74]. The anterior movement alters vector forces on the TM and scleral spur, causing them to move anteriorly and outward. The TM moves further into SC, reducing the TM lamellae tensile loading forces. Cataract surgery eliminates stresses pulling the ciliary muscle anteriorly. The new vector forces favor posterior and interior rotation of the scleral spur and ciliary body tendons [11]. These vector forces tend to pull the entire TM away from the external wall of SC, open intertrabecular spaces, and increase the tension or load on the trabecular lamellae (Figure 2).

9. Resistance: Physiology and Glaucoma Pathology

9.1. Little Resistance Is within the TM: Resistance Results from SC Collapse

The classic physiology studies of Grant and colleagues reveal that there is little resistance within the TM itself. Instead, their studies indicate that resistance results from TM motion that leads to SC wall closure and herniation into the entrances of CCs [8–11,36,67,68]. Grant's 1958–1963 studies [13,14] in ex vivo eyes used pressures far outside the normal range. The 25 mm Hg IOP represented the equivalent of an in vivo 33 mm Hg transtrabecular pressure gradient because of the absent 8 mm episcleral venous pressure. The contractile tone of the ciliary muscle was absent, and there was no histologic confirmation of the extent of tissue removal. Grant's group acknowledged and corrected these severe limitations in the later studies [8–11,36,67,68,78].

Unfortunately, the earlier work provided a simple, easily modeled TM doctrine, which was later demonstrated to be erroneous but entrenched in textbooks by that time. The ideology remains deeply embedded in the currently used investigative framework and permeates every aspect of research efforts. The typically declarative textbook and research reviews characterize control of outflow resistance as being isolated to a narrow region of the TM's outer wall. The passive model is not presented as provisional and needing further inquiry but as an issue that has been effectively resolved.

The selective absence of citations to the crucial literature does not permit readers themselves to grasp and process the evidence required to assess uncertainty in the declarative statements. Of greater concern, the declarative approach implies an area of settled science. The approach reduces the likelihood of early-stage investigators and busy clinicians challenging, exploring more broadly, or engaging in deeper inquiry, leading to treatment breakthroughs benefiting patients.

9.2. Isolation of Resistance to the TM: A Premise Inconsistent with the Best Evidence

Later studies by Grant's group refuted the premise that his widely cited earlier techniques can eliminate or even identify resistance limited to the TM. Complete removal of the external wall of SC, called sinusotomy, also removed 75% of the resistance. Many attachments were present between the TM and the external wall of SC, preventing isolation of tissue removal to either wall of the canal [10]. A repeat of the earlier studies, now followed by light and SEM examination, demonstrated that the removal technique damaged the TM-SC external wall connections that were torn and pulled away from the external wall of SC [10,11]. The numerous connections meant that there was no way to use the technique to truly separate TM and distal resistance.

Direct observation demonstrated that increasing IOP caused the TM to distend far into the scleral tunnel after removing the external wall of SC. The distension provided physical, directly observable evidence that the TM is mobile, and its distension can occlude SC [8]. A series of ingenious studies, illustrated in Figure 5, verified that resistance increases resulted from TM motion that caused SC collapse; of critical importance, the studies showed that ciliary body tension prevented SC collapse responsible for the increased resistance [8–11].

9.3. Trabecular Meshwork Stiffness Abnormalities as a Factor in Glaucoma

Ex vivo studies using multiple approaches have identified abnormal TM tissue biomechanics in glaucoma patients. One study used the elastic modulus with finite element modeling and found stiffness was modestly higher in glaucoma eyes. The elastic modulus is the ratio of the force exerted upon a substance to the resultant deformation.

Another parameter used to assess TM motion is the time-dependent shear modulus, a measure of ocular rigidity that assesses the outflow tissue's viscoelastic properties. The shear modulus is the ratio of shear stress to shear strain. Stress in this setting is the IOP, and strain is the tissue deformation. Recent studies found a highly significant reduction in both the long and short-term shear modulus of the ECM, collagen, and elastin in glaucoma vs. normal tissue. The authors concluded that the outflow tissues in glaucoma eyes are stiffer and less able to respond to dynamic IOP changes [79].

An additional stiffness parameter is load rate stiffening. Blinking, eye movement, and lid squeezing cause abrupt pressure increases that may be modified by load rate stiffening. In the outflow system, baseline tissue stiffness is tightly linked to the static loading force of IOP. The abrupt pressure transients require introducing another recently explored stiffness parameter, load rate-dependent stiffening with a time component.

With rapid movement, tissues stiffen more rapidly, reducing the overall tissue deformation. The stress of the same rise in IOP results in less deformation or strain compared with static conditions. The findings suggest that rate-dependent stiffening may protectively dampen tissue deformation from abrupt pressure transients in patients with normal tissue biomechanics [79].

Another method to assess both TM and CC tissue stiffness is real-time measurements of outflow pathway motion using high-resolution OCT. Evaluation of the complex motion curves using MANOVA demonstrated a significant reduction in movement of both the TM and tissues surrounding CCs in eyes with glaucoma [12].

10. Crucial Evidence: IOP, TM Removal, and Ciliary Muscle Tension: Impact on Outflow Facility

Figure 5A illustrates how crystalline lens backward movement dilates Schlemm's canal (SC) and reduces resistance [8,9,11,68]. The upper panel shows no lens depression. The trabecular meshwork (TM) is in extensive apposition to the external wall (EW) of SC causing the closure of the SC lumen (arrow). In the lower panel, with depression of the crystalline lens, the ciliary body (CB) and scleral spur (SS) rotate posteriorly, pulling the TM attachments away from the external wall of SC. The TM distends, and the SC lumen is large. The black arrow demonstrates the SC inlet valve extending from the TM to a hinged flap at a collector channel entrance.

Figure 5B shows that the corneal perfusion fitting contains a lens-depression device. The CB and SS move backward with lens depression, resulting in the opening of SC. As the lens moves backward, causing CB tension, resistance falls by over 50% (Figure 5C(1)). There is no iridectomy. Anterior chamber perfusion forces the lens backward, resulting in a reverse pupillary block phenomenon. The backward movement increases zonular tension that transmits to the ciliary body, scleral spur (SS), and TM tendons. The tension and vector forces cause the scleral spur and TM to move posteriorly and inward. In Figure 5C(2), with an iridectomy, pressure gradients equalize between the anterior and posterior chamber, eliminating posterior lens movement or ciliary body tension.

Figure 5D shows the outflow facility experimentally controlled at a series of steady-state intraocular pressures. The blue curve is the outflow facility with no ciliary body tension, as shown in the Figure 5C(2) protocol. The orange curve is the outflow facility with ciliary body tension resulting from the protocol, as shown in Figure 5C(1). Pressures in the abscissa need to be adjusted upward by 8 mm Hg to reflect transtrabecular in vivo pressure gradients because of the lack of episcleral venous pressure in the ex vivo setting. Ellingsen and Grant determined the reduction in outflow resistance from TM removal at each pressure, as noted in the blue curve shown in Figure 5C(2). As indicated by the boxed data, an effective IOP of 13, 18, and 33 mm Hg, trabeculotomy reduces resistance (R) by 14%, 27%, and 75%, respectively. The upward-pointing blue arrow and asterisk indicate the conditions of Grant's initial 1958 and 1963 studies. With simulated ciliary muscle tension as in condition C2, the outflow facility is initially higher than under condition C1. The facility of outflow remains high despite increasing IOP. The authors concluded that the apposition of the TM to the SC external wall caused increased resistance with increased pressure. They also concluded that ciliary muscle tension prevents SC wall apposition and associated reduction in outflow facility.

11. Identifying Outflow Structure Damage When Planning Surgical Intervention

11.1. Clinical Angiography: Office-Based Hemoglobin Video Editing

Pulsatile flow from the aqueous to the episcleral veins is readily visible using a slit lamp. Investigative studies with the technique provide clinicians with remarkable insights into physiologic outflow mechanisms [3,28]. Because it is very time-consuming, the slit lamp approach is of limited value in clinical settings.

Hemoglobin video imaging is a newly developed technique adapted for use at the slit lamp in a clinical environment. The technique provides noninvasive, real-time, high-resolution images. The approach can differentiate normal from glaucoma patients by quantifying the flow rate [80–83]. The hemoglobin absorption spectrum increases the contrast of red cells, improving the distinction between episcleral venous blood and aqueous. By studying flow patterns in the clinic, it may be possible to identify optimal MIGS placement locations before going to the OR.

11.2. Functional Outflow System Abnormality Assessment Using Phase-OCT

We lack knowledge of the crucially important IOP profile in individual patients. IOP measurements are inherently suboptimal. Office IOP readings occur at random times and are of brief duration, involving about 16 s of 31 million seconds in a year. Diurnal variation is not captured. In addition, there is unknown patient compliance, and the range of ocular transients is unknown.

In contrast, the outflow system's underlying biomechanical properties that permit it to maintain IOP homeostasis are intrinsic tissue properties. These biomechanical properties determine the TM's ability to distend and recoil. The PhS-OCT system enables identifying movement with a sensitivity of 20 nanometers with ~ a 1000 nanometer dynamic range. Tracking and quantitative measurements of real-time pulse-dependent TM motion are now possible in patients with the recently developed Phase-OCT system. The system identifies differences between glaucoma and normal patients, performing better than

IOP or tonography measurements [84]. The Phase-OCT technique also identifies diurnal pressure variability not captured in random office measurements.

11.3. Introduction of a Fluid Wave to Assess MIGS Placement and Surgical Success

During MIGS surgery, infusing a fluid bolus into the AC displaces blood in the episcleral veins, causing the clear fluid to create a pulsatile episcleral vein bolus and regional blanching. The pulsatile wave and blanching demonstrate patency of structural pathways from the AC to the aqueous and episcleral veins. These clinical findings are predictive of surgical success [85]. Other operating approaches introduce dyes into the AC or SC. These studies provide evidence of the pulsatile behavior of aqueous flow in both NH primates and humans. The approach shows promise in identifying the proper location for MIGS placement [86–88].

11.4. MIGS Reduction in IOP Is Not by Physiologic Mechanisms

Canal-based MIGS procedures avoid the risks of trabeculectomy surgery. The procedures represent a valuable interim contribution to glaucoma patient care while awaiting a more definitive problem resolution based on an improved understanding of outflow system physiology. Current MIGS procedures cannot restore physiologic pressure control mechanisms because they disrupt structures within SC involved in IOP control [4,36] (Figure 7). Nonetheless, the importance of MIGS is not diminished by their lack of targeting physiologic IOP control mechanisms.

Some SC-directed MIGS procedures remove much of the TM, and others cannulate the canal. The currently available cannulas are too large to fit within the confines of SC. These cannulas disrupt SC inner wall endothelium, simultaneously tearing the anterior and posterior walls at their attachment sites. A cannula passage also necessarily disrupts SIVs and attachments to SOV [6,10,11,15].

Well-defined structural features distal to the TM include SIV, septa and their hinged flaps at CCs, and the circumferentially oriented collapsible chamber surrounding SC. Such structural pathways are involved in regulating resistance distal to the TM. MIGS procedures ablate or disrupt these pressure-regulating structures at the TM and SC levels. However, TM flaps may be left behind, and the septa that maintain CDSP dimensions are not reliably removed. Even after circumferential trabeculotomy and canaloplasty, short-term IOP fluctuation may be high [89].

A recent study examined the effects of disrupting SIV linkage to the hinged flaps at SOV by injecting a fluid bolus into SC. The SOV channel dimensions were decreased after SIV connections to the TM were disrupted. Outflow tissue biomechanics were substantially altered, as illustrated by the quantitative changes in TM elastance [48]. Altered TM elastance necessitates alterations in physiologic pressure and pulse-dependent responses involved in IOP control.

12. Recovery of Normal Function—Requirements

12.1. Problem Identification as the First Step

In medicine, the nature of the problem must be identified before a rational solution can be implemented. Identification of the tissues causing IOP abnormality in glaucoma remains elusive. However, studies consistently show that alteration in stiffness/elastance of the TM-ciliary muscle complex is a primary factor

We reason that outflow tissues stiffen like other vascular tissues, such as the aorta subjected to constant oscillatory forces. Age-related tissue stiffening results from elastin fragmentation and replacement with collagen, which is 100 times less distensible than elastin. An illustration is age-related elastin replacement with collagen in the systemic vasculature, leading to the vessel wall stiffening that we call arteriolosclerosis. Aortic enlargement occurs due to vessel wall stiffening, leading to the inability to recoil. Pulsatile pressure subjects the aorta to continuous oscillations. The stiffening leads to aortic expansion and a 50% enlargement in diameter between ages 40 and 70 [29].

Elastin fragmentation and replacement with collagen is a systemwide age-related phenomenon likely to be shared by the TM lamellae. The TM lamellae are part of a vessel wall that we call SC. The lamellae experience constant pressure forces and oscillations like other vessel walls that result in progressive distention with aging. Vessel wall distention in the case of the TM results in outward movement into SC, narrowing its lumen. Such changes may result in persistent SC closure in glaucoma patients. When SC wall apposition persists, the TM loses its equipoise in 3D space. If the walls of SC become persistently appositional, the TM's ability to sense or respond to pressure changes is lost (Figure 2). In glaucoma, TM motion (Section 2.4) and pulsatile flow (Section 3.1) slow and then stop.

12.2. Problem Resolution as the Second Step

A reasonable goal for addressing the IOP problem in glaucoma is the restoration of a low, minimally fluctuating IOP. Current evidence indicates that optimized tissue elastance/stiffness restoration should restore homeostasis to normal. Techniques for identifying abnormal elastance and restoring it to normal are evolving [16,48,80–83].

12.3. Restoration of Normal Outflow System Elastance and IOP in Glaucoma

A practical illustration of restoration of elastance in glaucoma patients is the response to miotics. Prestress induced by IOP causes the entire outflow system to function as a tensionally unified complex. (Section 4.4). Ciliary muscle position and contractile properties control tensional loading forces, ensuring uniform distribution throughout the entire system from the TM to the level of the septa at CC entrances (Video 7) [4]. Ciliary muscle tension increases the loading force on the TM lamellae, causing them to move up the elastance curve, resulting in greater stiffness. At the same time, the TM moves toward the AC, enlarging SC [11,48,67,68].

Directly visible evidence of increased pulsatile flow in the aqueous veins can be correlated with known miotic-induced structural responses within the outflow system. Following the miotic-induced increase in pulsatile flow, IOP falls to a new temporary homeostatic setpoint. The increase in pulsatile flow followed by a reduction in IOP is compelling evidence of an elastance-related functional abnormality in glaucoma [1,3,26].

The miotic response provides robust evidence of the functional abnormality in glaucoma. It also furnishes clues to restoring normal outflow on a more permanent basis. Three techniques target the tension-dependent ciliary muscle or TM lamellae by introducing heat. ALT, SLT, and micropulse lasers are each designed to induce heat. Increased temperatures induce collagen shrinkage that can target the tension-dependent TM lamellae or ciliary muscle [90]. Cataract surgery and scleral expansion alter ciliary muscle tension and can lower IOP [91].

12.4. Cataract Surgery

One cataract-only control arm of a prospective randomized trial found a mean IOP reduction of 8.5 ± 4.3 mm Hg at 13 months. The OHTS study provided a rigorously controlled and characterized assessment of the effect of cataract surgery and found that IOP was reduced by greater than 4.0 mmHg (16%) [74,91,92].

A recently proposed explanation for the IOP reduction following cataract surgery is that it restores the aqueous outflow pump's sensory and motor properties that regulate IOP. Cataract surgery causes the AC to deepen, and the position of the residual lens capsule is posterior to SC. The new vector forces rotate the TM and scleral spur attachments backward in response to ciliary muscle tension, increasing tension in the trabecular tendons [74]. The new vector forces alter the effect of ciliary muscle tension. The TM interspaces enlarge, and SC's lumen volume increases, as shown in a recent OCT study in patients [93]. The restored configuration is more like that in youth, as revealed using high-resolution MRI [74,91]. The advantage of cataract removal is that no procedure-related outflow system structural damage occurs.

12.5. ALT, SLT, and Micropulse Laser as Elastance Improving Procedures

The TM lamellae–ciliary muscle complex is a tensionally integrated prestressed system. The trabecular lamellae are collagenous, and the ciliary muscle contains extensive fascial collagen components. Heating of collagen induces shrinkage. Heating that causes collagen shrinkage anywhere along the system necessarily transmits added tension to the entire complex. The elastin–collagen transition that diminishes elastance with age reduces the ability to respond to pressure gradients. Collagen shrinkage that induces tissue tightening may restore more normal IOP responses. Argon laser trabeculoplasty (ALT) causes heat-induced TM lamellar collagen shrinkage [94]. Selective laser trabeculoplasty (SLT) also heats outflow system tissues.

Pigmented cell death with cytokine release is a proposed mechanism for SLT's ability to reduce IOP. When heat is sufficient to kill cells, collagen shrinkage can also be expected. Histologic studies would not easily detect the small changes necessary to alter elastance [95]. Although subtle tissue shrinkage cannot be identified using histology, shrinkage can be identified using direct real-time same-sample imaging as achieved with a micropulse laser.

Cytokine release after an injury occurs rapidly and is of relatively brief duration. However, ALT and SLT effects on IOP often persist for many months to several years. Heat-induced tissue shrinkage during laser genioplasty is routinely observed and has a similar long-lasting effect. The relatively long duration of the SLT effect on IOP can be more easily explained by its ability to induce collagen shrinkage than the short-term effects of cytokine release [96].

The transscleral micropulse laser procedure causes ciliary muscle shrinkage and a change in TM configuration that is remarkably similar to the effects of miotics. It is essential to differentiate the micropulse technique from traditional procedures that use high energy to destroy the secretory ciliary endothelium. The laser penetration is too limited with the micropulse technique, so damage to the ciliary epithelium does not occur because the laser does not penetrate to its depth [97,98].

The micropulse procedure may prove attractive as a noninvasive means for restoring normal outflow function in glaucoma. Technique improvements can improve the success rate and reproducibility. Targets for parameter improvements include beam focus, wavelength, duty cycle, energy, and the development of a highly reproducible laser delivery system.

13. Limitations

Our report's crucial limitation is its reliance on studies from experimental platforms developed in our laboratories. Independent confirmation of the presence of the distal circumferential channels able to act as valves is lacking. The new awareness of the Ramirez group's work provides confirmatory evidence. It establishes the circumferential "outer collectors" as normally occurring structures in humans with anatomic and functional significance [50].

Another of this report's limitations was our use of controlled reverse perfusion of SC to study the dynamics of transtrabecular pressure gradients that had not been validated by an independent group. However, recently, another group successfully used the SC perfusion technique to study outflow system dynamics [79]. Their study demonstrated the platform's ability to explore the outflow pathway, finding a rate-dependent loading boundary with large fluctuations consistent with our findings.

Although anatomy, structural relationships, and motion are becoming clearer, much more work is needed to refine the tissue motion details. Our (Video 9) animation depicts one possible sequence of pulsatile flow, but it is only one of many scenarios and remains a wide-open question that is not easily resolvable with current technologies. The need to continually update the model illustrates our conceptual framework's evolving and provisional nature. We accept the need to maintain a degree of uncertainty and expect the model to undergo substantial modifications as new imaging technologies provide a more detailed picture of the outflow system's dynamic behavior.

14. Summary

The aqueous outflow system is a vascular circulatory loop. We present evidence leading to the conclusion that physiologic mechanisms in the rest of the vasculature also control aqueous outflow and intraocular pressure. In support of our conclusions, we consider readily verifiable reality-based knowledge from direct observation of pulsatile flow and its abnormalities in humans.

We describe pulsatile tissue motion, chambers, and valves that act synchronously to control the stroke volume of aqueous discharge into the venous system. We proposed that the outflow tissues function as a pump–conduit system similar to lymphatics. Our work introduces physiologic mechanisms involving pulse-dependent tissue and cellular motion as a sensory stimulus providing constant feedback to maintain a genomically determined intraocular pressure setpoint.

Our development of the pump conduit model also introduced the concept of pulse-dependent shear stress to regulate outflow pathway diameters through NO/endothelin pathways. We also introduced the role of the glycocalyx as a shear stress sensor, a barrier to prevent fluid passage across SC endothelium, and a means of ensuring load-bearing properties of the endothelium that enable its pressure-dependent deformation

We further introduced evidence of cellular attachments of the SC endothelium to the TM lamellae. The attachments permit us to introduce principles from vascular physiology, including pressure-dependent tensional integration and prestress central to mechanotransduction mechanisms that maintain homeostatic pressures throughout the vascular system. The constellation of findings leads us to conclude that the proposed behavior provides a rational basis to explain the regulation of aqueous outflow and intraocular pressure.

Author Contributions: Conceptualization M.J., C.X., E.M. and R.W.; methodology M.J., C.X., E.M. and R.W.; investigation M.J., C.X., E.M. and R.W.; original draft preparation M.J., C.X. and R.W. All authors have read and agreed to the published version of the manuscript.

Funding: This work was supported in part by research grants from the Public Health Service Center Grant PO1-EY000292, Training Grant TO1-EY-00018, and research grant RO1EY00002, R01EY0190601 from the National Eye Institute, the W. H. Coulter Foundation Translational Research Partnership Program, an Unrestricted Grant from Research to Prevent Blindness, and the Office of Research Infrastructure Programs of the National Institutes of Health through Grant No. P51OD010425 at the Washington National Primate Research Center and Carl Zeiss Meditec Inc.

Acknowledgments: The content is solely the responsibility of the authors and does not necessarily represent the official views of the grant-giving bodies. The funders had no role in the study design, data collection, analysis, publication decision, or manuscript preparation. Part of this work was conducted at the University of Washington Nanotech User Facility, a member of the NSF National Nanotechnology Infrastructure Network, the Biology Imaging Facility, and the Keck Microscopy Center at the University of Washington. The SightLife Eye Bank and the Oregon Vision Gift Eye Bank provided human tissues.

Conflicts of Interest: Chen Xin, Elizabeth Martin, and Ruikang Wang declare no financial conflict other than those listed under funding sources. Murray Johnstone serves as a consultant for Alcon and Elios Vision.

Abbreviations

trabecular meshwork (TM), Schlemm's canal (SC), SC inlet valve (SIV), SC outlet valve (SOV), optical coherence tomography (OCT), phase OCT (PhS-OCT), spectral domain OCT (SD-OCT), scanning electron microscopy (SEM), minimally invasive glaucoma surgery (MIGS), circumferential vascular channel (CVC), circumferential deep scleral plexus (CDSP), episcleral vein pressure (EVP), aqueous vein pressure (AVP).

References

1. Ascher, K.W. Aqueous Veins II. Local pharmacologic effects on aqueous veins III. Glaucoma and aqueous veins. *Am. J. Ophth.* **1942**, *25*, 1301–1315. [CrossRef]
2. Ascher, K.W. Physiologic importance of the visible elimination of intraocular fluid. *Am. J. Ophth.* **1942**, *25*, 1174–1209. [CrossRef]
3. Ascher, K.W. *The Aqueous Veins: Biomicroscopic Study of the Aqueous Humor Elimination*; Charles C. Thomas: Springfield, IL, USA, 1961; pp. 1–269.
4. Johnstone, M.; Xin, C.; Tan, J.; Martin, E.; Wen, J.; Wang, R.K. Aqueous outflow regulation–21st century concepts. *Prog. Retin. Eye Res.* **2021**, *83*, 100917. [CrossRef] [PubMed]
5. Johnstone, M.A. The aqueous outflow system as a mechanical pump: Evidence from examination of tissue and aqueous movement in human and non-human primates. *J. Glaucoma* **2004**, *13*, 421–438. [CrossRef] [PubMed]
6. Martin, E.A.; Johnstone, M.A. A Novel Technique Identifies Valve-Like Pathways Entering and Exiting Schlemm's Canal in Macaca nemestrina Primates With Similarities to Human Pathways. *Front. Cell Dev. Biol.* **2022**, *10*, 868029. [CrossRef] [PubMed]
7. Hariri, S.; Johnstone, M.; Jiang, Y.; Padilla, S.; Zhou, Z.; Reif, R.; Wang, R.K. Platform to investigate aqueous outflow system structure and pressure-dependent motion using high-resolution spectral domain optical coherence tomography. *J. Biomed. Opt.* **2014**, *19*, 106013. [CrossRef] [PubMed]
8. Ellingsen, B.A.; Grant, W.M. Influence of intraocular pressure and trabeculotomy on aqueous outflow in enucleated monkey eyes. *Investig. Ophthalmol.* **1971**, *10*, 705–709.
9. Ellingsen, B.A.; Grant, W.M. The relationship of pressure and aqueous outflow in enucleated human eyes. *Investig. Ophthalmol.* **1971**, *10*, 430–437.
10. Ellingsen, B.A.; Grant, W.M. Trabeculotomy and sinusotomy in enucleated human eyes. *Investig. Ophthalmol.* **1972**, *11*, 21–28.
11. Van Buskirk, E.M. Anatomic correlates of changing aqueous outflow facility in excised human eyes. *Investig. Ophthalmol. Vis. Sci.* **1982**, *22*, 625–632.
12. Johnstone, M.; Xin, C.; Acott, T.; Vranka, J.; Wen, J.; Martin, E.; Wang, R.K. Valve-Like Outflow System Behavior With Motion Slowing in Glaucoma Eyes: Findings Using a Minimally Invasive Glaucoma Surgery-MIGS-Like Platform and Optical Coherence Tomography Imaging. *Front. Med.* **2022**, *9*, 815866. [CrossRef] [PubMed]
13. Grant, W.M. Further studies on facility of flow through the trabecular meshwork. *Arch. Ophthal.* **1958**, *60*, 523–533. [CrossRef] [PubMed]
14. Grant, W.M. Experimental Aqueous Perfusion in Enucleated Human Eyes. *Arch. Ophthal.* **1963**, *69*, 783–801. [CrossRef] [PubMed]
15. Johnstone, M.A. Pressure-dependent changes in configuration of the endothelial tubules of Schlemm's canal. *Am. J. Ophthalmol.* **1974**, *78*, 630–638. [CrossRef] [PubMed]
16. Gao, K.; Song, S.; Johnstone, M.A.; Zhang, Q.; Xu, J.; Zhang, X.; Wang, R.K.; Wen, J.C. Reduced pulsatile trabecular meshwork motion in eyes with primary open angle glaucoma using phase-sensitive optical coherence tomography. *Investig. Ophthalmol. Vis. Sci.* **2020**, *61*, 21. [CrossRef] [PubMed]
17. Johnson, M.; Chan, D.; Read, A.T.; Christensen, C.; Sit, A.; Ethier, C.R. The pore density in the inner wall endothelium of Schlemm's canal of glaucomatous eyes. *Investig. Ophthalmol. Vis. Sci.* **2002**, *43*, 2950–2955.
18. Ethier, C.R.; Coloma, F.M.; Sit, A.J.; Johnson, M. Two pore types in the inner-wall endothelium of Schlemm's canal. *Investig. Ophthalmol. Vis. Sci.* **1998**, *39*, 2041–2048.
19. Sit, A.J.; Coloma, F.M.; Ethier, C.R.; Johnson, M. Factors affecting the pores of the inner wall endothelium of Schlemm's canal. *Investig. Ophthalmol. Vis. Sci.* **1997**, *38*, 1517–1525.
20. Grierson, I.; Lee, W.R.; Abraham, S.; Howes, R.C. Associations between the cells of the walls of Schlemm's canal. *Albrecht Von Graefes Arch. Klin. Exp. Ophthalmol.* **1978**, *208*, 33–47. [CrossRef]
21. Popper, K. *The Logic of Scientific Discovery*; Routledge: Oxfordshire, UK, 2005; pp. 1–544.
22. Allingham, R.R.; de Kater, A.W.; Ethier, C.R.; Anderson, P.J.; Hertzmark, E.; Epstein, D.L. The relationship between pore density and outflow facility in human eyes. *Investig. Ophthalmol. Vis. Sci.* **1992**, *33*, 1661–1669.
23. Stamer, W.D.; Braakman, S.T.; Zhou, E.H.; Ethier, C.R.; Fredberg, J.J.; Overby, D.R.; Johnson, M. Biomechanics of Schlemm's canal endothelium and intraocular pressure reduction. *Prog. Retin. Eye Res.* **2015**, *44*, 86–98. [CrossRef] [PubMed]
24. Stamer, W.D.; Ethier, C.R. Cellular Mechanisms Regulating Conventional Outflow of Aqueous Humor. In *Albert and Jakobiec's Principles and Practice of Ophthalmology*; Springer International Publishing: Cham, Switzerland, 2020; pp. 1–29.
25. Freddo, T.F.; Civan, M.; Gong, H. Aqueous Humor and the Dynamics of Its Flow: Mechanisms and Routes of Aqueous Humor Drainage. In *Albert and Jakobiec's Principles and Practice of Ophthalmology*; Springer International Publishing: Cham, Switzerland, 2021; pp. 1–46.
26. De Vries, S. *De Zichtbare Afvoer Van Het Kamerwater*; Drukkerij Kinsbergen: Amsterdam, The Netherlands, 1947; p. 1.
27. Stepanik, J. Der sichtbare Kammerwasserabfluss. Eine kinematographische Studie. *Klin. Monatsbl. Augenh.* **1957**, *130*, 208.
28. Stepanik, J. Measuring velocity of flow in aqueous veins. *Am. J. Ophthal.* **1954**, *37*, 918. [CrossRef] [PubMed]
29. Levick, J.R. *Introduction to Cardiovascular Physiology*; Hodder Education, a Hachette UK Comp.: London, UK, 2010; p. 325.
30. Coleman, D.J.; Trokel, S. Direct-Recorded Intraocular Pressure Variations in a Human Subject. *Arch. Ophthalmol.* **1969**, *82*, 637–640. [CrossRef]
31. Kaufmann, C.; Bachmann, L.M.; Robert, Y.C.; Thiel, M.A. Ocular pulse amplitude in healthy subjects as measured by dynamic contour tonometry. *Arch. Ophthalmol.* **2006**, *124*, 1104–1108. [CrossRef] [PubMed]

32. Turner, D.C.; Edmiston, A.M.; Zohner, Y.E.; Byrne, K.J.; Seigfreid, W.P.; Girkin, C.A.; Morris, J.S.; Downs, J.C. Transient intraocular pressure fluctuations: Source, magnitude, frequency, and associated mechanical energy. *Investig. Ophthalmol. Vis. Sci.* **2019**, *60*, 2572–2582. [CrossRef]
33. Schirmer, K.E. Reflux of blood in the canal of Schlemm quantitated. *Can. J. Ophthalmol.* **1969**, *4*, 40–44. [PubMed]
34. Suson, E.B.; Schultz, R.O. Blood in schlemm's canal in glaucoma suspects. A study of the relationship between blood-filling pattern and outflow facility in ocular hypertension. *Arch. Ophthalmol.* **1969**, *81*, 808–812. [CrossRef]
35. Schirmer, K.E. Gonioscopic assessment of blood in Schlemm's canal. Correlation with glaucoma tests. *Arch. Ophthalmol.* **1971**, *85*, 263–267. [CrossRef]
36. Johnstone, M.A.; Grant, W.M. Pressure-dependent changes in structure of the aqueous outflow system in human and monkey eyes. *Am. J. Ophthalmol.* **1973**, *75*, 365–383. [CrossRef]
37. Smith, R. Blood in the canal of Schlemm. *Br. J. Ophth.* **1956**, *40*, 358. [CrossRef] [PubMed]
38. Phelps, C.D.; Asseff, C.F.; Weisman, R.L.; Podos, S.M.; Becker, B. Blood reflux into Schlemm's canal. *Arch. Ophthalmol.* **1972**, *88*, 625–631. [CrossRef]
39. Kleinert, H. The compensation maximum: A new glaucoma sign in aqueous veins. *Arch. Ophth.* **1951**, *46*, 618–624. [CrossRef]
40. Stambaugh, J.; Fuhs, J.; Ascher, K.W. Study of the compensation-maximum test on aqueous veins. *AMA Arch. Ophth.* **1954**, *51*, 24. [CrossRef]
41. Kaufman, P.L.; Barany, E.H. Loss of acute pilocarpine effect on outflow facility following surgical disinsertion and retrodisplacement of the ciliary muscle from the scleral spur in the cynomolgus monkey. *Investig. Ophthalmol.* **1976**, *15*, 793–807.
42. Kaufman, P.L. Deconstructing aqueous humor outflow–The last 50 years. *Exp. Eye Res.* **2020**, *197*, 108105. [CrossRef] [PubMed]
43. Hogan, M.J.; Alvarado, J.; Weddell, J.E. *Histology of the Human Eye, and Atlas and Textbook*; Saunders: Philadelphia, PA, USA, 1971.
44. Grierson, I.; Lee, W.R. Changes in the monkey outflow apparatus at graded levels of intraocular pressure: A qualitative analysis by light microscopy and scanning electron microscopy. *Exp. Eye Res.* **1974**, *19*, 21–33. [CrossRef]
45. Grierson, I.; Lee, W.R. Junctions between the cells of the trabecular meshwork. *Albrecht Von Graefes Arch. Klin. Exp. Ophthalmol.* **1974**, *192*, 89–104. [CrossRef]
46. Lee, W.R.; Grierson, I. Relationships between intraocular pressure and the morphology of the outflow apparatus. *Trans. Ophthalmol. Soc. U. K.* **1974**, *94*, 430–449.
47. Johnstone, M.A. Pressure-dependent changes in nuclei and the process origins of the endothelial cells lining Schlemm's canal. *Investig. Ophthalmol. Vis. Sci.* **1979**, *18*, 44–51.
48. Xin, C.; Johnstone, M.; Wang, N.; Wang, R.K. OCT Study of Mechanical Properties Associated with Trabecular Meshwork and Collector Channel Motion in Human Eyes. *PLoS ONE* **2016**, *11*, e0162048. [CrossRef] [PubMed]
49. Carreon, T.; van der Merwe, E.; Fellman, R.L.; Johnstone, M.; Bhattacharya, S.K. Aqueous outflow-A continuum from trabecular meshwork to episcleral veins. *Prog. Retin. Eye Res.* **2017**, *57*, 108–133. [CrossRef] [PubMed]
50. Ramírez, J.M.; Ramírez, A.I.; Salazar, J.J.; Rojas, B.; De Hoz, R.; Triviño, A. Schlemm's canal and the collector channels at different developmental stages in the human eye. *Cells Tissues Organs.* **2004**, *178*, 180–185. [CrossRef] [PubMed]
51. Ashton, N. Anatomical study of Schlemm's canal and aqueous veins by means of neoprene casts-Part II. Aqueous Veins (continued). *Br. J. Ophth.* **1952**, *36*, 265. [CrossRef] [PubMed]
52. Lim, R. The surgical management of glaucoma: A review. *Clin. Exp. Ophthalmol.* **2022**, *50*, 213–231. [CrossRef] [PubMed]
53. Grierson, I.; Lee, W.R. Pressure-induced changes in the ultrastructure of the endothelium lining Schlemm's canal. *Am. J. Ophthalmol.* **1975**, *80*, 863–884. [CrossRef] [PubMed]
54. Grierson, I.; Lee, W.R. The fine structure of the trabecular meshwork at graded levels of intraocular pressure. (1) Pressure effects within the near-physiological range (8–30 mmHg). *Exp. Eye Res.* **1975**, *20*, 505–521. [CrossRef]
55. Grierson, I.; Lee, W.R. The fine structure of the trabecular meshwork at graded levels of intraocular pressure. (2) Pressures outside the physiological range (0 and 50 mmHg). *Exp. Eye Res.* **1975**, *20*, 523–530. [CrossRef]
56. Stamer, W.D.; Lei, Y.; Boussommier-Calleja, A.; Overby, D.R.; Ethier, C.R. eNOS, a pressure-dependent regulator of intraocular pressure. *Investig. Ophthalmol. Vis. Sci.* **2011**, *52*, 9438–9444. [CrossRef]
57. Lei, Y.; Stamer, W.D.; Wu, J.; Sun, X. Endothelial nitric oxide synthase-related mechanotransduction changes in aged porcine angular aqueous plexus cells. *Investig. Ophthalmol. Vis. Sci.* **2014**, *55*, 8402–8408. [CrossRef]
58. Ashpole, N.E.; Overby, D.R.; Ethier, C.R.; Stamer, W.D. Shear stress-triggered nitric oxide release from Schlemm's canal cells. *Investig. Ophthalmol. Vis. Sci.* **2014**, *55*, 8067–8076. [CrossRef] [PubMed]
59. Zhou, J.; Li, Y.-S.; Chien, S. Shear stress–initiated signaling and its regulation of endothelial function. *Arterioscler. Thromb. Vasc. Biol.* **2014**, *34*, 2191–2198. [CrossRef] [PubMed]
60. Chang, J.Y.; Stamer, W.D.; Bertrand, J.; Read, A.T.; Marando, C.M.; Ethier, C.R.; Overby, D.R. Role of nitric oxide in murine conventional outflow physiology. *Am. J. Physiol. Cell Physiol.* **2015**, *309*, C205–C214. [CrossRef] [PubMed]
61. McDonnell, F.; Dismuke, W.M.; Overby, D.R.; Stamer, W.D. Pharmacological regulation of outflow resistance distal to Schlemm's canal. *Am. J. Physiol. Cell Physiol.* **2018**, *315*, C44–C51. [CrossRef] [PubMed]
62. Waxman, S.; Wang, C.; Dang, Y.; Hong, Y.; Esfandiari, H.; Shah, P.; Lathrop, K.L.; Loewen, R.T.; Loewen, N.A. Structure-Function Changes of the Porcine Distal Outflow Tract in Response to Nitric Oxide. *Investig. Ophthalmol. Vis. Sci.* **2018**, *59*, 4886–4895. [CrossRef] [PubMed]

63. McDonnell, F.; Perkumas, K.M.; Ashpole, N.E.; Kalnitsky, J.; Sherwood, J.M.; Overby, D.R.; Stamer, W.D. Shear Stress in Schlemm's Canal as a Sensor of Intraocular Pressure. *Sci. Rep.* **2020**, *10*, 5804. [CrossRef] [PubMed]
64. Madekurozwa, M.; Stamer, W.D.; Reina-Torres, E.; Sherwood, J.M.; Overby, D.R. The ocular pulse decreases aqueous humor outflow resistance by stimulating nitric oxide production. *Am. J. Physiol. Cell Physiol.* **2021**, *320*, C652–C665. [CrossRef] [PubMed]
65. Reina-Torres, E.; De Ieso, M.L.; Pasquale, L.R.; Madekurozwa, M.; van Batenburg-Sherwood, J.; Overby, D.R.; Stamer, W.D. The vital role for nitric oxide in intraocular pressure homeostasis. *Prog. Retin. Eye Res.* **2021**, *83*, 100922. [CrossRef]
66. Rohen, J.W.; Lutjen, E.; Barany, E. The relation between the ciliary muscle and the trabecular meshwork and its importance for the effect of miotics on aqueous outflow resistance. A study in two contrasting monkey species, Macaca irus and Cercopithecus aethiops. *Albrecht Von Graefes Arch. Klin. Exp. Ophthalmol.* **1967**, *172*, 23–47. [CrossRef]
67. Van Buskirk, E.M.; Grant, W.M. Lens depression and aqueous outflow in enucleated primate eyes. *Am. J. Ophthalmol.* **1973**, *76*, 632–640. [CrossRef]
68. Van Buskirk, E.M. Changes in facility of aqueous outflow induced by lens depression and intraocular pressure in excised human eyes. *Am. J. Ophthalmol.* **1976**, *82*, 736–740. [CrossRef]
69. Van Buskirk, E.M. The canine eye: Lens depression and aqueous outflow. *Investig. Ophthalmol. Vis. Sci.* **1980**, *19*, 789–792.
70. Tamm, E.R.; Flugel, C.; Stefani, F.H.; Lutjen-Drecoll, E. Nerve endings with structural characteristics of mechanoreceptors in the human scleral spur. *Investig. Ophthalmol. Vis. Sci.* **1994**, *35*, 1157–1166.
71. Tamm, E.R.; Koch, T.A.; Mayer, B.; Stefani, F.H.; Lütjen-Drecoll, E. Innervation of myofibroblast-like scleral spur cells in human monkey eyes. *Investig. Ophthalmol. Vis. Sci.* **1995**, *36*, 1633–1644.
72. Tamm, E.R.; Flügel-Koch, C.; Mayer, B.; Lütjen-Drecoll, E. Nerve cells in the human ciliary muscle: Ultrastructural and immunocytochemical characterization. *Investig. Ophthalmol. Vis. Sci.* **1995**, *36*, 414–426.
73. Flügel-Koch, C.; Neuhuber, W.L.; Kaufman, P.L.; Lütjen-Drecoll, E. Morphologic indication for proprioception in the human ciliary muscle. *Investig. Ophthalmol. Vis. Sci.* **2009**, *50*, 5529–5536. [CrossRef] [PubMed]
74. Strenk, S.A.; Strenk, L.M.; Guo, S. Magnetic resonance imaging of the anteroposterior position and thickness of the aging, accommodating, phakic, and pseudophakic ciliary muscle. *J. Cataract Refract. Surg.* **2010**, *36*, 235–241. [CrossRef] [PubMed]
75. Lutjen-Drecoll, E.; Kaufman, P.L.; Barany, E.H. Light and electron microscopy of the anterior chamber angle structures following surgical disinsertion of the ciliary muscle in the cynomolgus monkey. *Investig. Ophthalmol. Vis. Sci.* **1977**, *16*, 218–225.
76. Lutjen-Drecoll, E.; Tamm, E.; Kaufman, P.L. Age-related loss of morphologic responses to pilocarpine in rhesus monkey ciliary muscle. *Arch. Ophthalmol.* **1988**, *106*, 1591–1598. [CrossRef] [PubMed]
77. Tamm, E.; Lütjen-Drecoll, E.; Jungkunz, W.; Rohen, J.W. Posterior attachment of ciliary muscle in young, accommodating old, presbyopic monkeys. *Investig. Ophthalmol. Vis. Sci.* **1991**, *32*, 1678–1692.
78. Rosenquist, R.; Epstein, D.; Melamed, S.; Johnson, M.; Grant, W.M. Outflow resistance of enucleated human eyes at two different perfusion pressures and different extents of trabeculotomy. *Curr. Eye Res.* **1989**, *8*, 1233–1240. [CrossRef]
79. Karimi, A.; Khan, S.; Razaghi, R.; Rahmati, S.M.; Gathara, M.; Tudisco, E.; Aga, M.; Kelley, M.J.; Jian, Y.; Acott, T.S. Developing an experimental-computational workflow to study the biomechanics of the human conventional aqueous outflow pathway. *Acta Biomater.* **2023**, *164*, 346–362. [CrossRef] [PubMed]
80. Khatib, T.Z.; Meyer, P.A.R.; Lusthaus, J.; Manyakin, I.; Mushtaq, Y.; Martin, K.R. Hemoglobin Video Imaging Provides Novel In Vivo High-Resolution Imaging and Quantification of Human Aqueous Outflow in Patients with Glaucoma. *Ophthalmol. Glaucoma* **2019**, *2*, 327–335. [CrossRef] [PubMed]
81. Lusthaus, J.A.; Khatib, T.Z.; Meyer, P.A.R.; McCluskey, P.; Martin, K.R. Aqueous outflow imaging techniques and what they tell us about intraocular pressure regulation. *Eye* **2020**, *35*, 216–235. [CrossRef]
82. Lusthaus, J.A.; Meyer, P.A.R.; Khatib, T.Z.; Martin, K.R. The Effects of Trabecular Bypass Surgery on Conventional Aqueous Outflow, Visualized by Hemoglobin Video Imaging. *J. Glaucoma* **2020**, *29*, 656–665. [CrossRef]
83. Lusthaus, J.A.; Meyer, P.A.R.; McCluskey, P.J.; Martin, K.R. Hemoglobin Video Imaging Detects Differences in Aqueous Outflow between Eyes with and without Glaucoma During the Water Drinking Test. *J. Glaucoma* **2022**, *31*, 511–522. [CrossRef] [PubMed]
84. Gao, K.; Song, S.; Johnstone, M.A.; Wang, R.K.; Wen, J.C. Trabecular meshwork motion in normal compared with glaucoma eyes. *Investig. Ophthalmol. Vis. Sci.* **2019**, *60*, 4824.
85. Fellman, R.L.; Grover, D.S. Episcleral venous fluid wave: Intraoperative evidence for patency of the conventional outflow system. *J. Glaucoma* **2014**, *23*, 347–350. [CrossRef] [PubMed]
86. Huang, A.S.; Camp, A.; Xu, B.Y.; Penteado, R.C.; Weinreb, R.N. Aqueous Angiography: Aqueous Humor Outflow Imaging in Live Human Subjects. *Ophthalmology* **2017**, *124*, 1249–1251. [CrossRef]
87. Huang, A.S.; Li, M.; Yang, D.; Wang, H.; Wang, N.; Weinreb, R.N. Aqueous Angiography in Living Nonhuman Primates Shows Segmental, Pulsatile, and Dynamic Angiographic Aqueous Humor Outflow. *Ophthalmology* **2017**, *124*, 793–803. [CrossRef]
88. Huang, A.S.; Saraswathy, S.; Dastiridou, A.; Begian, A.; Mohindroo, C.; Tan, J.C.H.; Francis, B.A.; Hinton, D.R.; Weinreb, R.N. Aqueous Angiography-Mediated Guidance of Trabecular Bypass Improves Angiographic Outflow in Human Enucleated Eyes. *Investig. Ophthalmol. Vis. Sci.* **2016**, *57*, 4558–4565. [CrossRef] [PubMed]
89. Wang, H.; Xin, C.; Han, Y.; Shi, Y.; Ziaei, S.; Wang, N. Intermediate outcomes of ab externo circumferential trabeculotomy and canaloplasty in POAG patients with prior incisional glaucoma surgery. *BMC Ophthalmol.* **2020**, *20*, 389. [CrossRef] [PubMed]
90. Kaufman, P.; Gabelt, B. Production and Flow of Aqueous Humor. In *Adler's Physiology of the Eye*; Kaufman, P.L., Levin, L.A., Alm A., Nilsson, S.F.E., Ver Hoeve, J., Eds.; Elsevier Health Sciences: New York, NY, USA, 2011; pp. 274–307.

91. Poley, B.J.; Lindstrom, R.L.; Samuelson, T.W.; Schulze, R. Intraocular pressure reduction after phacoemulsification with intraocular lens implantation in glaucomatous and nonglaucomatous eyes: Evaluation of a causal relationship between the natural lens and open-angle glaucoma. *J. Cataract Refract. Surg.* **2009**, *35*, 1946–1955. [CrossRef] [PubMed]
92. Mansberger, S.L.; Gordon, M.O.; Jampel, H.; Bhorade, A.; Brandt, J.D.; Wilson, B.; Kass, M.A.; Ocular Hypertension Treatment Study Group. Reduction in intraocular pressure after cataract extraction: The Ocular Hypertension Treatment Study. *Ophthalmology* **2012**, *119*, 1826–1831. [CrossRef] [PubMed]
93. Zhao, Z.; Zhu, X.; He, W.; Jiang, C.; Lu, Y. Schlemm's Canal Expansion After Uncomplicated Phacoemulsification Surgery: An Optical Coherence Tomography Study. *Investig. Ophthalmol. Vis. Sci.* **2016**, *57*, 6507–6512. [CrossRef] [PubMed]
94. Wise, J.B.; Witter, S.L. Argon laser therapy for open-angle glaucoma. A pilot study. *Arch. Ophthalmol.* **1979**, *97*, 319–322. [CrossRef] [PubMed]
95. Latina, M.A.; Tumbocon, J.A. Selective laser trabeculoplasty: A new treatment option for open angle glaucoma. *Curr. Opin. Ophthalmol.* **2002**, *13*, 94–96. [CrossRef] [PubMed]
96. Lowenstein, A.; Geyer, O.; Goldstein, M.; Lazar, M. Argon laser gonioplasty in the treatment of angle-closure glaucoma. *Am. J. Ophthalmol.* **1993**, *115*, 399–400. [CrossRef]
97. Moussa, K.; Feinstein, M.; Pekmezci, M.; Lee, J.H.; Bloomer, M.; Oldenburg, C.; Sun, Z.; Lee, R.K.; Ying, G.-S.; Han, Y. Histologic Changes Following Continuous Wave and Micropulse Transscleral Cyclophotocoagulation: A Randomized Comparative Study. *Transl. Vis. Sci. Technol.* **2020**, *9*, 22. [CrossRef]
98. Maslin, J.S.; Chen, P.P.; Sinard, J.; Nguyen, A.T.; Noecker, R. Histopathologic changes in cadaver eyes after MicroPulse and continuous wave transscleral cyclophotocoagulation. *Can. J. Ophthalmol.* **2020**, *55*, 330–335. [CrossRef]

Disclaimer/Publisher's Note: The statements, opinions and data contained in all publications are solely those of the individual author(s) and contributor(s) and not of MDPI and/or the editor(s). MDPI and/or the editor(s) disclaim responsibility for any injury to people or property resulting from any ideas, methods, instructions or products referred to in the content.

Article

Comparison between Intraocular Pressure Profiles over 24 and 48 h in the Management of Glaucoma

Philip Keye [1,*], Daniel Böhringer [1], Alexandra Anton [1,2], Thomas Reinhard [1] and Jan Lübke [1]

1. Eye Center, Medical Center–University of Freiburg, Faculty of Medicine, University of Freiburg, 79106 Freiburg, Germany
2. ADMEDICO Augenzentrum, Fährweg 10, 4600 Olten, Switzerland
* Correspondence: philip.keye@uniklinik-freiburg.de; Tel.: +49-(0)761-270-40010

Abstract: (1) Background: Due to significant variation, sporadic IOP measurements often fail to correctly assess the IOP situation in glaucoma patients. Thus, diurnal-nocturnal IOP profiles can be used as a diagnostic tool. The purpose of this study is to determine the additional diagnostic value of prolonged IOP profiles. (2) Methods: All diagnostic 48 h IOP profiles from a large university hospital, between 2017 and 2019, were reviewed. Elevated IOP > 21 mmHg, IOP variation > 6 mmHg and nocturnal IOP peaks were defined as IOP events of interest and counted. The analysis was repeated for the first 24 h of every IOP profile only. The Chi^2 test was used for statistical analysis. (3) Results: 661 IOP profiles were included. Specifically, 59% of the 48 h IOP profiles revealed IOP values above 21 mmHg, and 87% showed IOP fluctuation greater than 6 mmHg. Nocturnal peaks in the supine position could be observed in 51% of the patients. In the profiles censored for the first 24 h, the fractions were 50%, 71% and 48%, ($p < 0.01$, $p < 0.01$ and $p = 0.12$) respectively. (4) Conclusions: the 48 h IOP profiles identified more patients with IOP events of interest than the 24 h IOP profiles. The additional diagnostic value must be weighed against the higher costs.

Keywords: glaucoma; IOP; diurnal; nocturnal; fluctuation; variation

1. Introduction

Glaucoma is characterized by a progressive loss of retinal ganglion cells and represents one of the leading causes of blindness worldwide [1–3]. Several risk factors for the emergence and progression of glaucoma have been described, including older age, a family history of glaucoma, exfoliation, lower systolic blood pressure and elevated intraocular pressure (IOP) [4,5]. Among these, elevated IOP is the most important, since lowering the IOP has been shown to be the only therapeutic approach to reduce the risk of progressive loss of ganglion cells, and therefore, visual field loss [6]. In healthy humans, the IOP usually ranges from 10 to 21 mmHg and shows a significant fluctuation over a period of 24 h [7,8] The role of IOP fluctuation has been the subject of debate in recent years, with some studies suggesting that intraocular IOP fluctuation is an independent risk factor for the progression of glaucoma, and some studies suggesting otherwise [9]. For example, Tajunisah et al reported a mean IOP amplitude of 6 mmHg in glaucoma suspects compared to 4 mmHg in healthy eyes [10]. It has been shown that IOP frequently peaks at night. This is usually attributed to a supine sleeping position and the circadian rhythm [11].

With IOP being the only modifiable risk factor for visual field loss in glaucoma patients it is of utmost importance that high IOP values are detected and that those patients who should be considered for IOP-lowering therapeutic measures are identified. IOP is usually measured within normal office hours in an outpatient setting. However, it has been shown that sporadic IOP measurements often fail to reproduce IOP mean values, due to IOP fluctuation and the diurnal and nocturnal changes [12]. In many places, glaucoma patients with suspected progressive visual field loss and seemingly normal IOP values are hospitalized, and the IOP is measured repeatedly in order to approach the true mean IOP and rule out considerable IOP peaks that might contribute to the progression of glaucomatous damage [13]. Having knowledge of the individual IOP situation of a patient is valuable when it comes to deciding what therapeutic measures are best suited for that particular patient. The diagnostic value is largely independent of concurrent glaucoma medication or past glaucoma surgery, because IOP remains the only truly modifiable risk factor across all stages of glaucoma. If the IOP profile reveals an uncontrolled IOP situation as the cause of glaucoma progression, lowering the IOP is necessary irrespective of present glaucoma medication or past glaucoma surgery. It has been shown that diurnal pressure patterns show poor repeatability both in healthy controls and glaucoma patients [14,15]. Fischer et al. reported IOP profile data of a cohort of 80 patients who received a diurnal and nocturnal IOP profile, suggesting that both the maximum and mean IOP differed between day 1 and day 2 of the profile [16]. In recent years, a lot of effort has been put into the development of continuous IOP monitoring devices and the advances in this field are substantial. The desire for continuous IOP monitoring, e.g., over 24 h, arose from the limitations of singular IOP measurements: IOP fluctuation and IOP peaks could be detected more reliably without creating an artificial measuring situation, ideally at the patient's home. Both invasive and non-invasive approaches have been tested. Intraocular sensors (e.g., EYEMATE, Implandata Ophthalmic Products GmbH, Hannover, Germany) must be implanted into the eye, while most non-invasive approaches incorporate different designs for corneal contact lenses (e.g., Triggerfish CLS, Sensimed AG, Lausanne, Switzerland). Both technologies face difficulties. The implantation of an intraocular sensor carries a disproportionate risk of intraocular infections. Additionally, combined cataract surgery is usually required. Non-invasive contact lens technologies, on the other hand, are prone to measuring inaccuracies due to confounding factors, such as corneal curvature [17]. Due to these challenges, continuous IOP monitoring is not yet broadly incorporated into the clinical routine of glaucoma management, and therefore, "classical" measuring of the IOP remains of major importance.

In this study, we aim to determine the additional value of IOP profiles over 48 h, compared to IOP profiles over 24 h, regarding the ability to identify patients with elevated IOP values and significant IOP fluctuation. Additionally, we analyze whether potential nocturnal peaks are more frequently detected when measuring the IOP over 48 h. Since our goal was to obtain findings that are as universally valid as possible and of as much practical use as possible, all our data are based on a "real world" cohort of hospitalized patients from a large eye hospital, comprising different underlying ophthalmic diseases from the glaucoma family.

2. Materials and Methods

This retrospective mono-center cohort study was approved by the local ethics committee (vote no. 21-1184).

We manually reviewed our hospital database from the years 2017 to 2019 and identified all patients who had been admitted for an IOP profile, as part of the diagnostic routine. The reason for admission was mainly confirmed glaucoma with suspected progression of visual field loss under therapy (conservative mono- or multitherapy and/or surgical therapy) or, less frequently, suspected glaucoma with normal pressure values at outpatient presentation. Glaucoma diagnosis was established by a glaucoma specialist in accordance with the latest guidelines by the European Glaucoma Society and based on clinical examination, visual field examination and optical coherence tomography (OCT) measurements. Clinical signs, such as optic disc hemorrhage or deterioration of visual acuity due to glaucoma, were considered as signs of progression. Analysis tools from the OCT device manufacturer (Heidelberg Engineering, Heidelberg, Germany) were used to detect progression in the OCT measurements and trend-based analysis tools were incorporated to detect progression of visual field loss. We did not further distinguish between different types of glaucoma. The IOP profile usually starts on the first day of hospitalization at noon and is conducted over 24 or 48 h. The time points of IOP measurements were 12:00, 16:00, 20:00, 00:00 and 07:00. This resulted in a total of 10 IOP measurements over the period of 48 h and 5 over the period of 24 h. The 12:00, 16:00 and 20:00 measurements were performed using Goldmann applanation tonometry (GAT) in a sitting position; the 00:00 and 07:00 measurements were performed using a handheld contact tonometer (iCare pro tonometer, iCare Finland Oy) in a supine position. Measurements with the iCare device were repeated five times. The IOP values were only accepted if the device's integrated quality control approved the measurement. At the start of every IOP profile, a comparison measurement was performed to see if the iCare IOP values matched the GAT IOP values. If differences were found, these were incorporated into the iCare measured values. For organizational reasons, not all measurements were performed by the same investigator. Patients were instructed to adhere to their usual sleeping schedule. In this study, only IOP profiles over 48 h were considered for further analysis. IOP profiles with missing IOP values were excluded from the analysis. Of all the IOP profiles, 661 profiles matched these criteria and were included in the analysis.

For this study, we operationalized clinically meaningful IOP events according to the following criteria:

1. At least one IOP measurement over 21 mmHg;
2. IOP fluctuation over 6 mmHg, over the course of the IOP profile;
3. The IOP maximum in one of the nocturnal measurements in the supine position.

In the first step, we analyzed what percentage of all 48 h IOP profiles met any of these criteria. In the second step, the analysis was repeated for the same dataset, albeit censored for the first 24 h only. The data were analyzed using the R platform [18]. A Chi^2 test was used to compare the event rates between the groups. The alpha level was set to 0.05. We did not correct for multiple testing.

3. Results

Approximately 43% of the IOP profiles were derived from male patients and 57% from female patients. The mean age at the time point of the IOP profile was 64 years (56/64/75 quartiles). The underlying diagnosis was primary or secondary open-angle glaucoma (including pseudoexfoliative glaucoma, normal-tension glaucoma and pigmentary glaucoma) in 49% of the patients. In 9%, the diagnosis was glaucoma suspect or ocular hypertension. The remaining 42% consisted of glaucoma secondary to eye trauma, inflammation, other eye disorders, drugs (e.g., corticosteroids) and other, not further specified, glaucomas.

The share of IOP profiles that showed an IOP above 21 mmHg at least once within 48 h was 59%. When only the first 24 h of every IOP profile were considered, this percentage was 50%. This means that 9% of the eyes showed elevated IOP values only during the second day of the IOP profile. The difference was statistically significant ($p < 0.01$).

In 87% of all the eyes, the IOP showed a fluctuation of above 6 mmHg over the period of 48 h, whereas this was the case in 71% of the profiles when only the first 24 h were considered. This result was statistically significant ($p < 0.01$).

We analyzed whether the peak IOP of every IOP profile was measured in one of the nocturnal measurements (00:00 or 07:00, supine position). This was the case in 51% of the profiles over the period of 48 h, and in 50% of the cases when only the first 24 h were considered. The difference was not statistically significant ($p = 0.12$).

All results are shown in Table 1.

Table 1. Fractions of IOP profiles that met the predefined criteria for the 24 h and the 48 h group.

	After 24 h	After 48 h	Chi^2 Test
$IOP_{max} > 21$ mmHg	50%	59%	$p < 0.01$
IOP fluctuation > 6 mmHg	71%	87%	$p < 0.01$
IOP peak in supine position	48%	51%	$p = 0.12$

4. Discussion

In this study, we present data from a comparatively large number of IOP profiles that were collected for diagnostic purposes from our hospital. While to date there is little evidence that IOP profiles are important to limit visual field loss in glaucoma, recent literature tends to recommend IOP measurements outside normal office hours to identify patients at risk [13,16,19]. However, the implementation of routine IOP measurements outside normal office hours can be challenging from a practical perspective and certain biases, such as different examiners or interruptions to the patient's normal routine, can hardly be avoided. In Germany, inpatient IOP profiles are incorporated into the diagnostic process, for example, when glaucoma progression is suspected, while the IOP is repeatedly within the therapeutic range at outpatient visits. Those IOP profiles are usually conducted over the course of a 24 or 48 h inpatient stay. For the IOP profile to meet its intended purpose, it is crucial to gather enough data, but the benefit of longer measurement periods must be weighed against the additional costs. In our analysis, 9% of the eyes showed IOP values above 21 mmHg exclusively in the second 24 h of measurement. This observation supports the already published data on the poor reproducibility of diurnal IOP patterns. However, missing and potentially relevant IOP events might bear the risk of undertreatment. Regarding IOP fluctuation, our data suggest that IOP profiles over 48 h will identify more patients with significant short-term IOP variation. Taken together, our analysis adds to the published data on IOP profiles over 48 h being more reliable than IOP profiles over 24 h, regarding the detection of IOP peaks and elevated IOP means [15,16]. Our data quantify the additional benefit of a longer IOP profile regrading certain IOP events. Importantly, our study does not allow conclusions to be drawn on the optimal duration of an IOP profile, nor on the general value of this diagnostic tool. Many of the disadvantages and structural biases of traditional IOP profiles could be overcome by using technologies that allow for continuous IOP monitoring over a certain time frame, such as implantable devices or non-invasive approaches. The ideal device would need to gather as many accurate IOP measurements as possible in a certain time frame, be safe for use on patients and be cost efficient. However, due to technical issues with measuring accuracy, safety concerns (e.g., infections) and high costs, none the present technologies have been brought into broader use in the management of glaucoma.

The socio-economic aspects of diagnostic efforts should also be considered. The global prevalence of glaucoma is expected to rise in the near future, and by the year 2040 nearly 112 million people could be affected by the disease [3]. In Germany, a large population-based prospective cohort study suggested a glaucoma prevalence of 1.44% in 2018 [20]. Based on a population with an estimated 83 million people, this results in roughly 1.2 million manifest glaucoma cases. The economic burden of glaucoma is significant. The direct medical costs include medication, consultations and hospital visits. Examples of direct non-medical costs are transportation and public financial aid programs for the blind. Moreover, indirect costs such as a loss of productivity of patients and the need for caregivers add to the total costs [21]. Direct medical costs alone were reported to exceed EUR 1000 per year in western European countries at the beginning of the century [22,23]. More recent data from the US suggested annual direct costs of approximately USD 2200 for stage 5 glaucoma patients [24]. In Germany, the second night of an inpatient IOP profile accounts for approximately EUR 300, which has to be covered by the patient's health insurance. Given the diagnostic advantage of 48 h IOP profiles that our data suggest, this expense might be well invested if follow-up costs resulting from disease progression can be avoided.

By design, this study has certain limitations. We cannot determine whether the incorporation of IOP profiles per se improves long-term glaucoma outcomes. Furthermore, IOP events were operationalized in a simple manner irrespective of the form of glaucoma or anti-glaucomatous therapy. This ignores the possibility that different forms of glaucoma may differ significantly in the nature of their IOP variation. However, the detection of an uncontrolled IOP is equally important in all types of primary and secondary glaucoma and higher IOP fluctuation has been discussed as a risk factor in primary and secondary open-angle glaucoma, as well as in normal-tension glaucoma. Due to the reimbursement criteria for health insurance, our cohort predominantly consisted of patients under extensive anti-glaucomatous therapy and patients who had already experienced surgical intervention to lower their IOP. The early stages of glaucoma might show different IOP patterns. The difference of 16% of patients experiencing IOP fluctuation between the 24 and 48 h analysis should be viewed with caution because nocturnal measurements are performed with a handheld tonometer, whereas diurnal measurements are performed using GAT. Additionally, not all GAT measurements were conducted by the same examiner.

5. Conclusions

On the basis of our data, gathered from a "real world" mix of glaucoma patients and glaucoma suspects, we tend to recommend a time frame of 48 h rather than 24 h when IOP profiles are used as a diagnostic tool, especially in cases where IOP values were normal during the first 24 h of the profile. However, larger and randomized clinical trials are warranted to evaluate the general diagnostic value of IOP profiles.

Author Contributions: Conceptualization, J.L.; Data curation, P.K.; Formal analysis, D.B.; Investigation, P.K. and J.L.; Project administration, J.L.; Software, D.B.; Supervision, T.R.; Writing—original draft, P.K.; Writing—review & editing, D.B., A.A., T.R. and J.L. All authors have read and agreed to the published version of the manuscript.

Funding: This research received no external funding.

Institutional Review Board Statement: The local ethics committee (Ethics Committee, University of Freiburg, Engelbergerstrasse 21, 79106 Freiburg, Germany) approved the conduction of this study (vote no. 21-1184).

Informed Consent Statement: According to the vote by the local ethics committee, written informed consent to participate was not needed as written informed consent was obtained via the treatment contract for inpatient care. According to the vote, consent for publication was not needed.

Data Availability Statement: The data are available on reasonable request.

Acknowledgments: We acknowledge support from the Open Access Publication Fund of the University of Freiburg.

Conflicts of Interest: The authors declare no conflict of interest.

References

1. Weinreb, R.N.; Aung, T.; Medeiros, F.A. The pathophysiology and treatment of glaucoma: A review. *JAMA* **2014**, *311*, 1901–1911 [CrossRef]
2. Bourne, R.R.; Stevens, G.A.; White, R.A.; Smith, J.L.; Flaxman, S.R.; Price, H.; Jonas, J.B.; Keeffe, J.; Leasher, J.; Naidoo, K.; et al Causes of vision loss worldwide, 1990–2010: A systematic analysis. *Lancet Glob. Health* **2013**, *1*, e339–e349. [CrossRef]
3. Tham, Y.C.; Li, X.; Wong, T.Y.; Quigley, H.A.; Aung, T.; Cheng, C.Y. Global prevalence of glaucoma and projections of glaucoma burden through 2040: A systematic review and meta-analysis. *Ophthalmology* **2014**, *121*, 2081–2090. [CrossRef]
4. Leske, M.C.; Heijl, A.; Hussein, M.; Bengtsson, B.; Hyman, L.; Komaroff, E. Early Manifest Glaucoma Trial Group Factors for glaucoma progression and the effect of treatment: The early manifest glaucoma trial. *Arch. Ophthalmol.* **1960**, *121*, 48–56 [CrossRef]
5. Leske, M.C.; Wu, S.Y.; Hennis, A.; Honkanen, R.; Nemesure, B.; BESs Study Group. Risk factors for incident open-angle glaucoma The Barbados Eye Studies. *Ophthalmology* **2008**, *115*, 85–93. [CrossRef]
6. Maier, P.C.; Funk, J.; Schwarzer, G.; Antes, G.; Falck-Ytter, Y.T. Treatment of ocular hypertension and open angle glaucoma Meta-analysis of randomised controlled trials. *BMJ* **2005**, *331*, 134. [CrossRef]
7. David, R.; Zangwill, L.; Briscoe, D.; Dagan, M.; Yagev, R.; Yassur, Y. Diurnal intraocular pressure variations: An analysis of 690 diurnal curves. *Br. J. Ophthalmol.* **1992**, *76*, 280–283. [CrossRef]
8. Barkana, Y.; Anis, S.; Liebmann, J.; Tello, C.; Ritch, R. Clinical utility of intraocular pressure monitoring outside of normal office hours in patients with glaucoma. *Arch. Ophthalmol.* **2006**, *124*, 793–797. [CrossRef]
9. Leidl, M.C.; Choi, C.J.; Syed, Z.A.; Melki, S.A. Intraocular pressure fluctuation and glaucoma progression: What do we know? *Br J. Ophthalmol.* **2014**, *98*, 1315–1319. [CrossRef]
10. Tajunisah, I.; Reddy, S.C.; Fathilah, J. Diurnal variation of intraocular pressure in suspected glaucoma patients and their outcome *Graefe Arch. Clin. Exp. Ophthalmol.* **2007**, *245*, 1851–1857. [CrossRef]

11. Kim, J.H.; Caprioli, J. Intraocular Pressure Fluctuation: Is It Important? *J. Ophthalmic Vis. Res.* **2018**, *13*, 170–174.
12. Konstas, A.G.; Kahook, M.Y.; Araie, M.; Katsanos, A.; Quaranta, L.; Rossetti, L.; Holló, G.; Detorakis, E.T.; Oddone, F.; Mikropoulos, D.G.; et al. Diurnal and 24-h Intraocular Pressures in Glaucoma: Monitoring Strategies and Impact on Prognosis and Treatment. *Adv. Ther.* **2018**, *35*, 1775–1804. [CrossRef]
13. Bhartiya, S.; Ichhpujani, P. The Need to maintain Intraocular Pressure over 24 Hours. *J. Curr. Glaucoma Pract.* **2012**, *6*, 120–123.
14. Realini, T.; Weinreb, R.N.; Wisniewski, S.R. Diurnal intraocular pressure patterns are not repeatable in the short term in healthy individuals. *Ophthalmology* **2010**, *117*, 1700–1704. [CrossRef]
15. Realini, T.; Weinreb, R.N.; Wisniewski, S. Short-term repeatability of diurnal intraocular pressure patterns in glaucomatous individuals. *Ophthalmology* **2011**, *118*, 47–51, Erratum in Ophthalmology 2011, 118, 434. [CrossRef]
16. Fischer, N.; Weinand, F.; Kügler, M.U.; Scheel, S.; Lorenz, B. Sinnhaftigkeit von Tages-/Nacht-Augeninnendruckmessungen über 48 h [Are diurnal and nocturnal intraocular pressure measurements over 48 h justified?]. *Ophthalmologe* **2013**, *110*, 755–760. (In German) [CrossRef]
17. Xu, J.; Li, R.; Xu, H.; Yang, Y.; Zhang, S.; Ren, T.-L. Recent progress of continuous intraocular pressure monitoring. *Nano Select* **2022**, *3*, 1. [CrossRef]
18. R Core Team. *R: A Language and Environment for Statistical Computing*; R Foundation for Statistical Computing: Vienna, Austria, 2021.
19. Mansouri, K.; Tanna, A.P.; De Moraes, C.G.; Camp, A.S.; Weinreb, R.N. Review of the measurement and management of 24-hour intraocular pressure in patients with glaucoma. *Surv. Ophthalmol.* **2020**, *65*, 171–186. [CrossRef]
20. Höhn, R.; Nickels, S.; Schuster, A.K.; Wild, P.S.; Münzel, T.; Lackner, K.J.; Schmidtmann, I.; Beutel, M.; Pfeiffer, N. Prevalence of glaucoma in Germany: Results from the Gutenberg Health Study. *Graefe Arch. Clin. Exp. Ophthalmol.* **2018**, *256*, 1695–1702. [CrossRef]
21. Varma, R.; Lee, P.P.; Goldberg, I.; Kotak, S. An assessment of the health and economic burdens of glaucoma. *Am. J. Ophthalmol.* **2011**, *152*, 515–522. [CrossRef]
22. Traverso, C.E.; Walt, J.G.; Kelly, S.P.; Hommer, A.H.; Bron, A.M.; Denis, P.; Nordmann, J.P.; Renard, J.P.; Bayer, A.; Grehn, F.; et al. Direct costs of glaucoma and severity of the disease: A multinational long term study of resource utilisation in Europe. *Br. J. Ophthalmol.* **2005**, *89*, 1245–1249. [CrossRef]
23. Grüb, M.; Rohrbach, J.M. Zur sozioökonomischen Bedeutung des Glaukoms [On the socio-economic relevance of glaucoma]. *Klin. Monbl. Augenheilkd.* **2006**, *223*, 793–795. (In German) [CrossRef]
24. Lee, P.P.; Walt, J.G.; Doyle, J.J.; Kotak, S.V.; Evans, S.J.; Budenz, D.L.; Chen, P.P.; Coleman, A.L.; Feldman, R.M.; Jampel, H.D.; et al. A multicenter, retrospective pilot study of resource use and costs associated with severity of disease in glaucoma. *Arch. Ophthalmol.* **2006**, *124*, 12–19. [CrossRef]

Disclaimer/Publisher's Note: The statements, opinions and data contained in all publications are solely those of the individual author(s) and contributor(s) and not of MDPI and/or the editor(s). MDPI and/or the editor(s) disclaim responsibility for any injury to people or property resulting from any ideas, methods, instructions or products referred to in the content.

Article

Anterior Segment Parameter Changes after Cataract Surgery in Open-Angle and Angle-Closure Eyes: A Prospective Study

Kangyi Yang [1,2,3,4,†], Zhiqiao Liang [1,2,3,4,†], Kun Lv [1,2,3,4], Yao Ma [1,2,3,4], Xianru Hou [1,2,3,4] and Huijuan Wu [1,2,3,4,*]

1. Department of Ophthalmology, Peking University People's Hospital, Beijing 100044, China
2. Eye Diseases and Optometry Institute, Beijing 100044, China
3. Beijing Key Laboratory of Diagnosis and Therapy of Retinal and Choroid Diseases, Beijing 100044, China
4. College of Optometry, Peking University Health Science Center, Beijing 100044, China
* Correspondence: dr_wuhuijuan@126.com; Tel.: +86-010-88325413
† These authors contributed equally to this work.

Abstract: Background: To investigate the anterior segment parameters before and after cataract surgery in open-angle eyes and different subtypes of primary angle-closure glaucoma (PACG) eyes and to further explore the potential relationship between the anterior rotation of the ciliary process and crystalline lens. Methods: An observational, prospective study was performed on 66 patients who had cataract surgery including 22 chronic PACG patients, 22 acute PACG patients, and 22 open-angle cataract patients. Anterior segment parameters including the trabecular-ciliary process distance, ciliary process area, trabecular-ciliary angle (TCA), maximum ciliary body thickness (CBTmax), and so on, were measured using ultrasound biomicroscopy preoperatively and 3 months postoperatively. Results: After the surgery, there were significant increases in TCA ($p < 0.001$) and CBTmax ($p < 0.05$) in all three groups, while there was no significant change in the trabecular-ciliary process distance ($p > 0.05$) in all three groups. No significant difference in the changes of ciliary process area, TCA, and CBTmax ($p > 0.05$) pre- and postoperatively among the three groups were identified. Conclusions: Extractions of crystalline lenses played similar roles in terms of decreasing the anterior rotation of ciliary processes in open-angle eyes and angle-closure eyes. A natural anatomical abnormality may be a more important factor in the anterior rotation of ciliary processes in PACG patients.

Keywords: primary angle-closure glaucoma; anterior rotation of ciliary processes; mechanisms; cataract surgery; ultrasound biomicroscopy

1. Introduction

Primary angle-closure glaucoma (PACG) is characterized by elevated intraocular pressure (IOP) and obstruction of aqueous outflow as a result of mechanical obstruction of the trabecular meshwork, which is one of the leading causes of global irreversible blindness [1,2]. PACG can be classified into acute PACG and chronic PACG according to the characteristics of clinical presentation [3]. During the acute attack stage of acute PACG, the iris quickly and completely occludes the entire trabecular meshwork, and by contrast, in chronic PACG, the iris slowly creeps over the trabecular meshwork [3].

The majority of PACG cases in China result from a combination of multiple mechanisms, including pupillary block factors and non-pupillary block factors, such as a thick peripheral iris, a plateau iris, anterior attachment and insertion of the iris root, a forward shift of the lens, and anterior rotation of the ciliary processes exist [4]. Quantitative measurements revealed that the characteristics of the ciliary processes are one of the most important differences between eyes with angle-closure and normal eyes [3]. The ciliary processes of angle-closure eyes rotated more anteriorly than that of open-angle eyes. Additionally, the crystalline lens was considered to be involved in the pathogenesis of PACG because of the continuous growth in lens volume and lens vault (LV) [5,6]. The relationship between the anterior rotation of ciliary processes and the crystalline lens was also discussed in previous studies. In some studies, it had been reported that cataract surgery can widen the anterior chamber angle not only by decreasing lens volume and relieving pupillary block, but also by attenuating anterior positioning of the ciliary processes in the eyes with PACG [5,7]. Man et al. [8] even demonstrated that after lens extraction and intraocular lens (IOL) implantation, all PACG eyes had significantly longer trabecular-ciliary process distance (TCPD) and deeper aqueous depth (AQD). On the other hand, Li et al. [9] found that although there was a significant increase in AQD in acute primary angle-closure patients after phacoemulsification, the difference in TCPD was not significant. Therefore, whether the anterior traction of the lens to ciliary processes plays a role in the anterior rotation of ciliary processes or not remains ambiguous.

In this study, ultrasound biomicroscopy (UBM) had been used to evaluate anterior segment parameters before and after phacoemulsification and IOL implantation in acute PACG, chronic PACG, and open-angle eyes and to further explore whether the anterior rotation of ciliary processes has a potential relationship with the crystalline lens or not, which may provide more detailed information related to the pathogenesis of PACG.

2. Materials and Methods

2.1. Study Design

This was an observational, prospective study of Chinese subjects approved by the Ethics Committee of Peking University People's Hospital (approval number 2022PHB256-001) and it followed the tenets of the Declaration of Helsinki. Written informed consent was obtained from all subjects prior to recruitment.

2.2. Patients

Subjects diagnosed with PACG were recruited from the glaucoma clinics of Peking University People's Hospital from June 2016 to August 2022 and were classified as acute PACG and chronic PACG. Patients who visited clinics due to age-related cataracts were enrolled as the control group and were characterized by an open anterior chamber angle. Accordingly, 68 eyes of 68 subjects were included, of which 2 eyes were excluded due to poor UBM image quality.

Eyes with acute PACG were defined as eyes with two of the following symptoms: ocular or periocular pain, headache, nausea and/or vomiting, blurred vision, and halos around lights; and the following ophthalmologic findings: an IOP of more than 30 mm Hg, conjunctival hyperemia, corneal epithelial edema, a shallow anterior chamber with angle-closure, iris bombe and mid-dilated pupil, along with glaucomatous optic neuropathy and visual field defect.

Eyes with chronic PACG were defined as eyes without symptoms or signs of a prior acute attack, including glaucomatous fleck, keratic precipitates, or iris atrophy. Patients had more than three cumulative hours of peripheral anterior synechia and a chronically elevated IOP (>21 mm Hg), along with glaucomatous optic neuropathy or visual field defect.

Exclusion criteria included (1) secondary angle closure such as iris neovascularization, trauma, tumor, uveitis, and lens subluxation, (2) prior intraocular surgery, such as cataract surgery, trabeculoplasty, and trabeculotomy, (3) inability to tolerate gonioscopy or UBM examinations, and (4) cataract patients with nuclear opalescence, nuclear color or cortical cataract of more than grade 3 (LOCS III classification).

2.3. Ophthalmologic Examinations

All patients underwent ophthalmologic examinations, including best corrected visual acuity (BCVA) measured by the Snellen visual chart, IOP measurement by Goldmann applanation tonometry (Haag-Streit, Koniz, Switzerland), and axial length measured by IOLMaster biometry (IOLMaster 700, Carl Zeiss Meditec, 137 Inc., Dublin, CA, USA). Gonioscopy was performed in a dimly lit room by a glaucoma specialist using a Zeiss-style four-mirror gonioscopy lens (Model G-4, Volk Optical, 154 Inc., Mentor, OH, USA) at 16× magnification with and without indentation. Optical coherence tomography (Spectralis HRA + OCT, Heidelberg Engineering, Heidelberg, Germany) was used to test retinal nerve fiber layer defect and a visual field test (Humphrey Field Analyzer, Carl Zeiss Meditec, Inc., Dublin, CA, USA) was performed to show characteristic glaucomatous visual field defects.

2.4. Ultrasound Biomicroscopy

The anterior chamber configuration was determined before and at 3 months after cataract surgery using UBM (Aviso, Quantel Medical, Inc., Bozeman, MT, USA) and a 50-MHz transducer probe by an experienced operator (Y.W.) who was masked to the clinical data. Examinations were performed under the same room illumination, with the patient in the supine position. After topical anesthesia by using 0.4% oxybuprocaine hydrochloride (Benoxil®; Santen, Tokyo, Japan) eye drops, a plastic eye cup containing physiologic saline was mounted on the globe. To minimize accommodation, patients were instructed to fixate with the contralateral eye on a distant ceiling target. Each subject's eyes were measured in the superior, inferior, temporal, and nasal quadrants, as well as nasal and temporal scans centered on the pupil to obtain complete images of the anterior segment. Analyses were limited to images that clearly showed the scleral spur (SS), iris, ciliary body, and anterior surface of the lens.

2.5. Image Analysis

The UBM Images of chronic PACG, acute PACG, and open-angle cataracts were measured quantitatively in all four quadrants using an in-built caliper in the UBM software by a single examiner masked to clinical data. The SS was identified based on the differential tissue density between the collagen fibers of the SS and the longitudinal muscle of the ciliary body as a crucial anatomical mark in the curvature of the inner surface of the angled wall. The anterior segment parameters [10–14] were measured according to the methods of our previous publication and other research. The parameters on full-view scans at the nasal-temporal position were as follows. (1) AQD: the distance between the posterior surface of the central cornea and the anterior surface of the crystalline lens or IOL in the midline of the pupil. (2) Pupil diameter (PD): the shortest distance between the pupil edges of the iris cross-sections. (3) LV: the perpendicular distance from the anterior pole of the lens to the horizontal line between the SS. (4) Anterior chamber width (ACW): the distance between the two SS's. (5) Iris area: the cumulative cross-sectional area of the full length (from spur to pupil) of the iris. (6) Ciliary sulcus diameter (CSD): the distance between the two horizontal diameters for the ciliary sulcus (Figure 1). Parameters [10–12,14] measured on the radial scans at the superior, nasal, inferior, and temporal positions were as follows (1) An iris thickness of 750 μm (IT 750) and 2000 μm (IT 2000): an iris thickness of 750 μm and 2000 μm from the SS. (2) An angle-opening distance of 500 μm (AOD 500) and 750 μm (AOD 750): the distance between the posterior corneal surface and the anterior iris surface on a line perpendicular to the trabecular meshwork at 500 μm and 750 μm from the SS. (3) A trabecular iris space area of 500 μm (TISA 500) and 750 μm (TISA 750): the area bounded anteriorly by AOD 500 and AOD 750, as determined posteriorly by a line drawn from the SS perpendicular to the plane of the inner scleral wall to the iris, superiorly by the inner corneoscleral wall, and inferiorly by the iris surface. (4) A trabecular iris angle of 500 μm (TIA 500) and 750 μm (TIA 750): the apex of the angle at the iris recess and the arms of the angle passing through a point on the trabecular meshwork at 500 μm and 750 μm from the SS and the point on the iris perpendicularly opposite. (5) A ciliary process area (CPA): the cross-sectional area of the ciliary process bounded laterally by a line connecting the insertion location of the iris into the ciliary body and the crosspoint of a line of 500 μm from the SS perpendicular to the plane of the inner scleral wall to the ciliary process, and internally by the ciliary process surface. (6) A trabecular-ciliary angle (TCA) the angle between the posterior corneal surface and the anterior surface of the ciliary body (7) TCPD: the length of the line extending from the corneal endothelium 500 mm from the SS perpendicularly through the posterior surface of the iris to the ciliary process. (8) The maximum ciliary body thickness (CBTmax): the thickest location of the ciliary body (Figure 2). The vitreous zonule (VZ) [13]: the bridging bundles of zonular fibers running from the region of the zonular plexus in the valleys of the posterior pars plicata toward the vitreous membrane in the region of the ora serrata (Figure 3).

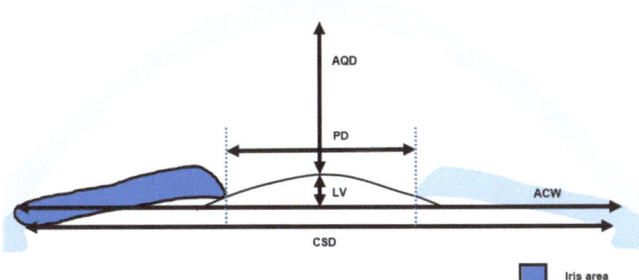

Figure 1. Anterior segment parameters on full-view scans at the nasal-temporal position measured by ultrasound biomicroscopy (UBM). (Illustrator: K.Y.). AQD: the distance between the posterior surface of the central cornea and the anterior surface of the crystalline lens or IOL in the midline of the pupil; PD: the shortest distance between the pupil edges of the iris cross-sections; LV: the perpendicular distance from the anterior pole of the lens to the horizontal line between the SS; ACW: the distance between the two SS's; iris area: the cumulative cross-sectional area of the full length (from spur to pupil) of the iris; CSD: the distance between the two horizontal diameters for the ciliary sulcus.

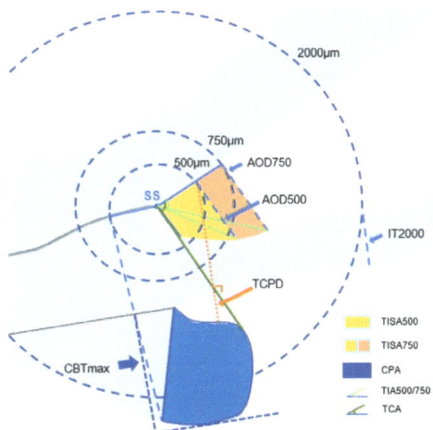

Figure 2. Anterior segment parameters on the radial scans at the superior, nasal, inferior, and temporal positions measured by ultrasound biomicroscopy (UBM). (Illustrator: K.Y.). IT 750/2000: iris thickness of 750 μm and 2000 μm from the SS; AOD 500/750: the distance between the posterior corneal surface and the anterior iris surface on a line perpendicular to the trabecular meshwork at 500 μm and 750 μm from the SS; TISA 500/750: the area bounded anteriorly by AOD 500 and AOD 750, as determined posteriorly by a line drawn from the SS perpendicular to the plane of the inner scleral wall to the iris, superiorly by the inner corneoscleral wall, and inferiorly by the iris surface; TIA 500/750: the apex of the angle at the iris recess and the arms of the angle passing through a point on the trabecular meshwork at 500 μm and 750 μm from the SS and the point on the iris perpendicularly opposite; CPA: the cross-sectional area of the ciliary process bounded laterally by a line connecting the insertion location of the iris into the ciliary body and the crosspoint of a line of 500 μm from the SS perpendicular to the plane of the inner scleral wall to the ciliary process, and internally by the ciliary process surface; TCA: the angle between the posterior corneal surface and the anterior surface of the ciliary body; TCPD: the length of the line extending from the corneal endothelium 500 mm from the SS perpendicularly through the posterior surface of the iris to the ciliary process; CBTmax: the thickest location of the ciliary body.

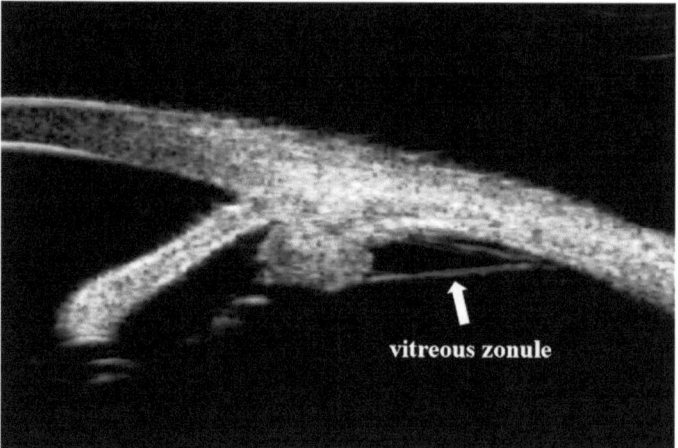

Figure 3. Vitreous zonule (arrows) visible in an ultrasound biomicroscopy (UBM) image of a 63-year-old acute PACG female.

2.6. Surgical Technique

All phacoemulsification and hydrophobic acrylic TECNIS ZA9003 IOL (Abbott Medical Optics Inc., Santa Ana, CA, USA.) implantation surgeries were performed by the same experienced surgeon (H.W.) and were then followed up by two ophthalmologists (Z.L. and H.W.). The pupil was dilated six times using 0.5% tropicamide phenylephrine (Santen, Osaka, Japan) 30 min prior to surgery. Phacoemulsification was performed under topical anesthesia using 0.4% oxybuprocaine hydrochloride. The corneal incision was performed at 11 o'clock. The chamber was immediately deepened using 1.7% sodium hyaluronate (Bausch & Lomb, Jinan, China). After continuous curvilinear capsulorhexis, the nucleus was removed with no intraoperative complications. An automated irrigation/aspiration apparatus was introduced into the anterior chamber to remove the cortical remnants and polish the posterior lens capsule. The intra-IOL was placed in the capsular bag. Postoperative treatment consisted of 0.5% tropicamide phenylephrine (Mydrin®-P; Santen, Osaka, Japan) administered once per night for 1 month, tobramycin and dexamethasone eye drops (Tobradex®; Alcon, Belgium) four times a day for 1 month, and 0.5% levofloxacin (Cravit®, Santen, Osaka, Japan) eye drops four times a day for 1 week after surgery.

2.7. Repeatability and Reproducibility

We performed repeatability and reproducibility analysis of UBM parameters. Five patients in each group were randomly selected for analysis. The first observer (K.Y.) measured parameters twice within two weeks to test intra-observer variability. A second observer (L.K.) measured the same images independently on a different day to decide inter-observer variability. The intra-observer and inter-observer variability were calculated using the coefficient of the intra-class coefficients.

2.8. Statistical Analysis

The results were analyzed using SPSS 22.0 (SPSS, Inc., Chicago, IL, USA). All data were calculated as a mean ± standard deviation. ANOVA tests or Kruskal–Wallis tests were used to compare the continuous variables (age, BCVA, IOP, axial length, AQD, PD, LV, ACW, CSD, iris area, IT 750/2000, AOD 500/750, TISA 500/750, TIA 500/750, CPA, TCA, TCPD, CBTmax, and the number of quadrants of VZ). The Shapiro–Wilk test was used to test whether the variables conform to normal distribution. The test showed that the data (age, CPA, TCPD, AQD, CSD, ACW, LV, IT 750, and iris area) conformed to normal distribution, therefore, analysis of Variance (ANOVA) tests were used to compare parametric variables. Alternatively, Kruskal–Wallis test, in the case of non-normally distributed variables, was used to compare non-parametric variables (BCVA, IOP, axial length, TCA, CBTmax, PD, IT 2000, AOD 500/750, TIA 500/750, TISA 500/750, and the number of quadrants of VZ). As for variance comparison among groups, the least significant difference (LSD) test was used for homogeneity, while the Tamhane test was used for heterogeneity. χ^2 tests were used to compare the categorical variables (gender) among the three groups. Paired contrast t-tests were used for the preoperative and postoperative comparison of AQD, PD, LV, ACW, CSD, iris area, IT 750/2000, AOD 500/750, TISA 500/750, TIA 500/750, CPA, TCA, TCPD, CBTmax, and the number of quadrants of VZ. A p-value of less than 0.05 was considered statistically significant.

3. Results

3.1. Demographics, Clinical Characteristics, and Preoperative Parameter Data

Sixty-six eyes of 66 patients including 22 chronic PACG eyes, 22 acute PACG eyes, and 22 open-angle cataract eyes were enrolled in this study. The demographic, clinical characteristics, and preoperative anterior segment UBM parameters are shown in Table 1. Among all participants, the mean ($\pm$ SD) age was 69.42 $\pm$ 7.82 years. Chronic PACG and acute PACG eyes had higher IOP and smaller axial length than open-angle eyes ($p < 0.05$). There was no significant difference in age, BCVA, and gender among the three groups ($p > 0.05$) (Table 1). Compared to open-angle eyes, chronic PACG and acute PACG eyes had smaller TCA, TCPD, CBTmax, AQD, ACW, TIA 500, TIA 750, AOD 500, AOD 750, TISA500, TISA 750, IT 750, a fewer number of quadrants of VZ, and larger CPA and LV preoperatively ($p < 0.05$). Chronic PACG eyes had larger AQD, and smaller LV and PD than acute PACG patients ($p < 0.05$). Acute PACG eyes had larger PD and a smaller iris area than open-angle cataract eyes ($p < 0.05$). No significant differences were found regarding CSD and IT 2000 preoperatively ($p > 0.05$).

Table 1. Comparison of demographics, clinical characteristics, and preoperative anterior segment UBM parameters among the three groups.

	Chronic PACG	Acute PACG	Open-Angle Cataract	p-Value *
Eyes	22	22	22	
Demographics and clinical characteristics				
Gender (male/female)	9/13	6/16	5/17	0.105
Age (years)	66.55 $\pm$ 7.07	70.73 $\pm$ 8.77	71.00 $\pm$ 7.03	0.394
BCVA (decimal)	0.38 $\pm$ 0.23	0.28 $\pm$ 0.30	0.35 $\pm$ 0.19	0.353
IOP (mmHg)	20.23 $\pm$ 9.16	23.68 $\pm$ 15.66	13.75 $\pm$ 2.09	0.001 *
Axial length (mm)	22.40 $\pm$ 0.65	22.58 $\pm$ 1.19	24.31 $\pm$ 1.79	0.000 *
Preoperative anterior segment parameters on UBM				
Preoperative CPA (mm^2)	0.60 $\pm$ 0.20	0.62 $\pm$ 0.17	0.41 $\pm$ 0.16	0.014 *
Preoperative TCA (degree)	54.98 $\pm$ 12.03	49.02 $\pm$ 11.04	83.94 $\pm$ 15.36	0.000 *
Preoperative TCPD (mm)	0.55 $\pm$ 0.14	0.50 $\pm$ 0.14	0.80 $\pm$ 0.18	0.000 *
Preoperative CBTmax (mm)	1.17 $\pm$ 0.11	1.16 $\pm$ 0.11	1.31 $\pm$ 0.12	0.000 *
Preoperative CSD (mm)	10.37 $\pm$ 0.63	10.42 $\pm$ 0.53	10.83 $\pm$ 0.98	0.069
Preoperative AQD (mm)	1.93 $\pm$ 0.23	1.56 $\pm$ 0.23	2.76 $\pm$ 0.41	0.000 *
Preoperative ACW (mm)	11.27 $\pm$ 0.48	11.30 $\pm$ 0.63	11.58 $\pm$ 0.75	0.020 *
Preoperative LV (mm)	0.84 $\pm$ 0.30	1.13 $\pm$ 0.25	0.34 $\pm$ 0.24	0.000 *
Preoperative PD (mm)	2.33 $\pm$ 0.61	4.04 $\pm$ 1.38	2.71 $\pm$ 0.54	0.007 *
Preoperative IT 750 (μm)	0.40 $\pm$ 0.09	0.39 $\pm$ 0.07	0.48 $\pm$ 0.06	0.024 *
Preoperative IT 2000 (μm)	0.45 $\pm$ 0.07	0.49 $\pm$ 0.10	0.52 $\pm$ 0.06	0.109
Preoperative TIA 500 (degree)	3.67 $\pm$ 4.48	2.57 $\pm$ 5.66	30.15 $\pm$ 11.18	0.000 *
Preoperative TIA 750 (degree)	3.69 $\pm$ 4.39	2.57 $\pm$ 5.78	29.23 $\pm$ 10.16	0.000 *
Preoperative AOD 500 (μm)	0.03 $\pm$ 0.04	0.02 $\pm$ 0.05	0.32 $\pm$ 0.15	0.000 *
Preoperative AOD 750 (μm)	0.05 $\pm$ 0.06	0.04 $\pm$ 0.08	0.45 $\pm$ 0.20	0.000 *
Preoperative TISA 500 (mm^2)	0.01 $\pm$ 0.01	0.01 $\pm$ 0.02	0.11 $\pm$ 0.06	0.000 *

Table 1. Cont.

	Chronic PACG	Acute PACG	Open-Angle Cataract	p-Value *
Preoperative TISA 750 (mm^2)	0.02 ± 0.02	0.02 ± 0.04	0.21 ± 0.10	0.000 *
Preoperative iris area (mm^2)	1.92 ± 0.17	1.68 ± 0.37	2.16 ± 0.28	0.002 *
Preoperative number of quadrants of VZ	1.55 ± 1.26	2.00 ± 1.07	2.73 ± 1.07	0.007 *

PACG = primary angle-closure glaucoma; BCVA = best corrected visual acuity; IOP = intraocular pressure; CPA = ciliary process area; TCA = trabecular-ciliary angle; TCPD = trabecular-ciliary process distance; CBTmax = maximum ciliary body thickness; CSD = ciliary sulcus diameter; AQD = aqueous depth; ACW = anterior chamber width; LV = lens vault; PD = pupil diameter; IT 750 = iris thickness at 750 µm; IT 2000 = iris thickness at 2000 µm; TIA 500 = trabecular iris angle at 500 µm; TIA 750 = trabecular iris angle at 750 µm; AOD 500 = angle-opening distance at 500 µm; AOD 750 = angle-opening distance at 750 µm; TISA 500 = trabecular iris space area at 500 µm; TISA 750 = trabecular iris space area at 750 µm; VZ= vitreous zonule. * χ^2 tests were used to compare gender; analysis of variance (ANOVA) tests or Kruskal–Wallis tests were used to compare age, AQD, PD, LV, ACW, CSD, iris area, IT 750/2000, AOD 500/750, TISA 500/750, TIA 500/750, CPA, TCA, TCPD, CBTmax, and the number of quadrants of VZ (n = 22).

3.2. Postoperative Parameter Data

There was a significant increase in TCA, CBTmax, AQD, LV, TIA 500, TIA 750, AOD 500, AOD 750, TISA 500, and TISA 750 ($p < 0.05$), while the number of quadrants of VZ was significantly decreased ($p < 0.05$) in all three groups 3 months after surgery. ACW, IT 750, and IT 2000 were significantly increased in chronic PACG eyes and acute PACG eyes postoperatively ($p < 0.05$). Compared to preoperative parameters, acute PACG eyes had smaller CPA, CSD, and a larger iris area ($p < 0.05$) postoperatively. Preoperative open-angle cataract eyes had smaller PD and a larger iris area 3 months after surgery ($p < 0.05$). No significant differences were found regarding TCPD in all three groups, respectively, 3 months after surgery ($p > 0.05$).

The comparisons of the changes in anterior segment parameters after cataract surgery among chronic PACG, acute PACG, and open-angle cataract groups are shown in Table 2. The extent of increase in AQD, LV, and IT 2000 was significantly larger in acute PACG eyes than in chronic PACG and open-angle cataract eyes after surgery ($p < 0.05$). Compared to open-angle cataract eyes, chronic PACG and acute PACG eyes had a larger increase in IT 750 postoperatively ($p < 0.05$). There was no significant difference in change in the CPA, TCA, TCPD, CBTmax, CSD, ACW, PD, TIA 500, TIA 750, AOD 500, AOD 750, TISA 500, TISA 750, iris area, and the number of quadrants of VZ among the three groups before and after surgery ($p > 0.05$).

Table 2. The comparisons of the changes in the anterior segment parameters after cataract surgery among the three groups.

Parameters	Chronic PACG	Acute PACG	Open-Angle Cataract	p-Value *
ΔCPA (mm^2)	−0.03 ± 0.15	−0.10 ± 0.17	−0.00 ± 0.12	0.182
ΔTCA (degree)	8.70 ± 9.57	12.38 ± 9.56	6.02 ± 7.92	0.096
ΔTCPD (mm)	0.05 ± 0.11 (n = 17)	0.04 ± 0.13 (n = 16)	0.05 ± 0.13 (n = 15)	0.904
ΔCBTmax (mm)	0.07 ± 0.14	0.06 ± 0.08	0.12 ± 0.12	0.155
ΔCSD (mm)	−0.23 ± 0.55	−0.29 ± 0.42	−0.17 ± 0.53	0.715
ΔAQD (mm)	1.45 ± 0.27	1.79 ± 0.43	1.37 ± 0.40	0.000 *
ΔACW (mm)	0.34 ± 0.51	0.12 ± 0.49	0.14 ± 0.43	0.204
ΔLV (mm)	−1.22 ± 0.31	−1.62 ± 0.35	−1.26 ± 0.35	0.000 *
ΔPD (mm)	−0.21 ± 0.64	−0.06 ± 0.94	−0.61 ± 0.58	0.054
ΔIT 750 (µm)	0.03 ± 0.05	0.07 ± 0.07	−0.01 ± 0.06	0.006 *
ΔIT 2000 (µm)	0.03 ± 0.05	0.08 ± 0.08	0.02 ± 0.06	0.004 *
ΔTIA 500 (degree)	13.41 ± 11.76	6.90 ± 9.22	11.33 ± 8.74	0.362
ΔTIA 750 (degree)	14.05 ± 11.33	7.19 ± 9.22	12.09 ± 8.32	0.264

Table 2. Cont.

Parameters	Chronic PACG	Acute PACG	Open-Angle Cataract	p-Value *
ΔAOD 500 (μm)	0.14 ± 0.13	0.07 ± 0.10	0.14 ± 0.11	0.101
ΔAOD 750 (μm)	0.22 ± 0.18	0.11 ± 0.14	0.22 ± 0.16	0.082
ΔTISA 500 (mm^2)	0.05 ± 0.04	0.02 ± 0.03	0.05 ± 0.04	0.103
ΔTISA 750 (mm^2)	0.09 ± 0.07	0.04 ± 0.06	0.10 ± 0.07	0.053
ΔIris area (mm^2)	0.21 ± 0.22	0.10 ± 0.28	0.09 ± 0.22	0.440
ΔNumber of quadrants of VZ	−0.73 ± 1.08	−0.82 ± 0.96	−1.27 ± 0.77	0.063

PACG = primary angle-closure glaucoma; Δ represents the difference between pre- and postoperative parameters (postoperative minus preoperative parameters); CPA = ciliary process area; TCA = trabecular-ciliary angle; TCPD = trabecular-ciliary process distance; CBTmax = maximum ciliary body thickness; CSD = ciliary sulcus diameter; AQD = aqueous depth; ACW = anterior chamber width; LV = lens vault; PD = pupil diameter; IT 750 = iris thickness at 750 μm; IT 2000 = iris thickness at 2000 μm; TIA 500 = trabecular iris angle at 500 μm; TIA 750 = trabecular iris angle at 750 μm; AOD 500 = angle-opening distance at 500 μm; AOD 750 = angle-opening distance at 750 μm; TISA 500 = trabecular iris space area at 500 μm; TISA 750 = trabecular iris space area at 750 μm; VZ = vitreous zonule. * Analysis of variance (ANOVA) tests or Kruskal–Wallis one-way ANOVA (k samples) tests (n = 22).

3.3. Intra-Class Coefficient Data

The intra-observer and inter-observer intra-class coefficients were 0.869–0.999 and 0.852–0.997, respectively (Table 3), which showed good repeatability and reproducibility of UBM parameters measured in this study.

Table 3. Intra-observer and inter-observer intra-class coefficients of the preoperative and postoperative parameters.

Parameters	Intra-Class Coefficients	
	Intra-Observer	Inter-Observer
Preoperative CPA (mm^2)	0.956	0.872
Postoperative CPA (mm^2)	0.913	0.852
Preoperative TCA (degree)	0.969	0.862
Postoperative TCA (degree)	0.982	0.927
Preoperative TCPD (mm)	0.967	0.869
Postoperative TCPD (mm)	0.968	0.914
Preoperative CBTmax (mm)	0.983	0.909
Postoperative CBTmax (mm)	0.970	0.876
Preoperative CSD (mm)	0.980	0.953
Postoperative CSD (mm)	0.973	0.980
Preoperative AQD (mm)	0.999	0.971
Postoperative AQD (mm)	0.999	0.997
Preoperative ACW (mm)	0.923	0.872
Postoperative ACW (mm)	0.916	0.873
Preoperative LV (mm)	0.968	0.933
Postoperative LV (mm)	0.950	0.885
Preoperative PD (mm)	0.998	0.988
Postoperative PD (mm)	0.988	0.963
Preoperative IT 750 (μm)	0.949	0.909
Postoperative IT 750 (μm)	0.906	0.873
Preoperative IT 2000 (μm)	0.913	0.876
Postoperative IT 2000 (μm)	0.975	0.934
Preoperative TIA 500 (degree)	0.974	0.940
Postoperative TIA 500 (degree)	0.988	0.954
Preoperative TIA 750 (degree)	0.974	0.966

Table 3. Cont.

Parameters	Intra-Class Coefficients	
	Intra-Observer	Inter-Observer
Postoperative TIA 750 (degree)	0.983	0.965
Preoperative AOD 500 (μm)	0.965	0.936
Postoperative AOD 500 (μm)	0.988	0.946
Preoperative AOD 750 (μm)	0.963	0.962
Postoperative AOD 750 (μm)	0.985	0.972
Preoperative TISA 500 (mm^2)	0.976	0.947
Postoperative TISA 500 (mm^2)	0.992	0.984
Preoperative TISA 750 (mm^2)	0.963	0.965
Postoperative TISA 750 (mm^2)	0.986	0.976
Preoperative iris area (mm^2)	0.991	0.910
Postoperative iris area (mm^2)	0.964	0.887
Preoperative number of quadrants of VZ	0.869	0.862
Postoperative number of quadrants of VZ	0.904	0.865

CPA = ciliary process area; TCA = trabecular-ciliary angle; TCPD = trabecular-ciliary process distance; CBTmax = maximum ciliary body thickness; CSD = ciliary sulcus diameter; AQD = aqueous depth; ACW = anterior chamber width; LV = lens vault; PD = pupil diameter; IT 750 = iris thickness at 750 μm; IT 2000 = iris thickness at 2000 μm; TIA 500 = trabecular iris angle at 500 μm; TIA 750 = trabecular iris angle at 750 μm; AOD 500 = angle-opening distance at 500 μm; AOD 750 = angle-opening distance at 750 μm; TISA 500 = trabecular iris space area at 500 μm; TISA 750 = trabecular iris space area at 750 μm; VZ = vitreous zonule.

4. Discussion

In this study, the anterior segment parameters before and after phacoemulsification and IOL implantation were investigated in open-angle eyes and different subtypes of PACG eyes. There was no significant difference identified between the three groups in the change of degree of anterior rotation of the ciliary body before and after cataract surgery. The effect of anterior traction by the crystalline lens on the anterior rotation of ciliary processes might be equal in open-angle eyes and angle-closure eyes. Hence, a natural anatomical structure abnormality might be another pathogenesis for anterior rotation of ciliary processes in PACG patients. To our knowledge, this is the first study to explore whether the anterior rotation of ciliary processes has a potential relationship with the crystalline lens or not in the pathogenesis of PACG by comparing the parameters in open-angle and angle-closure patients before and after phacoemulsification and IOL implantation.

Despite the increasing number of studies focusing on ciliary processes and crystalline lenses about their role in the pathogenesis of PACG recently [7–9,12,15,16], the relationship between them remains ambiguous. He et al. [14] proposed that healthy Chinese had smaller TCPD, TCA, and a thinner ciliary body thickness than healthy Caucasians. They suggested that the Chinese have a more anteriorly positioned lens, which may contribute to more anteriorly positioned ciliary processes and the thinner ciliary body might cause anterior positioning and thickening of the lens through the greater anterior positioning of the ciliary processes and the loosening of the zonules [14]. In the current study, the CBTmax of PACG groups was significantly thinner than the open-angle group, which is consistent with a previous study [14]. However, the results from our study demonstrated the extractions of crystalline lenses played similar roles in terms of decreasing the anterior rotation of ciliary processes in open-angle eyes and angle-closure eyes, which suggested that the anterior rotation of ciliary processes might be a natural anatomical structure in PACG patients rather than due to a lens-related reason. Ünsal et al. [12] found TCPD and CBTmax increased at 2 months after surgery in 36 cataract eyes. However, the difference did not reach significance. Pereira et al. [17] suggested that TCPD did not change after cataract surgery in eyes with an open-angle. Li et al. [9] also found TCPD increased with no significant difference in acute primary angle-closure eyes after phacoemulsification, and suggested that the lack of significant change in TCPD after surgery may be due to a small change in the position of the ciliary process as a result of cataract extraction. However Nonaka et al. [7] described TCPD increased significantly after cataract surgery in eyes with primary angle-closure or PACG and proposed that lens extraction can reposition the ciliary processes in a more posterior location. Unfortunately, the above studies did not compare patients with open-angle and closed-angle in the same study. Moreover, in contrast to previous studies demonstrating that TCPD increased dramatically in PACG eyes that received lens extraction [8,18], the result of the current study was that there was no significant TCPD increase in all groups postoperatively, which did not support the hypothesis of anterior rotation of ciliary processes resulting from anterior traction of the crystalline lens. In addition to TCPD, TCA could also reflect the anterior positioning of the ciliary processes. In the current study, the changes in TCA and TCPD among open-angle eyes and different subtypes of PACG eyes were not statistically significant postoperatively, which indicated that the attenuate effects of lens extraction were consistent in all three groups. Compared to open-angle eyes, PACG eyes maintained a narrower TCA and smaller TCPD after cataract surgery, indicating that anteriorly rotated ciliary processes was not completely eliminated by lens extraction in the PACG eyes. Therefore, the forward traction of crystalline lens can lead to the anterior rotation of the ciliary processes, but is not the only factor.

Previous studies demonstrated that the size of the anterior ciliary body might be related to the crystalline lens [16]. The ciliary muscle contraction caused forward and inward rotation of the ciliary body and increased the thickness of the anterior ciliary body [19]. Theoretically, if the anterior rotation of ciliary processes in patients with PACG was due to the crystalline lens anterior pulling of ciliary processes, CPA would decrease after cataract extraction. However, in the current study, there were no significant differences in the changes of CPA after cataract surgery among the three groups, which was the evidence to show that lens removal did not narrow the gap in the size of the anterior ciliary body between closed- and open-angle eyes in terms of CPA. Therefore, the forward traction of the crystalline lens has little effect on the shape of the ciliary processes in both PACG eyes and open-angle eyes.

An experimental study found after VZ lysis, the ciliary body moved forward which narrowed the anterior chamber angle [13]. Shon et al. [20] described the relationship between VZ and anterior chamber angle characteristics in two clusters of PAC and PACG eyes and demonstrated that eyes with no VZ appeared to have smaller TCA, TCPD, AOD 500, AOD 750, TISA 500, and TISA 750 than eyes with visible VZ. In the current study, chronic PACG eyes and acute PACG eyes had a smaller number of quadrants of VZ, narrower angle, and more anterior rotation of ciliary processes than open-angle eyes before surgery. Anatomically, PACG eyes lacking VZ may play a potential role in angle closure. Weakened zonular fibers may rupture during surgery [21], which could explain the significant decrease in VZ in all three groups after surgery. Thus, the loss of VZ may have counterbalanced the posterior movement of the ciliary process caused by cataract extraction. Hence, further explorations about VZ and cataract extraction with larger sample sizes are warranted.

Modesti et al. [22] proposed that there was a decrease in the ciliary ring diameter and CSD, as well as changes in the shape of ciliary processes, resulting from the absence of zonular fiber tension after lens extraction. In the current study, acute PACG eyes had smaller CSD postoperatively. Though the changes in CSD among open-angle eyes and different subtypes of PACG eyes were not statistically significant postoperatively, chronic PACG and acute PACG eyes had smaller postoperative CSD than open-angle eyes exposed persistent anterior rotation of ciliary processes in PACG eyes. Further research is needed to investigate the correlation between CSD and ciliary processes in PACG eyes.

In the current study, we showed that as a natural anatomical abnormality, the anterior rotation of ciliary processes in PACG patients may not be associated with the lens factor. It is important to increase our understanding of the pathogenesis of PACG, to urge us to further explore the cause of anterior rotation of ciliary processes, such as the association with the presence of vitreous zonule. Reducing the volume of the ciliary body or relieving the anterior rotation of ciliary processes may further help us to carry out new treatments for PACG patients, such as cyclophotocoagulation.

Several limitations need to be noted in the present study. Firstly, the sample size was relatively small and there was no comparison with another imaging modality. Secondly, although miotics and mydriatics were not used before UBM examination, some angle-closure eyes used other anti-glaucoma drugs before cataract surgery. The potential effect of these drugs on anterior segment structure is not clear. Finally, since all patients had some degree of cataracts, we are unable to explore the potential relationship between the ciliary body and transparent lens at the moment.

5. Conclusions

This study demonstrates that extractions of crystalline lenses played similar roles in terms of decreasing the anterior rotation of ciliary processes in open-angle eyes and angle-closure eyes, and the anterior rotation of ciliary processes could not be eradicated completely postoperatively in angle-closure eyes. More attention should be paid to the natural anatomical abnormality of anterior rotation of ciliary processes, as it may provide more detailed information related to the pathogenesis of PACG.

Author Contributions: Conceptualization, H.W.; methodology, K.Y. and Z.L.; data curation, H.W., X.H., K.L. and Y.M.; writing—original draft preparation, Z.L.; writing—review and editing, K.Y.; funding acquisition, H.W. All authors have read and agreed to the published version of the manuscript.

Funding: This research was funded by the Beijing Science and Technology Plan Project, grant number Z191100007619045, the National Natural Science Foundation of China, grant number 61634006, and the National Key R&D Program of China, grant number 2020YFC2008200.

Institutional Review Board Statement: The study was conducted in accordance with the Declaration of Helsinki and was approved by the Ethics Committee of Peking University People's Hospital (protocol code 2022PHB256-001).

Informed Consent Statement: Informed consent was obtained from all subjects involved in the study.

Data Availability Statement: Data presented in this study are available from the corresponding author upon request.

Acknowledgments: The authors thank Y.W. for performing UBM for patients.

Conflicts of Interest: The authors declare no conflict of interest.

References

1. Xu, B.Y.; Chiang, M.; Chaudhary, S.; Kulkarni, S.; Pardeshi, A.A.; Varma, R. Deep Learning Classifiers for Automated Detection of Gonioscopic Angle Closure Based on Anterior Segment OCT Images. *Am. J. Ophthalmol.* **2019**, *208*, 273–280. [CrossRef] [PubMed]
2. Tham, Y.C.; Li, X.; Wong, T.Y.; Quigley, H.A.; Aung, T.; Cheng, C.Y. Global prevalence of glaucoma and projections of glaucoma burden through 2040: A systematic review and meta-analysis. *Ophthalmology* **2014**, *121*, 2081–2090. [CrossRef]
3. Sun, X.; Dai, Y.; Chen, Y.; Yu, D.-Y.; Cringle, S.J.; Chen, J.; Kong, X.; Wang, X.; Jiang, C. Primary angle closure glaucoma: What we know and what we don't know. *Prog. Retin. Eye Res.* **2017**, *57*, 26–45. [CrossRef] [PubMed]
4. Wang, F.; Wang, D.; Wang, L. Exploring the Occurrence Mechanisms of Acute Primary Angle Closure by Comparative Analysis of Ultrasound Biomicroscopic Data of the Attack and Fellow Eyes. *Biomed. Res. Int.* **2020**, *2020*, 8487907. [CrossRef] [PubMed]
5. Senthil, S.; Rao, H.L.; Choudhari, N.; Garudadri, C. Phacoemulsification versus Phacotrabeculectomy in Medically Controlled Primary Angle Closure Glaucoma with Cataract in an Indian Cohort: A randomized controlled trial. *Int. Ophthalmol.* **2021**, *42*, 35–45. [CrossRef]
6. Potop, V.; Corbu, C. The role of clear lens extraction in angle closure glaucoma. *Rom. J. Ophthalmol.* **2017**, *61*, 244–248. [CrossRef] [PubMed]
7. Nonaka, A.; Kondo, T.; Kikuchi, M.; Yamashiro, K.; Fujihara, M.; Iwawaki, T.; Yamamoto, K.; Kurimoto, Y. Angle Widening and Alteration of Ciliary Process Configuration after Cataract Surgery for Primary Angle Closure. *Ophthalmology* **2006**, *113*, 437–441. [CrossRef]
8. Man, X.; Chan, N.C.Y.; Baig, N.; Kwong, Y.Y.Y.; Leung, D.Y.L.; Li, F.C.H.; Tham, C.C.Y. Anatomical effects of clear lens extraction by phacoemulsification versus trabeculectomy on anterior chamber drainage angle in primary angle-closure glaucoma (PACG) patients. *Graefes. Arch. Clin. Exp. Ophthalmol.* **2015**, *253*, 773–778. [CrossRef]

9. Li, S.; Chen, Y.; Wu, Q.; Lu, B.; Wang, W.; Fang, J. Angle parameter changes of phacoemulsification and combined phacotrabeculectomy for acute primary angle closure. *Int. J. Ophthalmol.* **2015**, *8*, 742–747. [CrossRef]
10. You, S.; Liang, Z.; Yang, K.; Zhang, Y.; Oatts, J.; Han, Y.; Wu, H. Novel Discoveries of Anterior Segment Parameters in Fellow Eyes of Acute Primary Angle Closure and Chronic Primary Angle Closure Glaucoma. *Investig. Ophthalmol. Vis. Sci.* **2021**, *62*, 6. [CrossRef]
11. Oh, J.; Shin, H.H.; Kim, J.H.; Kim, H.M.; Song, J.S. Direct Measurement of the Ciliary Sulcus Diameter by 35-Megahertz Ultrasound Biomicroscopy. *Ophthalmology* **2007**, *114*, 1685–1688. [CrossRef] [PubMed]
12. Ünsal, E.; Eltutar, K.; Muftuoglu, İ.K. Morphologic Changes in the Anterior Segment using Ultrasound Biomicroscopy after Cataract Surgery and Intraocular Lens Implantation. *Eur. J. Ophthalmol.* **2016**, *27*, 31–38. [CrossRef] [PubMed]
13. Lütjen-Drecoll, E.; Kaufman, P.L.; Wasielewski, R.; Ting-Li, L.; Croft, M.A. Morphology and Accommodative Function of the Vitreous Zonule in Human and Monkey Eyes. *Investig. Ophthalmol. Vis. Sci.* **2010**, *51*, 1554–1564. [CrossRef] [PubMed]
14. He, N.; Wu, L.; Qi, M.; He, M.; Lin, S.; Wang, X.; Yang, F.; Fan, X. Comparison of Ciliary Body Anatomy between American Caucasians and Ethnic Chinese Using Ultrasound Biomicroscopy. *Curr. Eye Res.* **2015**, *41*, 485–491. [CrossRef] [PubMed]
15. Park, K.-A.; Yun, J.-H.; Kee, C. The Effect of Cataract Extraction on the Contractility of Ciliary Muscle. *Am. J. Ophthalmol.* **2008**, *146*, 8–14. [CrossRef]
16. Fayed, A.A.E. Ultrasound biomicroscopy value in evaluation of restoration of ciliary muscles contractility after cataract extraction. *Clin. Ophthalmol.* **2017**, *11*, 855–859. [CrossRef]
17. Pereira, F.A.; Cronemberger, S. Ultrasound biomicroscopic study of anterior segment changes after phacoemulsification and foldable intraocular lens implantation. *Ophthalmology* **2003**, *110*, 1799–1806. [CrossRef]
18. Tham, C.C.; Leung, D.Y.; Kwong, Y.Y.; Li, F.C.; Lai, J.S.; Lam, D.S. Effects of Phacoemulsification Versus Combined Phaco-trabeculectomy on Drainage Angle Status in Primary Angle Closure Glaucoma (PACG). *J. Glaucoma.* **2010**, *19*, 119–123. [CrossRef]
19. Ma, J.; Chen, X. Dynamic changes of configuration and position of human ciliary body during accommodation. *Zhonghua Yan Ke Za Zhi* **2004**, *40*, 590–596.
20. Shon, K.; Sung, K.R.; Kwon, J.; Hye Jo, Y. Vitreous Zonule and its Relation to Anterior Chamber Angle Characteristics in Primary Angle Closure. *J. Glaucoma.* **2019**, *28*, 1048–1053. [CrossRef]
21. Bassnett, S. Zinn's zonule. *Prog. Retin. Eye Res.* **2021**, *82*, 100902. [CrossRef] [PubMed]
22. Modesti, M.; Pasqualitto, G.; Appolloni, R.; Pecorella, I.; Sourdille, P. Preoperative and postoperative size and movements of the lens capsular bag: Ultrasound biomicroscopy analysis. *J. Cataract. Refract. Surg.* **2011**, *37*, 1775–1784. [CrossRef] [PubMed]

Disclaimer/Publisher's Note: The statements, opinions and data contained in all publications are solely those of the individual author(s) and contributor(s) and not of MDPI and/or the editor(s). MDPI and/or the editor(s) disclaim responsibility for any injury to people or property resulting from any ideas, methods, instructions or products referred to in the content.

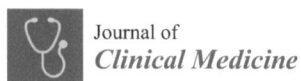

Journal of
Clinical Medicine

Article

Association between Optic Nerve Sheath Diameter and Lamina Cribrosa Morphology in Normal-Tension Glaucoma

Seung Hyen Lee [1], Tae-Woo Kim [2,*], Eun Ji Lee [2] and Hyunkyung Kil [3]

[1] Department of Ophthalmology, Nowon Eulji Medical Center, Eulji University College of Medicine, Seoul 01830, Republic of Korea
[2] Department of Ophthalmology, Seoul National University Bundang Hospital, Seoul National University College of Medicine, Seongnam 13620, Republic of Korea
[3] Department of Ophthalmology, Bundang Jesaeng General Hospital, Seongnam 13590, Republic of Korea
* Correspondence: twkim7@snu.ac.kr

Abstract: (1) Background: To compare optic nerve sheath diameter (ONSD) in normal-tension glaucoma (NTG) and healthy eyes and to investigate the association between ONSD and lamina cribrosa (LC) morphology. (2) Methods: This cross-sectional study included 69 NTG eyes and 69 healthy eyes matched for age, axial length, and intraocular pressure. The LC curvature index (LCCI) was measured from horizontal Cirrus HD-OCT B-scan images from five uniformly divided positions vertically of the optic nerve. The average LCCI was defined as the mean of the measurements at these five locations. ONSD was measured as the width of the optic nerve sheath at the site perpendicular 3 mm behind the posterior globe. LCCI and ONSD were compared in eyes with NTG and healthy eyes. The clinical factors that could affect LCCI were analyzed. (3) Results: NTG eyes had significantly smaller mean ONSD (4.55 ± 0.69 mm vs. 4.97 ± 0.58 mm, $p < 0.001$) and larger average LCCI (11.61 ± 1.43 vs. 7.58 ± 0.90, $p < 0.001$) than matched healthy control eyes. LCCI was significantly correlated with smaller ONSD, higher intraocular pressure, thinner global retinal nerve fiber thickness, and worse visual field loss in all subjects (all Ps ≤ 0.022). (4) Conclusions: NTG eyes had smaller ONSD and greater LCCI than healthy control eyes. In addition, a negative correlation was observed between ONSD and LCCI. These findings suggest that cerebrospinal fluid pressure, which ONSD indirectly predicts, may affect LC configuration. Changes in the retrolaminar compartment may play a role in glaucoma pathogenesis.

Keywords: optic nerve sheath diameter; normal-tension glaucoma; lamina cribrosa curvature

Citation: Lee, S.H.; Kim, T.-W.; Lee, E.J.; Kil, H. Association between Optic Nerve Sheath Diameter and Lamina Cribrosa Morphology in Normal-Tension Glaucoma. *J. Clin. Med.* 2023, 12, 360. https://doi.org/10.3390/jcm12010360

Academic Editor: Kevin Gillmann

Received: 7 December 2022
Revised: 28 December 2022
Accepted: 29 December 2022
Published: 2 January 2023

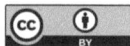

Copyright: © 2023 by the authors. Licensee MDPI, Basel, Switzerland. This article is an open access article distributed under the terms and conditions of the Creative Commons Attribution (CC BY) license (https://creativecommons.org/licenses/by/4.0/).

1. Introduction

Glaucoma is characterized by progressive optic neuropathy and equivalent visual field defects. In the pathophysiology of glaucoma, the most crucial independent risk factor is well known as the mechanical stress associated with an increase in intraocular pressure (IOP) [1,2]. However, glaucomatous optic nerve damage can develop and progress even when the IOP is in the normal range, a condition called normal-tension glaucoma (NTG). The pathophysiology of NTG, however, has not been fully determined.

The lamina cribrosa (LC) structurally supports the pathway of retinal ganglion cell axons and divides the optic nerve into two parts: the intraocular space anteriorly and the retrobulbar space posteriorly [3]. Experimental and clinical studies have shown that the LC morphology changes depending on the magnitude of IOP [4,5]. In an experimental model of glaucoma, it has been found that an IOP elevation induced the LC to curve posteriorly [4]. In contrast, the LC became less bowed when the IOP was lowered by IOP reduction treatment [5]. In addition to the effect of IOP on the LC, increase of cerebrospinal fluid (CSF) pressure also raised the strain of LC and retrolaminar neural tissue [6,7]. These findings indicate that the translaminar pressure gradient (TLPG) between the intraocular and retrobulbar space/tissue can induce LC deformation. Interestingly, the greater degree of backward LC bowing observed in eyes with high tension glaucoma, relative to healthy eyes, was also observed in eyes with NTG [8,9]. This finding suggests that TLPG may be still greater in eyes with NTG than in healthy eyes.

Since the optic nerve is surrounded by CSF, CSF pressure is closely related to retrolaminar tissue pressure [10]. However, invasive methods are required to measure CSF pressure. An alternative noninvasive approach, measurement of optic nerve sheath diameter (ONSD) by ultrasonography, is proposed as a surrogate parameter to estimate CSF pressure [11,12]. ONSD was found to be smaller in NTG eyes than in healthy control eyes in several previous studies, suggesting that CSF pressure is likely lower in NTG than in healthy subjects [13,14]. This finding gives an explanation that TLPG may be high in eyes with NTG, despite IOP being within the normal range. We hypothesized that, if low CSF pressure plays a significant role in generating high TLPG in NTG, thereby promoting posterior deformation of the LC, there would be a significant relationship between ONSD and the degree of backward LC bowing.

The purpose of this study was to compare ONSD in eyes with NTG and healthy control eyes and to investigate the relationship between LC morphology and ONSD in eyes with NTG.

2. Materials and Methods

The electronic medical records of all subjects who visited Bundang Jesaeng Hospital Glaucoma Clinic between February 2017 and December 2020 were retrospectively reviewed. The IRB of Bundang Jesaeng Hospital approved this study, which was conducted in accordance with the Helsinki Declaration.

2.1. Study Subjects

All subjects received general ophthalmic examinations as described elsewhere [15]. Stereo disc photography with a CR-2 Plus AF (Canon Inc., Tokyo, Japan), Cirrus HD-OCT (Carl Zeiss-Meditec, Jena, Germany), immersion B-scan ultrasonography (Quantel Medical compact II; Quantel Medical), central corneal thickness (Orbscan II), axial length (IOL Master 500; Carl Zeiss Meditec Ltd, Jena, Germany) and 24-2 Humphrey perimetry (Carl Zeiss Meditec, Jena, Germany) were also performed.

Eyes included in this study needed to have a best-corrected visual acuity 20/40 or better, −6.0D or higher and +3.0D or lower spherical refraction, −3.0 to +3.0 D for cylinder correction, normally open anterior chamber angle, and reliable visual field tests. The following eyes were excluded; (1) optic nerve tilt [16,17] or torsion [17,18] to remove the possibility that the LC may be deformed by other reasons, (2) intraocular surgery history excluding cataract operation, (3) diagnosis other than normal-tension glaucoma (e.g., secondary glaucoma), (4) neurologic disorders that can affect visual field loss, (5) low-quality image (i.e., signal strength < 7) caused by media opacity or patient incorporation, (6) ill-defined anterior surface of the central LC.

NTG was defined as having of glaucomatous optic neuropathy with a corresponding glaucomatous visual field defect; the maximum IOP without medications ≤21 mmHg; open angle on gonioscopy, and no secondary cause of glaucoma. A glaucomatous visual field defect was confirmed in two consecutive tests as described elsewhere [15].

The healthy control subjects were defined as eyes with normal IOP (≤21 mmHg) without an increase in IOP, no glaucomatous optic disc, no obvious retinal nerve fiber layer (RNFL) defects, a circumpapillary RNFL thickness measured by OCT in the normal range (within the 95th percentile of the normal data) and a normal visual field results (without glaucomatous or neurologic field defects).

One eye was randomly selected when both eyes met the inclusion criteria. Age, axial length, and IOP were matched between NTG and healthy control eyes using a frequency matching method.

Baseline IOP was defined as the average of the values measured 5 or more times prior to the initiation of IOP-lowering therapy and scan IOP was measured on the day of taking Cirrus HD-OCT images.

2.2. Cirrus High-Definition Optical Coherence Tomography Imaging of the Optic Nerve Head

Images of the optic nerve head of all subjects was obtained by a single well-trained technician using the Cirrus HD OCT 6000. Subjects with high-quality scans were included for analysis. High-quality OCT images were defined as those with a signal strength ≥ 7 (maximum, 10) without any motion artifacts, involuntary saccades, apparent decentration misalignment, or algorithm segmentation error. Optic disc images were obtained using an optic disc cube protocol of a 6×6 mm^2 area composed of 40,000 points (200×200 axial scans) and 21-HD line raster scans (9 mm length in enhanced depth imaging [EDI] mode). The built-in analysis algorithm (software version 11.5; Carl Zeiss Meditec, Jena, Germany) detects the center of the optic disc and calculates the peripapillary RNFL thickness at the 3.46 mm diameter circle automatically from the dataset consisting of 256 A-scans.

2.3. Lamina Cribrosa Curvature Index Measurement

LC morphology was quantified by a measurement of the LC curvature index (LCCI). The LCCI was determined how curved the LC is, as described previously [8,15]. Briefly, the line connecting two points that descend vertically from the two Bruch's membrane opening points until the anterior border of the LC was defined as the LC surface line. Lamina cribrosa curve depth (LCCD) was the maximal depth from LC surface line to LC surface and the width (W) was defined as the length of this LC surface line. The LCCI was estimated as followed: LCCI = (LCCD/W) $\times$ 100 (Figure 1B) [19].

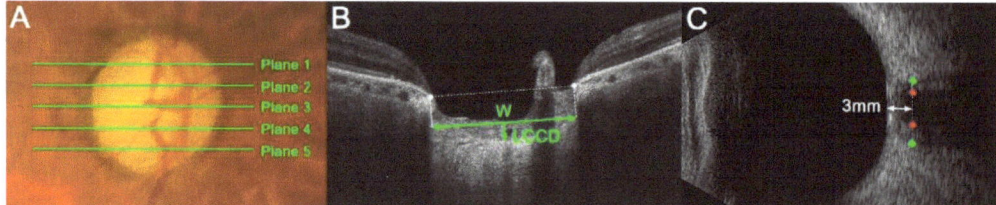

Figure 1. Measurements of the lamina cribrosa (LC) curvature index (LCCI), optic nerve sheath diameter (ONSD) and optic nerve diameter (OND). (**A**) Stereoscopic optic disc photograph image The five horizontal green lines indicate the locations where the measurements were performed. (**B**) Cirrus HD OCT B-scan images were obtained at plane 4 as shown in (**A**). The LCCI was measured by dividing the LC curve depth (LCCD) by the length of the LC surface reference line (W) within Bruch's membrane opening (BMO) and multiplying by 100. (**C**) Transorbital ultrasonographic image The ONSD (distance between green dots) and OND (red dots) were assessed perpendicular to the scanning place 3 mm behind the globe.

The measurement of LCCIs was performed at five locations dividing the optic nerve into 5 equal parts vertically using the built-in caliper of the viewer program (software version 11.5; Carl Zeiss Meditec, Jena, Germany) twice by a single experienced observer (SHL) blinded to the clinical information. The analysis used average of the two values measured twice. The average LCCI was defined as the mean values of measurements at the five locations.

2.4. Measurement of Optic Nerve Sheath Diameter and Optic Nerve Diameter

B-scan images were acquired by a single experienced technician who was blinded to the study protocol using transorbital ultrasonography with a linear 10-MHz probe. The patient lied in a supine position, followed by placement of sterile gel and probing slightly without pressure on the eyelid to prevent eye damage. The transverse view of the globe and retrobulbar part was obtained by holding the probe with the axial plane on the eyelid.

The ONSD and OND were defined as the optic nerve sheath width and the optic nerve width perpendicular to the vertical axis of the scanning site 3 mm behind the globe (Figure 1C), respectively. A position 3 mm behind the eyeball was a site that is susceptible to expansion due to rises in intracranial pressure (ICP) [20,21]. It was also the site of the greatest ultrasound contrast and the optimal distensibility of the optic nerve sheath in terms of CSF dynamics [20]. The ONSD and OND in all eyes were measured twice by a single glaucoma specialist (LSH) using Image J software (version 1.50 e; National Institutes of Health, Bethesda, MD, USA) in a masked manner, with the average of the two measured values used for the analysis.

2.5. Statistical Analysis

The intra-observer agreement between LCCI, ONSD and OND measurements was assessed using Bland-Altman limits of agreement and intra-class correlation coefficients. Independent t-tests (for continuous variables) and chi-square tests (for categorical variables) were performed in the comparison between the two groups. Bonferroni's correction was applied to t-tests based on the number of locations. Linear regression analyses were conducted to evaluate the factors related to LCCI. Fisher's z transformation was used to evaluate difference in the correlation coefficient between groups. p values < 0.05 were considered as statistically significant. The Statistical Package for Social Sciences was used in all statistical analyses (ver. 22.0, SPSS, Inc. Chicago, IL, USA).

3. Results

3.1. Demographic and Clinical Characteristics

This retrospective study initially involved 117 healthy control eyes and 98 eyes with NTG. Of these eyes, eight healthy control and 19 NTG eyes were excluded because of poor quality of OCT images, in which the anterior LC contour cannot be clearly distinguished even in one of five images of disc scan. In addition, two healthy control and five NTG eyes were excluded due to poor ultrasonographic image quality that did not allow a clear delineation of the optic nerve sheath margin. After matching the groups for age, IOP and axial length, 69 eyes of 69 NTG patients and 69 eyes of 69 healthy control subjects were finally included.

Table 1 presents the demographic characteristics of the study subjects. There were significant differences in mean deviation and pattern standard deviation on visual field tests, global RNFL thickness and ONSD (all $p \leq 0.002$, Table 1). ONSD was significantly lower in eyes with NTG than in healthy control eyes (4.55 ± 0.69 mm vs. 4.97 ± 0.58 mm, $p < 0.001$). The 95% Bland-Altman limits of agreement were −1.12 mm to 1.07 mm, −0.74 mm to 0.61 mm and −1.49 to 1.62, for the measurements of ONSD, OND and LCCI, respectively. The intra-class correlation coefficients for the interobserver reproducibility in measuring the ONSD, OND, and LCCI were 0.975, 0.987, and 0.967, respectively.

3.2. Comparison of LCCI in the Two Groups

Table 2 compares LCCI in NTG and healthy control eyes. The average LCCI in NTG eyes was 11.61 ± 1.43. In all five planes, the LCCI was significantly larger in NTG than in healthy control eyes (all $p < 0.001$).

3.3. Factors Associated with LCCIs

Univariate analysis showed that higher scan IOP, thinner global RNFL thickness, worse visual field loss and smaller ONSD were significantly associated with average LCCI (all Ps ≤ 0.019. In order to exclude multicollinearity between global RNFL thickness and visual field MD (variance inflation factor [VIF] = 4.000 and 3.972, respectively) and obtain reliable results, multivariate analysis was performed using two models. The average LCCI showed significant negative association with ONSD, global RNFL thickness, and visual field loss (all Ps < 0.001, Table 3) and significant positive correlation with scan IOP (Ps ≤ 0.022) in all subjects (Table 3; Figure 2) in both models. There was no significant difference of correlation coefficient between NTG and healthy groups (z score = 1.36, p = 0.087).

Table 1. Demographic characteristics of the study subjects.

Variables	Healthy Control Eyes (n = 69)	NTG Eyes (n = 69)	p Value
Demographic characteristics			
Age, years	67.8 ± 10.2	67.8 ± 9.8	0.986
Female, n (%)	33 (47.8)	36 (52.2)	0.734
Diabetes mellitus, n (%)	17 (24.6)	18 (26.1)	0.845
Hypertension, n (%)	35 (50.7)	34 (49.3)	0.865
Ophthalmic characteristics			
Baseline IOP, mmHg	16.9 ± 2.1	n/a	
Scan IOP, mmHg	14.9 ± 2.7	14.8 ± 2.5	0.718
Spherical error, diopters	−0.41 ± 2.25	−1.11 ± 2.86	0.111
Axial length, mm	23.75 ± 0.96	23.86 ± 1.18	0.543
Central corneal thickness, μm	547.1 ± 37.4	534.7 ± 29.0	0.124
VF MD, dB	−1.18 ± 2.30	−10.59 ± 8.24	**<0.001**
VF PSD, dB	1.59 ± 2.80	6.71 ± 3.76	**0.002**
Global RNFL thickness, μm	88.0 ± 8.9	68.2 ± 12.7	**<0.001**
ONSD, mm	4.97 ± 0.58	4.55 ± 0.69	**<0.001**
OND, mm	3.29 ± 0.35	3.21 ± 0.36	0.174

NTG = normal tension glaucoma; IOP = intraocular pressure; VF = visual field; MD = mean deviation; dB = decibel; PSD = pattern standard deviation; RNFL = retinal nerve fiber layer; ONSD = optic nerve sheath diameter; OND = optic nerve diameter. Data are reported as mean ± standard deviation or as number (percent), with statistically significant p values in boldface.

Table 2. Comparison of LCCI in healthy and NTG eyes.

	Healthy Eyes (n = 69)	NTG Eyes (n = 69)	p Value
Plane 1	7.88 ± 1.09	12.07 ± 1.78	**<0.001**
Plane 2	7.71 ± 1.28	11.77 ± 1.77	**<0.001**
Plane 3	6.89 ± 1.29	10.55 ± 1.68	**<0.001**
Plane 4	7.60 ± 1.38	11.34 ± 2.00	**<0.001**
Plane 5	7.85 ± 1.25	12.08 ± 2.06	**<0.001**
Average	7.58 ± 0.90	11.61 ± 1.43	**<0.001**

LCCI = lamina cribrosa curvature index; NTG = normal-tension glaucoma. Data are mean ± standard deviation values. Bonferroni correction was applied to raw data for measurements in the five planes. Values significant after Bonferroni correction (p < 0.01; 0.05/5) are shown in bold.

Table 3. Factors associated with LCCI in all subjects.

	All Subjects (n = 138)						
	Univariate		Multivariate Model 1			Multivariate Model 2		
Variables	Beta	p	Beta	p	VIF	Beta	p	VIF
Age, per 1-year older	0.008	0.706						
Gender, female	−0.299	0.455						
Diabetes mellitus	0.230	0.617						
Hypertension	−0.207	0.606						
Scan IOP, mmHg	0.182	**0.019**	0.129	**0.022**	1.019	0.151	**0.012**	1.019
Spherical equivalent, diopter	−0.142	0.166						
Axial length, mm	0.127	0.498						
Central cornea thickness, μm	−0.004	0.663						
Global RNFL thickness, μm	−0.096	**<0.001**	−0.083	**<0.001**	1.059			
Visual field MD, dB	−0.169	**<0.001**				−0.147	**<0.001**	1.052
ONSD, mm	−1.666	**<0.001**	−1.168	**<0.001**	1.078	−1.253	**<0.001**	1.066

IOP = intraocular pressure; RNFL = retinal nerve fiber layer; MD = mean deviation; dB = decibel; ONSD = optic nerve sheath diameter. Only variables with p < 0.1 on univariate analysis were included in the multivariate model. Statistically significant factors are shown in boldface.

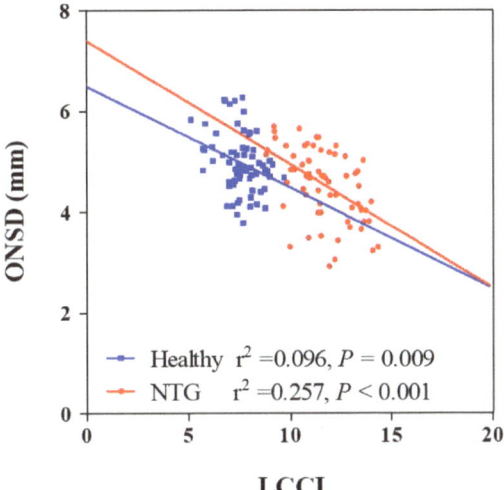

Figure 2. Scatterplots showing the relationship between lamina cribrosa curvature index and clinical parameters. Solid lines represent trend lines.

3.4. Representative Subjects

Figure 3 shows two eyes, a healthy control eye (Figure 3A–D) and a glaucomatous eye (Figure 3E–H). The healthy eye had a relatively flat LC with wide ONSD, whereas the glaucomatous eye had a curved LC with a narrow ONSD. Note that LCCI was larger and ONSD was smaller in the NTG than in the healthy eye.

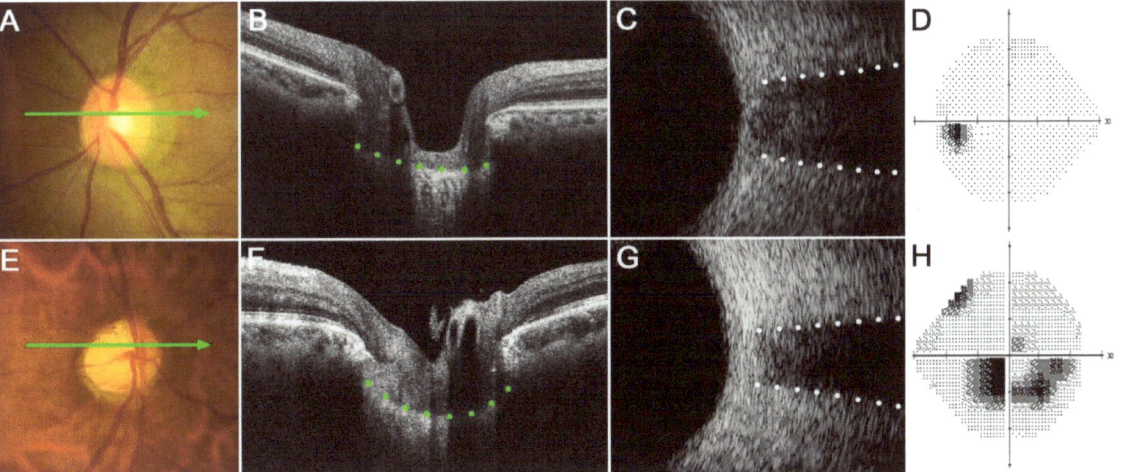

Figure 3. Representative eyes showing the relationship between the lamina cribrosa curvature index (LCCI) and optic nerve sheath diameter (ONSD). (**A–D**) A healthy left eye of a 63-year-old woman with a relatively flat LC and wide ONSD. (**E–H**) A glaucomatous right eye of a 59-year-old man with curved LC and narrow ONSD. (**A,E**) Stereoscopic optic disc photograph images. (**B,F**) Cirrus HD OCT B-scan images obtained at the locations indicated by light green arrows in (**A,E**), respectively. (**C,G**) Transorbital ultrasound images showing that ONSD was larger in the healthy eye (**C**) than in the glaucomatous eye (**G**). Note that LCCI is considerably larger in (**F**) than in (**B**), whereas the ONSD is notably larger in (**C**) than in (**G**). The comparison of these two representative eyes indicates a negative correlation between LCCI and ONSD.

4. Discussion

The present findings demonstrated that NTG eyes have smaller ONSD and larger LCCI than healthy control eyes, with a significant negative correlation between ONSD and LCCI. To our knowledge, this study is the first to investigate the relationship between ONSD and LC morphology.

In accordance with previous findings, the present study found that average LCCI was significantly larger in eyes with NTG than in healthy control eyes [15]. This finding suggests that TLPG is still relatively high in NTG eyes despite IOP being within the normal range.

Methods that measure CSF pressure, such as lumbar puncture, are limited in clinical practice because of their invasiveness. In contrast, ultrasound-based assessment of ONSD is a noninvasive method used clinically to detect increases in ICP in emergency and intensive care units [11,22,23]. The subarachnoid space surrounding the optic nerve does not directly communicate [10,24], but still connected with the rest of the CSF space [25]. Therefore, CSF pressure has been shown to generally correlate with ONSD in several previous studies [11,12,26]. Since the optic nerve sheath is elastic, ONSD may increase when the CSF pressure is increased [27]. Conversely, ONSD is reduced in patients with intracranial hypotension [28,29]. Therefore, measurements of ONSD have been used to investigate the role of CSF pressure in the pathophysiology of glaucoma [13,14,30,31].

The present study found that ONSD was significantly smaller in NTG eyes than in healthy control eyes matched for age, IOP and axial length. Given that ONSD indirectly represents CSF pressure, these results suggest that CSF pressure is lower in NTG than in healthy eyes. Until now, it is inconclusive whether CSF pressure is high or low in the NTG [32,33]. These present findings are consistent with previous experimental and clinical studies showing that CSF pressure is abnormally decreased in NTG [33–36]. These observations are also in agreement with previous studies that the subarachnoid space is narrower in NTG eyes than in high-tension glaucoma and healthy control eyes [13,14]. Taken together, these findings indicate that low CSF pressure plays a significant role in NTG.

The response of the LC according to the TLPG would be inevitably affected by the material properties of the LC. Until now, LC properties such as rigidity cannot be directly measured. It is generally known that the LC stiffens with age [37], and the LC becomes thinner as the axial length increases [38]. We tried to minimize the effect of these LC properties on LC morphology by matching age and axial length between two groups.

It is noteworthy that there was a negative correlation between average LCCI and ONSD in all subjects. LC curvature may be determined by the net effect of the TLPG and material properties. Therefore, not only IOP but also retrolaminar tissue pressure may contribute to the configuration of the LC. Although the material properties of the LC are also related, the correlation between LCCI and ONSD in NTG eyes suggests that low CSF pressure is related to the greater LCCI in NTG than in healthy eyes (Figure 4).

The average ONSDs measured in healthy control (4.97 ± 0.58 mm) and NTG (4.55 ± 0.69 mm) eyes in the present study are comparable to those previously reported in studies that measured ONSD using ultrasound [13,39] and magnetic resonance imaging [14]. In addition, a recent meta-analysis found that ONSD cut-off values for assessing intracranial hypertension varied from 4.80 to 6.30 mm [40].

The present study had limitations. First, this study did not consider several parameters potentially associated with the response of the LC, such as LC thickness and the material properties of the laminar and peripapillary scleral connective tissue [41]. These parameters however, are difficult or impossible to measure currently. As new technology advances make these parameters measurable, a more reliable relationship between LC morphology and postlaminar compartment will be obtained. Second, actual measurement of CSF pressure was not performed in the present study, then it could not be definitely concluded that the smaller ONSD would be correlated with lower CSF pressure. However, the validity of using ONSD as a surrogate to CSF pressure has been suggested in multiple studies [12,42,43]. Third, a tilted or torted optic disc were not included, therefore our results cannot be applicable to these eyes directly. Forth, LCCI measurements using OCT were performed in the sitting position, and ONSD measurements using ultrasonography were made in the supine position. Since CSF pressure may vary depending on body posture, it is possible that the result was affect by a difference in body position. However, modalities of the two measurement methods were unified in each setting, it would not have had a significant effect on the results.

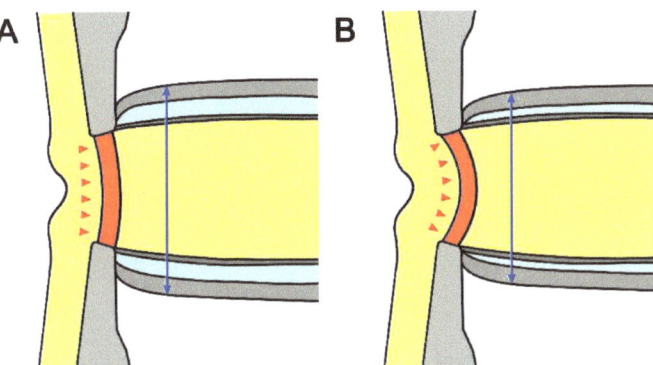

Figure 4. Schematic diagram of the optic nerve in healthy (**A**) and glaucomatous (**B**) eyes. Note that smaller ONSD and more posteriorly curved LC in NTG suggested that low cerebrospinal fluid pressure may induce a relatively higher TLPG in NTG than in healthy eyes. The double headed blue arrows indicate ONSD and the red arrows represent the morphology of LC.

In conclusion, ONSD was smaller and LCCI was larger in NTG than in healthy control eyes. These findings are consistent with the concept that lower CSF pressure may play a significant role in the pathogenesis of glaucomatous optic neuropathy in NTG.

Author Contributions: Conceptualization, S.H.L. and T.-W.K.; methodology, S.H.L. and H.K.; validation, S.H.L., T.-W.K., E.J.L. and H.K.; formal analysis, S.H.L. and E.J.L.; investigation, S.H.L. and E.J.L.; resources, S.H.L.; data curation, S.H.L. and H.K.; writing—original draft preparation, S.H.L. and T.-W.K.; writing—review and editing, S.H.L., T.-W.K. and E.J.L.; visualization, S.H.L.; supervision, T.-W.K.; project administration, S.H.L. and T.-W.K.; funding acquisition, S.H.L. and T.-W.K. All authors have read and agreed to the published version of the manuscript.

Funding: This research was supported by Eulji University, grant number EJRG-22-02.

Institutional Review Board Statement: The study was conducted in accordance with the Declaration of Helsinki, and approved by the Institutional Review Board of Bundang Jesaeng Hospital (protocol code 2021-01-007).

Informed Consent Statement: Patient consent was waived due to the retrospective study nature.

Data Availability Statement: The data presented in this study are available on request from the corresponding author. The data are not publicly available due to privacy issues.

Conflicts of Interest: The authors declare no conflict of interest. The funders had no role in the design of the study; in the collection, analyses, or interpretation of data; in the writing of the manuscript.

References

1. Leske, M.C.; Connell, A.M.; Wu, S.Y.; Hyman, L.G.; Schachat, A.P. Risk factors for open-angle glaucoma. The Barbados Eye Study. *Arch. Ophthalmol.* **1995**, *113*, 918–924. [CrossRef] [PubMed]
2. Burgoyne, C.F.; Downs, J.C.; Bellezza, A.J.; Suh, J.K.; Hart, R.T. The optic nerve head as a biomechanical structure: A new paradigm for understanding the role of IOP-related stress and strain in the pathophysiology of glaucomatous optic nerve head damage. *Prog. Retin. Eye Res.* **2005**, *24*, 39–73. [CrossRef] [PubMed]
3. Radius, R.L.; Gonzales, M. Anatomy of the lamina cribrosa in human eyes. *Arch. Ophthalmol.* **1981**, *99*, 2159–2162. [CrossRef] [PubMed]
4. Bellezza, A.J.; Rintalan, C.J.; Thompson, H.W.; Downs, J.C.; Hart, R.T.; Burgoyne, C.F. Deformation of the lamina cribrosa and anterior scleral canal wall in early experimental glaucoma. *Investig. Ophthalmol. Vis. Sci.* **2003**, *44*, 623–637. [CrossRef] [PubMed]

5. Lee, S.H.; Yu, D.A.; Kim, T.W.; Lee, E.J.; Girard, M.J.; Mari, J.M. Reduction of the Lamina Cribrosa Curvature After Trabeculectomy in Glaucoma. *Investig. Ophthalmol. Vis. Sci.* **2016**, *57*, 5006–5014. [CrossRef] [PubMed]
6. Feola, A.J.; Coudrillier, B.; Mulvihill, J.; Geraldes, D.M.; Vo, N.T.; Albon, J.; Abel, R.L.; Samuels, B.C.; Ethier, C.R. Deformation of the Lamina Cribrosa and Optic Nerve Due to Changes in Cerebrospinal Fluid Pressure. *Investig. Ophthalmol. Vis. Sci.* **2017**, *58*, 2070–2078. [CrossRef]
7. Morgan, W.H.; Chauhan, B.C.; Yu, D.-Y.; Cringle, S.J.; Alder, V.A.; House, P.H. Optic disc movement with variations in intraocular and cerebrospinal fluid pressure. *Investig. Ophthalmol. Vis. Sci.* **2002**, *43*, 3236–3242.
8. Lee, S.H.; Kim, T.W.; Lee, E.J.; Girard, M.J.; Mari, J.M.; Ritch, R. Ocular and Clinical Characteristics Associated with the Extent of Posterior Lamina Cribrosa Curve in Normal Tension Glaucoma. *Sci. Rep.* **2018**, *8*, 961. [CrossRef] [PubMed]
9. Kim, J.-A.; Kim, T.-W.; Lee, E.J.; Girard, M.J.; Mari, J.M. Comparison of lamina cribrosa morphology in eyes with ocular hypertension and normal-tension glaucoma. *Investig. Ophthalmol. Vis. Sci.* **2020**, *61*, 4. [CrossRef] [PubMed]
10. Morgan, W.H.; Yu, D.Y.; Alder, V.A.; Cringle, S.J.; Cooper, R.L.; House, P.H.; Constable, I.J. The correlation between cerebrospinal fluid pressure and retrolaminar tissue pressure. *Investig. Ophthalmol. Vis. Sci.* **1998**, *39*, 1419–1428.
11. Soldatos, T.; Chatzimichail, K.; Papathanasiou, M.; Gouliamos, A. Optic nerve sonography: A new window for the non-invasive evaluation of intracranial pressure in brain injury. *Emerg. Med. J.* **2009**, *26*, 630–634. [CrossRef]
12. Hansen, H.C.; Helmke, K. Validation of the optic nerve sheath response to changing cerebrospinal fluid pressure: Ultrasound findings during intrathecal infusion tests. *J. Neurosurg.* **1997**, *87*, 34–40. [CrossRef] [PubMed]
13. Liu, H.; Yang, D.; Ma, T.; Shi, W.; Zhu, Q.; Kang, J.; Wang, N. Measurement and Associations of the Optic Nerve Subarachnoid Space in Normal Tension and Primary Open-Angle Glaucoma. *Am. J. Ophthalmol.* **2018**, *186*, 128–137. [CrossRef]
14. Wang, N.; Xie, X.; Yang, D.; Xian, J.; Li, Y.; Ren, R.; Peng, X.; Jonas, J.B.; Weinreb, R.N. Orbital cerebrospinal fluid space in glaucoma: The Beijing intracranial and intraocular pressure (iCOP) study. *Ophthalmology* **2012**, *119*, 2065–2073. [CrossRef] [PubMed]
15. Lee, S.H.; Kim, T.W.; Lee, E.J.; Girard, M.J.; Mari, J.M. Diagnostic Power of Lamina Cribrosa Depth and Curvature in Glaucoma. *Investig. Ophthalmol. Vis. Sci.* **2017**, *58*, 755–762. [CrossRef] [PubMed]
16. Jonas, J.B.; Papastathopoulos, K.I. Optic disc shape in glaucoma. *Graefes Arch. Clin. Exp. Ophthalmol.* **1996**, *234* (Suppl. 1), S167–S173. [CrossRef]
17. Vongphanit, J.; Mitchell, P.; Wang, J.J. Population prevalence of tilted optic disks and the relationship of this sign to refractive error. *Am. J. Ophthalmol.* **2002**, *133*, 679–685. [CrossRef]
18. Samarawickrama, C.; Mitchell, P.; Tong, L.; Gazzard, G.; Lim, L.; Wong, T.Y.; Saw, S.M. Myopia-related optic disc and retinal changes in adolescent children from singapore. *Ophthalmology* **2011**, *118*, 2050–2057. [CrossRef]
19. Lee, S.H.; Kim, T.W.; Lee, E.J.; Girard, M.J.; Mari, J.M. Lamina Cribrosa Curvature in Healthy Korean Eyes. *Sci. Rep.* **2019**, *9*, 1756 [CrossRef]
20. Liu, D.; Kahn, M. Measurement and relationship of subarachnoid pressure of the optic nerve to intracranial pressures in fresh cadavers. *Am. J. Ophthalmol.* **1993**, *116*, 548–556. [CrossRef]
21. Helmke, K.; Hansen, H.C. Fundamentals of transorbital sonographic evaluation of optic nerve sheath expansion under intracranial hypertension. I. Experimental study. *Pediatr. Radiol.* **1996**, *26*, 701–705. [CrossRef] [PubMed]
22. Kimberly, H.H.; Shah, S.; Marill, K.; Noble, V. Correlation of optic nerve sheath diameter with direct measurement of intracranial pressure. *Acad. Emerg. Med.* **2008**, *15*, 201–204. [CrossRef] [PubMed]
23. Dubourg, J.; Javouhey, E.; Geeraerts, T.; Messerer, M.; Kassai, B. Ultrasonography of optic nerve sheath diameter for detection of raised intracranial pressure: A systematic review and meta-analysis. *Intensive Care Med.* **2011**, *37*, 1059–1068. [CrossRef] [PubMed]
24. Killer, H.; Jaggi, G.; Flammer, J.; Miller, N.R.; Huber, A.; Mironov, A. Cerebrospinal fluid dynamics between the intracranial and the subarachnoid space of the optic nerve. Is it always bidirectional? *Brain* **2007**, *130*, 514–520. [CrossRef]
25. Lenfeldt, N.; Koskinen, L.-O.D.; Bergenheim, A.T.; Malm, J.; Eklund, A. CSF pressure assessed by lumbar puncture agrees with intracranial pressure. *Neurology* **2007**, *68*, 155–158. [CrossRef]
26. Ragauskas, A.; Matijosaitis, V.; Zakelis, R.; Petrikonis, K.; Rastenyte, D.; Piper, I.; Daubaris, G. Clinical assessment of noninvasive intracranial pressure absolute value measurement method. *Neurology* **2012**, *78*, 1684–1691. [CrossRef]
27. Raspanti, M.; Marchini, M.; Della Pasqua, V.; Strocchi, R.; Ruggeri, A. Ultrastructure of the extracellular matrix of bovine dura mater, optic nerve sheath and sclera. *J. Anat.* **1992**, *181*, 181.
28. Watanabe, A.; Horikoshi, T.; Uchida, M.; Ishigame, K.; Kinouchi, H. Decreased diameter of the optic nerve sheath associated with CSF hypovolemia. *AJNR Am. J. Neuroradiol.* **2008**, *29*, 863–864. [CrossRef]
29. Rohr, A.; Jensen, U.; Riedel, C.; van Baalen, A.; Fruehauf, M.C.; Bartsch, T.; Hedderich, J.; Doerner, L.; Jansen, O. MR imaging of the optic nerve sheath in patients with craniospinal hypotension. *AJNR Am. J. Neuroradiol.* **2010**, *31*, 1752–1757. [CrossRef]
30. Abegão Pinto, L.; Vandewalle, E.; Pronk, A.; Stalmans, I. Intraocular pressure correlates with optic nerve sheath diameter in patients with normal tension glaucoma. *Graefes Arch. Clin. Exp. Ophthalmol.* **2012**, *250*, 1075–1080. [CrossRef]
31. Jaggi, G.P.; Miller, N.R.; Flammer, J.; Weinreb, R.N.; Remonda, L.; Killer, H.E. Optic nerve sheath diameter in normal-tension glaucoma patients. *Br. J. Ophthalmol.* **2012**, *96*, 53–56. [CrossRef] [PubMed]
32. Lindén, C.; Qvarlander, S.; Jóhannesson, G.; Johansson, E.; Östlund, F.; Malm, J.; Eklund, A. Normal-tension glaucoma has normal intracranial pressure: A prospective study of intracranial pressure and intraocular pressure in different body positions. *Ophthalmology* **2018**, *125*, 361–368. [CrossRef] [PubMed]

33. Ren, R.; Jonas, J.B.; Tian, G.; Zhen, Y.; Ma, K.; Li, S.; Wang, H.; Li, B.; Zhang, X.; Wang, N. Cerebrospinal fluid pressure in glaucoma: A prospective study. *Ophthalmology* **2010**, *117*, 259–266. [CrossRef] [PubMed]
34. Berdahl, J.P.; Allingham, R.R.; Johnson, D.H. Cerebrospinal fluid pressure is decreased in primary open-angle glaucoma. *Ophthalmology* **2008**, *115*, 763–768. [CrossRef] [PubMed]
35. Berdahl, J.P.; Fautsch, M.P.; Stinnett, S.S.; Allingham, R.R. Intracranial pressure in primary open angle glaucoma, normal tension glaucoma, and ocular hypertension: A case-control study. *Investig. Ophthalmol. Vis. Sci.* **2008**, *49*, 5412–5418. [CrossRef] [PubMed]
36. Jonas, J.B.; Ritch, R.; Panda-Jonas, S. Cerebrospinal fluid pressure in the pathogenesis of glaucoma. *Prog. Brain Res.* **2015**, *221*, 33–47. [CrossRef] [PubMed]
37. Albon, J.; Purslow, P.P.; Karwatowski, W.S.; Easty, D.L. Age related compliance of the lamina cribrosa in human eyes. *Br. J. Ophthalmol.* **2000**, *84*, 318–323. [CrossRef] [PubMed]
38. Ren, R.; Wang, N.; Li, B.; Li, L.; Gao, F.; Xu, X.; Jonas, J.B. Lamina cribrosa and peripapillary sclera histomorphometry in normal and advanced glaucomatous Chinese eyes with various axial length. *Investig. Ophthalmol. Vis. Sci.* **2009**, *50*, 2175–2184. [CrossRef]
39. Cardim, D.; Czosnyka, M.; Chandrapatham, K.; Badenes, R.; Bertuccio, A.; Noto, A.D.; Donnelly, J.; Pelosi, P.; Ball, L.; Hutchinson, P.J. Effects of age and sex on optic nerve sheath diameter in healthy volunteers and patients with traumatic brain injury. *Front. Neurol.* **2020**, *11*, 764. [CrossRef] [PubMed]
40. Robba, C.; Santori, G.; Czosnyka, M.; Corradi, F.; Bragazzi, N.; Padayachy, L.; Taccone, F.S.; Citerio, G. Optic nerve sheath diameter measured sonographically as non-invasive estimator of intracranial pressure: A systematic review and meta-analysis. *Intensive Care Med.* **2018**, *44*, 1284–1294. [CrossRef]
41. Downs, J.C.; Suh, J.K.; Thomas, K.A.; Bellezza, A.J.; Hart, R.T.; Burgoyne, C.F. Viscoelastic material properties of the peripapillary sclera in normal and early-glaucoma monkey eyes. *Investig. Ophthalmol. Vis. Sci.* **2005**, *46*, 540–546. [CrossRef] [PubMed]
42. Schroeder, C.; Katsanos, A.H.; Richter, D.; Tsivgoulis, G.; Gold, R.; Krogias, C. Quantification of optic nerve and sheath diameter by transorbital sonography: A systematic review and metanalysis. *J. Neuroimaging* **2020**, *30*, 165–174. [CrossRef] [PubMed]
43. Chen, L.-M.; Wang, L.-J.; Hu, Y.; Jiang, X.-H.; Wang, Y.-Z.; Xing, Y.-Q. Ultrasonic measurement of optic nerve sheath diameter: A non-invasive surrogate approach for dynamic, real-time evaluation of intracranial pressure. *Br. J. Ophthalmol.* **2019**, *103*, 437–441. [CrossRef] [PubMed]

Disclaimer/Publisher's Note: The statements, opinions and data contained in all publications are solely those of the individual author(s) and contributor(s) and not of MDPI and/or the editor(s). MDPI and/or the editor(s) disclaim responsibility for any injury to people or property resulting from any ideas, methods, instructions or products referred to in the content.

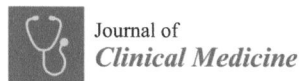 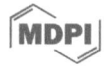

Comment

Could Young Cerebrospinal Fluid Combat Glaucoma? Comment on Lee et al. Association between Optic Nerve Sheath Diameter and Lamina Cribrosa Morphology in Normal-Tension Glaucoma. *J. Clin. Med.* 2023, 12, 360

Peter Wostyn

Department of Psychiatry, PC Sint-Amandus, 8730 Beernem, Belgium; wostyn.peter@skynet.be;
Tel.: +32-472713719; Fax: +32-50-819720

Citation: Wostyn, P. Could Young Cerebrospinal Fluid Combat Glaucoma? Comment on Lee et al. Association between Optic Nerve Sheath Diameter and Lamina Cribrosa Morphology in Normal-Tension Glaucoma. *J. Clin. Med.* 2023, 12, 360. *J. Clin. Med.* **2023**, 12, 3285. https://doi.org/10.3390/jcm12093285

Academic Editor: Kevin Gillmann

Received: 25 January 2023
Accepted: 16 April 2023
Published: 5 May 2023

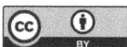

Copyright: © 2023 by the author. Licensee MDPI, Basel, Switzerland. This article is an open access article distributed under the terms and conditions of the Creative Commons Attribution (CC BY) license (https://creativecommons.org/licenses/by/4.0/).

I enjoyed reading the article by Lee et al. [1] entitled "Association between Optic Nerve Sheath Diameter and Lamina Cribrosa Morphology in Normal-Tension Glaucoma" published recently in *Journal of Clinical Medicine*. I would like to congratulate the authors for performing this cross-sectional study with findings of great importance for our understanding of the pathophysiology of normal-tension glaucoma (NTG), and I would appreciate the opportunity to make a comment on possible therapeutic implications.

The authors compared optic nerve sheath diameter (ONSD) in eyes with NTG and healthy control eyes and investigated the relationship between ONSD and lamina cribrosa (LC) morphology. They demonstrated that NTG eyes have smaller ONSDs and larger LC curvature indexes (LCCIs) than healthy control eyes, with a significant negative correlation between ONSD and LCCI. Given that NTG eyes had smaller ONSDs and that this may reflect lower cerebrospinal fluid (CSF) pressure, and given the greater degree of backward LC bowing observed in NTG eyes compared with healthy eyes, the authors concluded that lower CSF pressure may play a significant role in the pathogenesis of glaucomatous optic neuropathy in NTG. The authors also nicely reviewed additional evidence from previous studies suggesting that reduced CSF pressure may be involved in the pathogenesis of NTG.

Taken together, the above observations call for targeted research aiming to prevent or slow glaucomatous optic nerve damage via safe strategies that modulate intracranial pressure (ICP). Such treatment strategies could provide a protective effect for the optic nerve by increasing the ICP within the safe range, and thus by decreasing the trans-lamina cribrosa pressure difference, i.e., the difference between intraocular pressure and orbital subarachnoid space (SAS) pressure [2]. As discussed below, I believe research related to alterations in CSF composition could further open avenues for new approaches to the treatment of NTG.

The optic nerve is a white matter tract of the central nervous system (CNS) that is enveloped by all three meningeal layers and is surrounded by CSF in the SAS [3,4]. Growing evidence in the literature provides strong support for the concept that not only low CSF pressure [5] but also altered CSF composition [6–8] within the optic nerve SAS is involved in NTG pathogenesis. Indeed, the compartmentation of the optic nerve SAS with disturbed CSF dynamics has been shown to be associated with NTG [6–8]. In this context, not only interventions targeting ICP but also approaches targeting CSF dynamics could be new directions in glaucoma treatment. Such interventions could improve CSF circulation around the optic nerve, leading to the enhanced removal of potentially neurotoxic waste products that accumulate in the optic nerve [2].

Furthermore, advanced knowledge of age-related changes in CSF composition is essential to better understand age-associated neurodegenerative diseases and might further open up new therapeutic strategies for NTG. CSF contains a complex mix of substances, including vitamins, peptides, nucleosides and growth factors, that are crucial for CNS health [9]. However, CSF protein composition changes dramatically with age [10]. For example, there is a decrease in growth factors such as brain-derived neurotrophic factor (BDNF) [10]. Studies revealed that BDNF plays an essential role in maintaining the health of retinal ganglion cells and that the deprivation of BDNF leads to the induction of their apoptosis [11,12]. The reduced retrograde axonal transport of BDNF from the brain to the retina has been suggested as a likely mechanism of glaucomatous optic neuropathy [11,12]. Intriguingly, a new study conducted by Iram et al. [10] discovered that the intracerebroventricular infusion of young CSF into aged mice has rejuvenating effects on the brain. It was found that infusing young CSF directly into aged brains improves memory function, which occurs along with an increase in oligodendrocyte progenitor cell proliferation and hippocampal myelination. Fibroblast growth factor 17, whose levels decrease with age in human CSF, was identified as a major component of the rejuvenating effects of young CSF. Given the altered CSF protein composition in aging [10], and given that NTG is a neurodegenerative disease associated with increased age, the question is whether such age-related changes in the composition of CSF within the optic nerve SAS contribute to the pathogenesis of glaucomatous optic neuropathy. If confirmed, it would be worthwhile to further explore whether the intrathecal administration (or administration via other routes such as topical and intravitreal) of factors present in young CSF might be a therapeutic strategy for glaucoma, given the significant number of patients experiencing this devastating disease for whom existing treatment options are ineffective. Intrathecal infusion pumps are already widely used for the management of chronic pain (morphine pump) and spasticity (baclofen pump) [13,14]. If the intrathecal administration of such CSF factors was proven to be effective in treating glaucoma, this new treatment, if enriched with brain rejuvenating factors, could also protect against age-related cognitive decline, as reported by Iram et al. [10]. The latter is especially important for patients with NTG, who have been shown to have a significantly higher risk of developing Alzheimer's disease [15].

Conflicts of Interest: Peter Wostyn is named as an inventor on patents filed by P&X Medical NV relating to glaucoma treatment using an intrathecal cerebrospinal fluid pump system.

References

1. Lee, S.H.; Kim, T.-W.; Lee, E.J.; Kil, H. Association between optic nerve sheath diameter and lamina cribrosa morphology in normal-tension glaucoma. *J. Clin. Med.* **2023**, *12*, 360. [CrossRef] [PubMed]
2. Wostyn, P.; Van Dam, D.; De Deyn, P.P. Intracranial pressure and glaucoma: Is there a new therapeutic perspective on the horizon? *Med. Hypotheses* **2018**, *118*, 98–102. [CrossRef] [PubMed]
3. London, A.; Benhar, I.; Schwartz, M. The retina as a window to the brain—From eye research to CNS disorders. *Nat. Rev. Neurol.* **2013**, *9*, 44–53. [CrossRef] [PubMed]
4. Killer, H.E.; Jaggi, G.P.; Flammer, J.; Miller, N.R.; Huber, A.R. The optic nerve: A new window into cerebrospinal fluid composition? *Brain* **2006**, *129*, 1027–1030. [CrossRef] [PubMed]
5. Berdahl, J.P.; Allingham, R.R. Intracranial pressure and glaucoma. *Curr. Opin. Ophthalmol.* **2010**, *21*, 106–111. [CrossRef] [PubMed]
6. Killer, H.E.; Miller, N.R.; Flammer, J.; Meyer, P.; Weinreb, R.N.; Remonda, L.; Jaggi, G.P. Cerebrospinal fluid exchange in the optic nerve in normal-tension glaucoma. *Br. J. Ophthalmol.* **2012**, *96*, 544–548. [CrossRef] [PubMed]
7. Pircher, A.; Montali, M.; Wostyn, P.; Pircher, J.; Berberat, J.; Remonda, L.; Killer, H.E. Impaired cerebrospinal fluid dynamics along the entire optic nerve in normal-tension glaucoma. *Acta Ophthalmol.* **2018**, *96*, e562–e569. [CrossRef] [PubMed]
8. Pircher, A.; Neutzner, A.; Montali, M.; Huber, A.; Scholl, H.P.N.; Berberat, J.; Remonda, L.; Killer, H.E. Lipocalin-type prostaglandin D synthase concentration gradients in the cerebrospinal fluid in normal-tension glaucoma patients with optic nerve sheath compartmentation. *Eye Brain* **2021**, *13*, 89–97. [CrossRef] [PubMed]
9. Johanson, C.E.; Duncan, J.A., 3rd; Klinge, P.M.; Brinker, T.; Stopa, E.G.; Silverberg, G.D. Multiplicity of cerebrospinal fluid functions: New challenges in health and disease. *Cereb. Fluid Res.* **2008**, *5*, 10. [CrossRef] [PubMed]
10. Iram, T.; Kern, F.; Kaur, A.; Myneni, S.; Morningstar, A.R.; Shin, H.; Garcia, M.A.; Yerra, L.; Palovics, R.; Yang, A.C.; et al. Young CSF restores oligodendrogenesis and memory in aged mice via Fgf17. *Nature* **2022**, *605*, 509–515. [CrossRef] [PubMed]
11. Lambuk, L.; Mohd Lazaldin, M.A.; Ahmad, S.; Lezhitsa, I.; Agarwal, R.; Uskoković, V.; Mohamud, R. Brain-derived neurotrophic factor-mediated neuroprotection in glaucoma: A review of current state of the art. *Front. Pharmacol.* **2022**, *13*, 875662. [CrossRef] [PubMed]
12. Gupta, V.; You, Y.; Li, J.; Gupta, V.; Golzan, M.; Klistorner, A.; van den Buuse, M.; Graham, S. BDNF impairment is associated with age-related changes in the inner retina and exacerbates experimental glaucoma. *Biochim. Biophys. Acta* **2014**, *1842*, 1567–1578. [CrossRef] [PubMed]

13. Bruel, B.M.; Burton, A.W. Intrathecal Therapy for Cancer-Related Pain. *Pain Med.* **2016**, *17*, 2404–2421. [CrossRef] [PubMed]
14. Abou Al-Shaar, H.; Alkhani, A. Intrathecal baclofen therapy for spasticity: A compliance-based study to indicate effectiveness. *Surg. Neurol. Int.* **2016**, *7*, S539–S541. [PubMed]
15. Chen, Y.Y.; Lai, Y.J.; Yen, Y.F.; Shen, Y.C.; Wang, C.Y.; Liang, C.Y.; Lin, K.H.; Fan, L.W. Association between normal tension glaucoma and the risk of Alzheimer's disease: A nationwide population-based cohort study in Taiwan. *BMJ Open* **2018**, *8*, e022987. [CrossRef] [PubMed]

Disclaimer/Publisher's Note: The statements, opinions and data contained in all publications are solely those of the individual author(s) and contributor(s) and not of MDPI and/or the editor(s). MDPI and/or the editor(s) disclaim responsibility for any injury to people or property resulting from any ideas, methods, instructions or products referred to in the content.

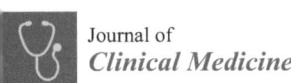

Reply

Reply to Wostyn, P. Could Young Cerebrospinal Fluid Combat Glaucoma? Comment on "Lee et al. Association between Optic Nerve Sheath Diameter and Lamina Cribrosa Morphology in Normal-Tension Glaucoma. *J. Clin. Med.* 2023, 12, 360"

Seung Hyen Lee [1], Tae-Woo Kim [2,*], Eun Ji Lee [2] and Hyunkyung Kil [3]

1. Department of Ophthalmology, Nowon Eulji Medical Center, Eulji University College of Medicine, Seoul 01830, Republic of Korea
2. Department of Ophthalmology, Seoul National University Bundang Hospital, Seoul National University College of Medicine, Seongnam 13620, Republic of Korea
3. Department of Ophthalmology, Bundang Jesaeng General Hospital, Seongnam 13590, Republic of Korea
* Correspondence: twkim7@snu.ac.kr; Tel.: +82-31-787-7374; Fax: +82-31-787-4057

We are pleased to see that Peter Wostyn has contributed a Comment: "Could Young Cerebrospinal Fluid Combat Glaucoma?" [1] in response to our paper published in the *Journal of Clinical Medicine*.

The author proposed a treatment strategy to control intracranial pressure (ICP) based on our findings that lower cerebrospinal fluid (CSF) pressure, which can be expected with a small optic nerve sheath diameter (ONSD), may be involved in the pathogenesis of normal-tension glaucoma (NTG) [2]. In particular, the author introduced an approach to glaucoma treatment by changing the CSF composition, assuming that not only CSF pressure but also altered CSF composition affects the pathophysiology of NTG.

Recent studies have suggested that changes in the composition of CSF may be involved in the pathogenesis of NTG. Wostyn et al. proposed an alternative pathogenesis of NTG in which CSF circulatory failure results in reduced neurotoxin clearance along the optic nerve [3]. Additionally, our group reported that increased T-tau protein in CSF is associated with thinner lamina cribrosa (LC) thickness [4]. This supports the common pathophysiology of glaucoma and Alzheimer's disease as neurodegenerative diseases [5–7]. Considering all of these, the altered composition of CSF may have a role in the pathophysiology of glaucoma. However, the specific differences in CSF composition in NTG patients and the specific role of these proteins in the development of NTG are still the subject of much debate.

Our study only indirectly speculated that a small ONSD was associated with a low CSF pressure [2] and did not prove it by measuring the actual CSF pressure. Moreover, it is beyond the scope of our study whether a small ONSD is associated with differing CSF composition or resulting in different CSF flow dynamics. Therefore, the result of our study cannot be used as supportive evidence for the potential benefit of refreshing CSF composition in NTG patients.

In conclusion, modifying the composition of CSF to treat glaucoma is an innovative and intriguing idea that warrants further investigation. However, it is questionable whether the small ONSD in NTG patients can justify such treatment. Further research is required to enhance insight into the role of CSF pressure and composition in the pathogenesis of NTG.

Author Contributions: S.H.L., writing—original draft preparation; T.-W.K., writing—review and editing; S.H.L., T.-W.K., E.J.L. and H.K. All authors have read and agreed to the published version of the manuscript.

Conflicts of Interest: This reply has no conflict of interest.

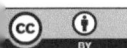

References

1. Wostyn, P. Could Young Cerebrospinal Fluid Combat Glaucoma? Comment on Lee et al. Association between Optic Nerve Sheath Diameter and Lamina Cribrosa Morphology in Normal-Tension Glaucoma. *J. Clin. Med.* 2023, *12*, 360. *J. Clin. Med.* **2023**, *12*, 3285. [CrossRef] [PubMed]
2. Lee, S.H.; Kim, T.-W.; Lee, E.J.; Kil, H. Association between Optic Nerve Sheath Diameter and Lamina Cribrosa Morphology in Normal-Tension Glaucoma. *J. Clin. Med.* **2023**, *12*, 360. [CrossRef] [PubMed]
3. Wostyn, P.; De Groot, V.; Van Dam, D.; Audenaert, K.; De Deyn, P.P. Senescent changes in cerebrospinal fluid circulatory physiology and their role in the pathogenesis of normal-tension glaucoma. *Am. J. Ophthalmol.* **2013**, *156*, 5–14.e2. [CrossRef] [PubMed]
4. Lee, E.J.; Kim, T.W.; Lee, D.S.; Kim, H.; Park, Y.H.; Kim, J.; Lee, J.W.; Kim, S. Increased CSF tau level is correlated with decreased lamina cribrosa thickness. *Alzheimers Res. Ther.* **2016**, *8*, 6. [CrossRef]
5. Hinton, D.R.; Sadun, A.A.; Blanks, J.C.; Miller, C.A. Optic-nerve degeneration in Alzheimer's disease. *N. Engl. J. Med.* **1986**, *315*, 485–487. [CrossRef] [PubMed]
6. Blanks, J.C.; Hinton, D.R.; Sadun, A.A.; Miller, C.A. Retinal ganglion cell degeneration in Alzheimer's disease. *Brain Res.* **1989**, *501*, 364–372. [CrossRef] [PubMed]
7. Sadun, A.A.; Bassi, C.J. Optic nerve damage in Alzheimer's disease. *Ophthalmology* **1990**, *97*, 9–17. [CrossRef] [PubMed]

Disclaimer/Publisher's Note: The statements, opinions and data contained in all publications are solely those of the individual author(s) and contributor(s) and not of MDPI and/or the editor(s). MDPI and/or the editor(s) disclaim responsibility for any injury to people or property resulting from any ideas, methods, instructions or products referred to in the content.

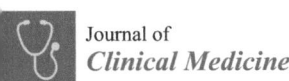

Brief Report

The Effectiveness of Pattern Scanning Laser Trabeculoplasty as an Additional Treatment for the Patients of Open-Angle Glaucoma Receiving Full Ocular Hypotensive Medications

Yosuke Ueno, Yusuke Haruna, Mami Tomita, Atsushi Sakai, Shogo Ogawa and Shigeru Honda *

Department of Ophthalmology and Visual Sciences, Graduate School of Medicine, Osaka Metropolitan University, Osaka 545-8585, Japan; m21679m@omu.ac.jp (Y.U.)
* Correspondence: shonda@omu.ac.jp

Abstract: Objectives: Our purpose was to examine the effectiveness of pattern scanning laser trabeculoplasty (PSLT) as an additional treatment for patients of open-angle glaucoma (OAG) receiving maximized ocular hypotensive medications (OHM). **Methods**: A total of 40 eyes of 33 patients (average age 72.7 ± 10.7 years) who had not previously undergone open glaucoma surgery or laser trabeculoplasty and were treated with maximized OHM between June 2018 and March 2022 were included. A 360-degree PSLT was conducted, and postoperative intraocular pressure (IOP) and survival curves at 1, 3, 6, 9, and 12 months were evaluated. **Results**: According to the Kaplan–Meier survival analysis, the average survival time was 8.1 months and the survival rate at 12 months was 0.55, with death defined as postoperative IOP reduction of less than 10% or requiring additional treatment. The average survival time was 4.9 months and the survival rate at 12 months was 0.28, with death defined as postoperative IOP reduction of less than 20% or requiring additional treatment. Nine eyes showed increased IOP (three eyes) or worsened visual field (six eyes) during the course and underwent additional open glaucoma surgery. In the 31 eyes which received no additional treatment after PSLT, the mean preoperative IOP was 18.5 ± 3.9 mmHg, which reduced to 15.3 ± 4.1 mmHg ($p = 1.62 \times 10^{-6}$), 15.5 ± 3.4 mmHg ($p = 1.51 \times 10^{-5}$), 15.7 ± 4.0 mmHg ($p = 1.75 \times 10^{-5}$), 14.7 ± 4.38 ($p = 2.89 \times 10^{-6}$), and 15.0 ± 4.0 mmHg ($p = 5.74 \times 10^{-9}$) at 1, 3, 6, 9, and 12 months after PSLT, respectively. The IOP reduction rate one year after PSLT was 18.7%. Of the 31 eyes, 13 (42%) achieved a 20% reduction in IOP compared to the baseline. **Conclusions**: Adjunctive treatment with PSLT in OAG patients receiving maximized OHM may be effective over 12 months of follow-up.

Keywords: glaucoma; pattern scanning laser trabeculoplasty; full ocular hypotensive medications

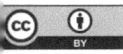

1. Introduction

Recently, various modalities have been developed for treating glaucoma [1], but glaucoma is still one of the most common causes of premature blindness. The only established treatment for glaucoma is to lower intraocular pressure (IOP). The initial treatments for open-angle glaucoma (OAG) are usually an application of ocular hypotensive medications (OHMs), and if the IOP fails to be controlled by several combinations of OHM, then surgical treatments are considered. Laser trabeculoplasty (LTP) is one of the surgical treatments for OAG that is often performed in clinical practice [2,3]. To date, there have been several modalities developed as LTP. Wise et al. introduced argon laser trabeculoplasty (ALT) in 1979 [4], and Latina et al. proposed selective laser trabeculoplasty (SLT) in 1995 [5]. Pattern scanning laser trabeculoplasty (PSLT) using the PASCAL® laser developed by TOPCON was proposed in 2006 [6]. PSLT is a treatment method that allows multiple coagulations to be made at once, and the irradiation area can be controlled by computer-based monitoring, which is likely easier than performing SLT. A pilot study reported an average IOP reduction rate of 24% 6 months after 532 nm wavelength PSLT [6]. Wong et al. reported that the IOP reduction rate 1 year after PSLT was 11.6% [7], and Mansouri et al. reported that the

IOP reduction rate 1 year after PSLT was estimated to be 14% [8]. Although SLT using a Q-switched laser is likely the most commonly performed LTP in current clinical practice [9], several reports have described that the IOP lowering rate of 577 nm wavelength PSLT and SLT was equivalent after 6 and 12 months [10], which encouraged the use of PSLT than SLT as adjunctive therapy for lowering IOP because of its easiness. However, most previous reports administrated LTP only after the OHM had been washed out, or at a stage where the number of OHMs was not maximized. Although it is common to perform open glaucoma surgery for patients using maximized OHM to decrease IOP and maintain the visual field [1], there might be some situations where surgery cannot be performed right away (e.g., financial and scheduling issues for the patient; systemic condition of the patients; hospital circumstances; and especially during the coronavirus pandemic, when there were cases where non-life emergent surgery is not possible at all). In such situations, LTP could be considered an adjunctive therapy in ordinary clinical practices. Thus, the effects of PSLT in this condition are likely worth evaluating.

Here, we retrospectively investigate the effectiveness of 577 nm wavelength PSLT as an additional treatment for OAG patients receiving maximized OHMs.

2. Subjects and Methods

This study was approved by the Institutional Review Board at the Osaka Metropolitan University Graduate School of Medicine (No. 2023-116) and was conducted following the Declaration of Helsinki. All cases in this study were Japanese individuals recruited from the Department of Ophthalmology at Osaka Metropolitan University Hospital in Japan. Written informed consent for the use of ordinary clinical data in the following retrospective studies was obtained from all subjects on their first visit to the hospital, and an opt-out for this study was indicated on the department website after approval of the study by the Institutional Review Board at the Osaka Metropolitan University Graduate School of Medicine.

The records of consecutive OAG patients who had not previously undergone any glaucoma surgery or LTP and who received maximized OHMs for glaucoma between June 2018 and March 2022 were reviewed in this study. The maximized OHMs consist of combinations of 3 or more eye drops, including prostaglandin $F_{2\alpha}$ analogs, beta-blockers, carbonic anhydrase inhibitors, α_2 adrenergic agonists, and Rho kinase inhibitors. The cases of OAG secondary to uveitis, steroid use, or neovascular glaucoma were excluded. Gonioscopically open angles were a requirement for study inclusion. All IOP measurements were performed using Goldmann applanation tonometry. Visual fields were assessed using a Humphrey field analyzer (HFA) in 21 eyes and Goldmann perimetry in 19 eyes every 3–6 months, or more frequently if a progression of visual field defects was suspected. The average MD in 21 eyes examined with HFA was -16.8 ± 8.2 dB before PSLT. Although the visual field measured with Goldmann perimetry could not be evaluated using MD values, they all exhibited visual field impairment with the V-4 isopter, which corresponds to a III or higher grade according to the Kosaki classification and, hence, did not fall under the early stage of glaucoma.

PSLT was performed as an additional treatment without reducing the number of OHMs used before the treatment. For PSLT, PASCAL Streamline 577® (wavelength 577 nm) (TOPCON, Tokyo, Japan) was used. The treatment procedure was carried out according to the company's instructions. A single mirror gonio laser lens (1× Indexing Lens; Ocular Instruments, Bellevue, WA, USA) was used to project and align the laser patterns onto the trabecular meshwork (TM). Laser power was titrated by placing a single laser spot (100 μm diameter) into the inferior quadrant at a 10 ms exposure duration. In all cases, a starting power level of 200 mW was chosen, and power was reduced or increased until a barely visible lesion (light blanching of TM) was achieved. In a majority of eyes, some degree of pigmentation was visible in the inferior chamber angle (where titration was performed). If there was no pigmentation, the PSLT procedure was performed with 400 mW. After titration, the power was maintained, but the pulse duration was automatically reduced to 5 ms to produce subvisible lesions. The 360° treatment of TM was administered in 32 steps, where each pattern was composed of 39 spots spanning 11.25° of the trabecular meshwork—three rows of 13 spots each (1152 in total), with zero spacing between the adjacent spots—and the contact lens was rotated every 11.25° after a segment was treated to maintain no overlap and no gaps in the treatment spots. Apraclonidine eye drops were administered 30 min before and after laser treatment to prevent a transient increase in IOP. Postoperatively, 0.1% fluorometholone eye drops were administered as an anti-inflammatory agent, and cases suspected of being steroid responders were given 0.1% bromfenac sodium hydrate eye drops for one week. PSLT was performed once and not repeated over 12 months of follow-up. The IOP was measured monthly, and if a high IOP (>21 mmHg) was found, it was measured again within a few weeks. If a continuous increase in IOP and/or a worsened visual field was found, additional open glaucoma surgery (trabeculotomy or trabeculectomy) was performed.

The primary outcome measure was the IOP reduction rate at 12 months postoperatively. Changes in the IOP values and survival curve at 1, 3, 6, 9, and 12 months postoperatively were also evaluated as the secondary outcomes. To investigate the changes in the IOP after PSLT, cases who underwent additional open glaucoma surgery during the follow-up period were excluded from the assessment.

For statistics, IBM, SPSS ver.24.0 software was used. Changes in the IOP were evaluated using a paired t-test. Survival analysis was assessed using the Kaplan–Meier survival analysis table. A p-value of less than 0.05 was considered to be statistically significant.

3. Results

The baseline characteristics of the participants are shown in Table 1. A total of 40 eyes of 33 patients were included in this study. The average age was 72.7 ± 10.7 years (57–89 years), 19 patients were male, and 14 patients were female. The disease types were as follows: 35 eyes had primary open-angle glaucoma (POAG) and 5 eyes had pseudoexfoliation glaucoma (PEG). The average preoperative IOP was 20.1 ± 4.9 mmHg, and the eye drop score (counting 1 for single agents, 2 for combination agents) was 4.1 ± 1.1. The PSLT irradiation conditions were as follows: the average number of coagulations was 1297, the average laser power was 338 mW, and the average irradiation energy was 1.69 mJ. As for postoperative complications, one patient (2.5%) showed a transient increase in IOP exceeding 5 mmHg compared to the preoperative level, and no other changes such as anterior iris adhesion were observed in any patient.

Table 1. Baseline characteristics of the patients.

Sex	male 19, female 14
Age (years)	72.7 ± 10.7 (range 57–89)
Type of glaucoma	POAG 35 eyes, PEG 5 eyes
Lens status	Phakic 17 eyes, IOL 23 eyes
IOP (mmHg)	20.1 ± 4.9
Eye drop score	4.1 ± 1.1

POAG: primary open angle glaucoma, PEG: pseudoexfoliation glaucoma, IOL: intraocular lens, IOP: intraocular pressure.

At 12 months after PSLT, 23 out of 40 eyes (57.5%) showed a reduction in IOP of 10% or more compared to the baseline, and 13 eyes (32.5%) showed a decrease of 20% or more. Of 40 eyes, 31 (77.5%) were followed up for one year without any changes in the eye drops or additional treatments such as open glaucoma surgery. The other nine eyes had increased IOP (three eyes) or a worsened visual field (six eyes) during the course and underwent additional open glaucoma surgery (trabeculotomy for 1 eye, Express® device insertion for 1 eye, and trabeculectomy for 7 eyes); hence, they were excluded from the subsequent analyses.

The results of Kaplan–Meier survival analysis of 40 eyes are shown in Table 2 and Figure 1. If death was defined as the point in time when the rate of decrease in IOP was less than 10% twice in a row, the survival rate gradually decreased over time, which resulted in an average survival time of 8.1 months, and the survival rate at 12 months was 0.55 (Table 2 and Figure 1A). If death was defined as the point in time when the rate of decrease in IOP was less than 20% on two consecutive occasions, the survival rate showed an acute decline to 0.52 a month after PSLT. Further, it decreased gradually until 12 months of follow-up was reached. Consequently, the average survival time was 4.9 months, and the survival rate at 12 months was 0.28 (Table 2 and Figure 1B).

Table 2. The mean survival time (months) when the rate of decrease in IOP was less than 10% (top) or 20% (bottom) on two consecutive occasions.

Estimate	Standard Error	95% Confidence Interval	
		Lower Bound	Upper Bound
8.125	0.779	6.599	9.651
Estimate	Standard Error	95% Confidence Interval	
		Lower Bound	Upper Bound
4.925	0.773	3.410	6.440

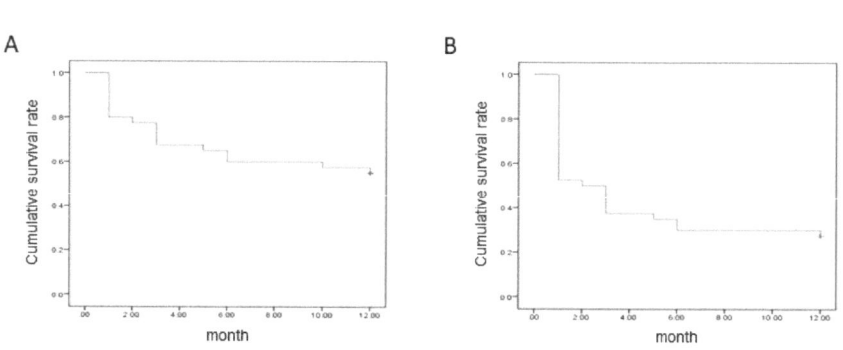

Figure 1. Results of Kaplan–Meier survival analysis if death was defined as the point in time when the rate of decrease in intraocular pressure was less than 10% (**A**) or 20% (**B**) twice in a row.

To compare the baseline parameters between the drop-out and non-drop-out groups, there was no difference in age or sex. However, the mean baseline IOPs in the drop-out and non-drop-out groups were 25.8 ± 3.5 and 18.5 ± 3.9 mmHg, respectively, which are significantly different ($p = 1.26 \times 10^{-5}$). Moreover, the mean eye drop scores before PSLT were 4.8 ± 0.4 and 4.0 ± 1.2 in the drop-out and non-drop-out groups, respectively, which are also significantly different ($p = 0.040$).

Figure 2 shows the chronological change in the IOP in the 31 eyes which did not require any change in eye drops or additional open glaucoma surgery after PSLT. In this group, the average IOP before PSLT was 18.5 ± 3.9 mmHg, and the average IOP and IOP reduction rate after PSLT were 15.3 ± 4.1 mmHg ($p = 1.62 \times 10^{-6}$), 17.3%; 15.5 ± 3.4 mmHg ($p = 1.51 \times 10^{-5}$), 16.2%; 15.7 ± 4.0 mmHg ($p = 1.75 \times 10^{-5}$), 15.1%; 14.7 ± 4.38 ($p = 2.89 \times 10^{-6}$), 20.5%; and 15.0 ± 4.0 mmHg ($p = 5.74 \times 10^{-9}$), 18.9% at 1, 3, 6, 9, and 12 months, respectively.

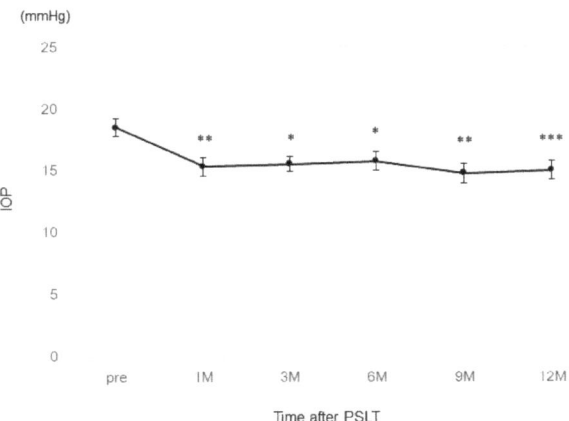

Figure 2. The chronological change in IOP in the 31 eyes which did not require any changes in eye drops or additional treatment after PSLT. * $p < 1 \times 10^{-4}$, ** $p < 1 \times 10^{-5}$, *** $p < 1 \times 10^{-8}$.

4. Discussions

In the present study, we have demonstrated that PSLT for the OAG cases receiving maximized OHM may have some treatment effects over 12 months. Namely, 58% of the eyes showed a 10% or greater reduction in IOP after PSLT, and 78% of the eyes avoided additional treatments after PSLT during this period.

A previous report mentioned that the IOP-lowering effect of PSLT was 24% after 6 months [6]. Another report showed that the IOP reduction rate 6 months after PSLT was approximately 19% [8]. They stated that the IOP reduction rate may have been modest due to the lower baseline IOP than that previously reported. In this study, the IOP reduction rate after PSLT was approximately 15% at 6 months and approximately 19% at 1 year in the eyes which required no additional treatments. The effect of PSLT on lowering IOP might be limited in the present study compared to the previous reports since we performed PSLT as an additional treatment for OAG patients who were being treated with maximized OHMs, who likely had more severe baseline conditions of glaucoma than those in the previous studies using PSLT. A previous report demonstrated that PSLT for uncontrolled ocular hypertension or POAG reduced the IOP from 20.3 mmHg to 15.9 mmHg (20.8% reduction) [11], which is consistent with our results. Kontić et al. reported that SLT reduced the mean IOP from 20.5 mmHg to 16.0 mmHg (21.9% reduction) at 12 months postoperatively in OAG patients receiving maximal medical therapy [12], which was almost equivalent to the result of this study. In contrast, 9 eyes out of 40 in the present study required additional glaucoma surgeries due to an elevation of IOP and/or a deterioration of visual field defects during the follow-up period, which likely affected the assessment of the mean IOP. Therefore, such cases were excluded from the analysis for the change in IOP after PSLT, and only 31 eyes could be assessed for the IOP reduction rate over 12 months. This might have caused a selection bias in calculating the IOP reduction rate after PSLT in this study. In the Kaplan–Meier survival analysis, the 12-month survival rate was 0.28 when death was defined as failure to reduce IOP by 20% or more below preoperative levels. Elahi et al. reported a better 1-year survival rate at 0.44 after PSLT using the same definition used in our study [10]. However, in the present study, PSLT was administrated in more advanced stages characterized by a larger number of OHMs and more progressed visual field impairment, while in the previous reports, the average mean defect (MD) was about 5 dB in HFA perimetry, which indicates a relatively early stage of glaucoma. Ahuja et al. found that 28% of patients with advanced glaucoma undergoing ab interno trabeculotomy using the trabectome required additional intervention compared to only 10% of patients with mild to moderate glaucoma [13]. In the advanced stage of glaucoma, additional open glaucoma surgeries are often required earlier when lowering IOP is not prompt or insufficient, which might have affected the survival rate in the present study. The drop-out group showed significantly higher baseline IOP and eye drop scores than the non-drop-out group, indicating that PSLT may be more suitable for those in less advanced stages.

For patients being treated with maximized OHM, open glaucoma surgery may be preferable and effective in lowering IOP and maintaining the visual field [1]. However, immediate open glaucoma surgery may not be possible in several situations, such as a poor systemic condition of the patient or the coronavirus pandemic, and PSLT is very important as an alternative intervention when open surgery cannot be performed immediately. Another advantage of PSLT is that there are relatively fewer complications with the procedure. In the present study, only one eye showed a transient increase in IOP exceeding 5 mmHg compared to the preoperative level, and no other adverse events, such as anterior iris adhesion, were observed in any patient. The present results showed that, although the effect of PSLT of lowering IOP by more than 20% was limited for the OAG patients receiving maximized OHMs, it could be expected to reduce IOP by more than 10% in 57.5% of the cases over 12 months. Hence, in certain cases, PSLT may be considered a stopgap until the next open surgery.

The limitations of this study are its research design, which was of a retrospective nature, and the small sample size. The results of the present study warrant a prospective study with a larger sample size. In addition, the cohort in this study included both primary OAG and secondary OAG (namely, PEG) cases, which did not distinguish the effects of PSLT on each phenotype. Moreover, a quantitative analysis in visual fields was not conducted, since half of the cases were measured for the visual field with Goldmann perimetry. Further studies are required in order to clarify those issues.

In conclusion, PSLT could be considered an adjunctive treatment for patients with advanced glaucoma stages who require many OHMs, although 22.5% of the treated eyes required subsequent surgical interventions.

Author Contributions: Conceptualization, Y.U. and Y.H.; methodology, Y.U.; software, Y.U.; validation, Y.H., M.T. and A.S.; formal analysis, Y.U.; investigation, Y.U., M.T., A.S. and S.O.; resources, Y.U.; data curation, Y.U.; writing—original draft preparation, Y.U.; writing—review and editing, S.H.; supervision, S.H. All authors have read and agreed to the published version of the manuscript.

Funding: This research received no external funding.

Institutional Review Board Statement: The study was conducted according to the guidelines of the Declaration of Helsinki and approved by the Institutional Review Board of Osaka Metropolitan University (protocol code 2023-116 and date of approval 14 December 2023).

Informed Consent Statement: Written informed consent for using ordinary clinical data in the following retrospective studies was obtained from all subjects on their first visit to the hospital, and an opt-out for this study was indicated on the department website after approval by the IRB.

Data Availability Statement: All data generated or analyzed during this study are included in this article.

Conflicts of Interest: The authors declare no conflicts of interest.

References

1. Jóhannesson, G.; Stille, U.; Taube, A.B.; Karlsson, M.; Kalaboukhova, L.; Bergström, A.; Peters, D.; Lindén, C. Guidelines for the management of open-angle glaucoma: National Program Area Eye Diseases, National Working Group Glaucoma. *Acta Ophthalmol.* **2024**, *102*, 135–150. [CrossRef] [PubMed]
2. Chang, T.C.; Vanner, E.A.; Fujino, D.; Kelly, S.; Parrish, R.K. Factors Associated with Laser Trabeculoplasty Response Duration Analysis of a Large Clinical Database (IRIS Registry). *J. Glaucoma* **2021**, *30*, 902–910. [CrossRef]
3. Rasmuson, E.; Bengtsson, B.; Lindén, C.; Heijl, A.; Aspberg, J.; Andersson-Geimer, S.; Jóhannesson, G. Long-term follow-up of laser trabeculoplasty in multi-treated glaucoma patients. *Acta Ophthalmol.* **2024**, *102*, 179–185. [CrossRef] [PubMed]
4. Wise, J.B. Long-term control of adult open-angle glaucoma by argon laser treatment. *Ophthalmology* **1981**, *88*, 197–202. [CrossRef]
5. Latina, M.A. Selective laser trabeculoplasty-180-degree treatment. *J. Glaucoma* **2007**, *16*, 274–275. [CrossRef] [PubMed]
6. Turati, M.; Gil-Carrasco, F.; Morales, A.; Quiroz-Mercado, H.; Andersen, D.; Marcellino, G.; Schuele, G.; Palanker, D. Patterned laser trabeculoplasty. *Ophthalmic Surg. Lasers Imaging Retin.* **2010**, *41*, 538–545. [CrossRef]

7. Wong, M.O.M.; Lai, I.S.; Chan, P.P.; Chan, N.C.; Chan, A.Y.; Lai, G.W.; Chiu, V.S.; Leung, C.K. Efficacy and safety of selective laser trabeculoplasty and pattern scanning laser trabeculoplasty: A randomised clinical trial. *Br. J. Ophthalmol.* **2021**, *105*, 514–520. [CrossRef] [PubMed]
8. Mansouri, K.; Shaarawy, T. Comparing pattern scanning laser trabeculoplasty to selective laser trabeculoplasty: A randomized controlled trial. *Acta Ophthalmol.* **2017**, *95*, e361–e365. [CrossRef]
9. Rolim-de-Moura, C.R.; Paranhos, A., Jr.; Loutfi, M.; Burton, D.; Wormald, R.; Evans, J.R. Laser trabeculoplasty for open-angle glaucoma and ocular hypertension. *Cochrane Database Syst. Rev.* **2022**, *8*, CD003919. [CrossRef] [PubMed]
10. Elahi, S.; Rao, H.L.; Paillard, A.; Mansouri, K. Outcomes of pattern scanning laser trabeculoplasty and selective laser trabeculoplasty: Results from the lausanne laser trabeculoplasty registry. *Acta Ophthalmol.* **2021**, *99*, e154–e159. [CrossRef]
11. Espinoza, G.; Castellanos-Castellanos, Y.A.; Pedraza-Concha, A.; Rodríguez-Una, I.; Acuña, M.F.; Parra, J.C. Mid-term results of patterned laser trabeculoplasty for uncontrolled ocular hypertension and primary open angle glaucoma. *Int. J. Ophthalmol.* **2021**, *14*, 1199–1204. [CrossRef] [PubMed]
12. Kontić, M.; Ristić, D.; Vukosavljević, M. Hypotensive effect of selective laser trabeculoplasty in patients with medically uncontrolled primary open-angle glaucoma. *Srp. Arh. Za Celok. Lek.* **2014**, *142*, 524–528. [CrossRef] [PubMed]
13. Ahuja, Y.; Ma Khin Pyi, S.; Malihi, M.; Hodge, D.O.; Sit, A.J. Clinical results of ab interno trabeculotomy using the trabectome for open-angle glaucoma: The Mayo Clinic series in Rochester, Minnesota. *Am. J. Ophthalmol.* **2013**, *156*, 927–935.e2. [CrossRef] [PubMed]

Disclaimer/Publisher's Note: The statements, opinions and data contained in all publications are solely those of the individual author(s) and contributor(s) and not of MDPI and/or the editor(s). MDPI and/or the editor(s) disclaim responsibility for any injury to people or property resulting from any ideas, methods, instructions or products referred to in the content.

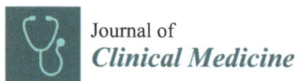

Systematic Review

Efficacy and Safety of Rho Kinase Inhibitors vs. Beta-Blockers in Primary Open-Angle Glaucoma: A Systematic Review with Meta-Analysis

Brenda Nana Wandji [1,2,*], Noélie Bacq [1] and Adèle Ehongo [1]

[1] Hôpital Universitaire de Bruxelles (HUB), CUB Hôpital Erasme, Service d'Ophtalmologie, Université Libre de Bruxelles (ULB), Route de Lennik 808, 1070 Bruxelles, Belgium
[2] Ecole de Santé Publique, Université Libre de Bruxelles, 1070 Brussels, Belgium
* Correspondence: nanawandjisandy4@gmail.com; Tel.: +32-4-70-18-40-55

Abstract: Background: In order to support the positioning of Rho kinase inhibitors (Rhokis) in the European market for the treatment of glaucoma, scientific evidence comparing the efficacy and safety of Rhokis and beta-blockers (β-βs) in the treatment of open-angle glaucoma after 3 months was assembled through a systematic review and meta-analysis (meta-A) of randomized controlled trials (RCTs). **Methods:** Relevant articles were searched for on PubMed, EMBASE, and the Cochrane Library. Of the 251 articles found, three met all eligibility criteria. These three articles were assessed for risk of bias. Data were extracted and a random effects meta-A was performed. The studies' methods were homogeneous but there was great heterogeneity within the data ($I^2 = 92–93\%$; $p < 0.001$). **Results:** All studies had low risk of bias. The meta-A showed statistically better efficacy of β-βs, resulting in an intraocular pressure (IOP) reduction mean difference of 1.73 (1.19–2.27) at 8 a.m., 0.66 (0.19–1.15) at 10 a.m. and 0.49 mmHg (0.001–0.98) at 4 p.m., compared to Rhokis. This difference is not clinically significant as intra-operator variability of IOP measurements varies from ±2 to ±3 mmHg The adverse effects of Rhokis were essentially topical, whereas β-βs mainly caused systemic side effects. **Conclusions:** This Meta-A showed that Rhokis are clinically non-inferior to beta-blockers in reducing IOP. Rhokis have a better safety profile.

Keywords: Rho kinase inhibitors; beta-blockers; intraocular pressure; glaucoma; adverse effects; adults; systematic review; meta-analysis; efficacy; alternative therapy

Citation: Nana Wandji, B.; Bacq, N.; Ehongo, A. Efficacy and Safety of Rho Kinase Inhibitors vs. Beta-Blockers in Primary Open-Angle Glaucoma: A Systematic Review with Meta-Analysis. *J. Clin. Med.* **2024**, *13*, 1747. https://doi.org/10.3390/jcm13061747

Academic Editor: Eun Ji Lee

Received: 7 February 2024
Revised: 11 March 2024
Accepted: 13 March 2024
Published: 18 March 2024

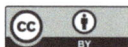

Copyright: © 2024 by the authors. Licensee MDPI, Basel, Switzerland. This article is an open access article distributed under the terms and conditions of the Creative Commons Attribution (CC BY) license (https://creativecommons.org/licenses/by/4.0/).

1. Introduction

Glaucoma refers to a group of progressive optic neuropathies characterized by excavation or cupping of the optic disc, apoptotic degeneration of retinal ganglion cells, and corresponding visual field defects [1,2]. Glaucoma is the leading cause of irreversible blindness, affecting around 57.5 million people worldwide in 2015 [3,4]. With the growing number and proportion of elderly people, it is projected that 111.8 million people will have glaucoma in 2040 [3,5]. It has a prevalence of 2.6% in Europe [6]. Glaucomas can be classified into open-angle glaucomas and angle-closure glaucomas to describe the anatomic status of the anterior chamber angle. Each of these is further divided into primary or secondary types, indicating the absence or presence of other clinically identifiable ocular or systemic disorders causing the glaucoma [2].

Glaucoma is a multifactorial disease and its pathogenesis is incompletely understood. Although there are a substantial number of cases of normal pressure glaucoma [7], the main objective in the management of glaucoma is still to reduce the intraocular pressure (IOP) [8] Several classes of drugs are used for this purpose, with prostaglandin F2α analogues and beta-blockers being the most widespread [9]. Beta-blockers have adverse cardiovascular and respiratory effects (bronchospasm, bradycardia, hypotension, arrhythmia, and reduced ventricular ejection fraction) in up to 13% of patients, and neurological effects (dizziness, hallucinations, and confusion) in three to 10% of patients [10]. These effects are even more serious in elderly patients with multiple comorbidities [11,12].

Over the past few years, new classes of drugs have been developed to reduce IOP, such as Rho kinase inhibitors. This therapeutic class has shown its efficacy in reducing IOP, both in monotherapy and combination therapy [13]. The added value of this group lies in their neuroprotective and vasoactive properties, such as cell survival and axon regeneration [14]. Moreover, Rho kinase inhibitors have mainly topical side effects, generally conjunctival hyperemia [15]. This new therapeutic class was approved in Japan in 2014 and in the USA in 2017 [16], but not in Europe, where studies have only been conducted, in Germany, since 2021 [17].

Studies providing high levels of scientific evidence would support arguments for the introduction of Rho kinase inhibitors to the European market. This would diversify the therapeutic options available for glaucoma patients, because Rho kinase inhibitors have also been shown to further reduce IOP in patients previously treated with drugs from other therapeutic classes [18]. Moreover, it is beneficial to have a wide therapeutic choice in case of side effects, intolerance, or allergies with other therapeutic classes, particularly for elderly patients and/or those with co-morbidities, in whom beta-blockers can be responsible for life threatening adverse effects [19–21].

So far, no meta-analysis of randomized controlled trials comparing Rho kinase inhibitors and beta-blockers in open-angle glaucoma is available in the published literature. Therefore, the main objective of this review was to assemble scientific evidence related to the efficacy and safety of Rho kinase inhibitors compared to beta-blockers in reducing IOP in patients with primary open-angle glaucoma.

2. Materials and Methods

A literature search was conducted using online databases (PubMed, EMBASE, Google scholar, and the Cochrane Library) for studies published from 2001 to 1 July 2023. Specific search strategies were developed for each database. This review was performed in accordance with the PRISMA (Preferred Reporting Items for Systematic Reviews and Meta-Analyses) guidelines [22].

Data were extracted from 1 May to 1 July 2023. The following search terms were used: "open angle glaucoma" for population; "Rho Kinase inhibitor" for intervention; "beta-blockers" for comparison; and "intraocular pressure" for outcome. Synonyms of search terms were combined using "OR," whereas population, intervention, comparison and outcome were combined by "AND."

An example of the research strategy for PubMed was: ("Rho associated Kinases"[MeSH Terms] OR ("Rho associated"[All Fields] AND "Kinases"[All Fields]) OR "Rho associated Kinases"[All Fields] OR ("Rho"[All Fields] AND "Kinase"[All Fields]) OR "Rho Kinase"[All Fields]) AND ("antagonists and inhibitors"[MeSH Subheading] OR ("antagonists"[All Fields] AND "inhibitors"[All Fields]) OR "antagonists and inhibitors"[All Fields] OR "inhibitors"[All Fields] OR "inhibitor"[All Fields] OR "inhibitor s"[All Fields]) AND ("beta-blocker"[All Fields] OR "beta-blockers"[All Fields] OR "betablocking"[All Fields]) AND ("glaucoma, open angle"[MeSH Terms] OR ("glaucoma"[All Fields] AND "open angle"[All Fields]) OR "open-angle glaucoma"[All Fields] OR ("open"[All Fields] AND "angle"[All Fields] AND "glaucoma"[All Fields]) OR "open angle glaucoma"[All Fields]).

The selection was based on the acronym "PICOS":

- Patients: performed on adults, 18 years old or more with a primary open-angle glaucoma diagnosis based on gonioscopy, OCT, and visual field defects with or without ocular hypertension.
- Intervention: Rho kinase inhibitors treatment with no additional concomitant therapy for at least 3 months.
- Comparison: beta-blockers treatment with no additional concomitant therapy for at least 3 months.

- Outcome: the reduction of IOP after a 3-month treatment was assessed by subtracting the IOP recorded at 3 months after medication from the IOP at baseline (ΔIOP = IOP at 3 months − IOP at baseline). A negative value of ΔIOP implies that the study drug is effective in lowering IOP. From each study, the mean difference of the IOP reduction was extracted at various times because IOP values can fluctuate through the day. The occurrences of systemic and topical adverse effects in both groups were also assessed.

Study design: randomized controlled trials (RCTs) published in English or French between 2001 (the publication year of the first studies on Rho kinase inhibitors for the treatment of glaucoma) and 2023 were included. The following were excluded:

- Case reports, systematic reviews, books, editorials, opinions, grey literature.
- Studies on types of glaucoma other than primary open-angle glaucoma.
- Studies in which additional therapies or surgical procedures for glaucoma management were also performed.
- Studies which did not specify the required data (IOP difference before and after treatment).

Titles and abstracts were assessed according to the eligibility criteria, then duplicates were excluded using Rayyan software (https://www.rayyan.ai/, Rayyan Systems Inc., Cambridge, MA, USA). The full texts of studies whose titles/abstracts contained insufficient information for a decision were also assessed. The studies that met the eligibility criteria were included in this systematic review and meta-analysis. A complementary search of the reference lists of studies included in this systematic review was performed manually.

Two researchers (BN and NB) extracted data from the included articles. The following data were extracted: authors/year of publication, study design, number of participants, characteristics of the samples (sex and participants' age), the name of the beta-blocker and Rho kinase inhibitor used, mean values and standard deviation for the IOP, the follow-up duration, and the proportions of local and general adverse effects. Disagreements between the two researchers were resolved with the aid of a third researcher (AE).

The risk analysis for bias was performed using a tool called ROB-2 [23]. The following fields are assessed by this tool: (1) bias arising from the randomization process, (2) deviations from intended interventions, (3) missing outcome data, (4) measurement of outcomes, and (5) selection of the reported results. Each item contains several questions, and the response to each question is used to classify the study in terms of low/moderate/high risk of bias. The total score of the item is reported according to the category in which most responses fall.

Two researchers (BN and NB) conducted the analysis independently, and the results were compared until a consensus was reached.

Data were analyzed using Stata version 17 (StataCorp. 2021. Stata Statistical Software Release 17. College Station, TX: StataCorp LLC, College Station, TX, 77845 USA). A meta-analysis with random effects model was used. The effect size was estimated using Cohen's d (since the sample for each study was >10) with the corresponding 95% confidence interval We calculated the I^2 statistics with the following classification of degree of heterogeneity: <25% (low heterogeneity), 25–50% (moderate heterogeneity), >50% (high heterogeneity) We assessed H^2 as the ratio of the variance of the estimated overall effect size from a random-effects meta-analysis compared to the variance from a fixed-effects meta-analysis There was perfect homogeneity across studies when H^2 equaled 1, and the greater the value of H^2, the greater was the heterogeneity. p values of less than 0.05 were considered statistically significant.

3. Results

3.1. Study Selection

The electronic searches identified 251 studies, of which 20 duplicates were removed. Three articles were included in this systematic review and meta-analysis. The article selection process is presented in Figure 1.

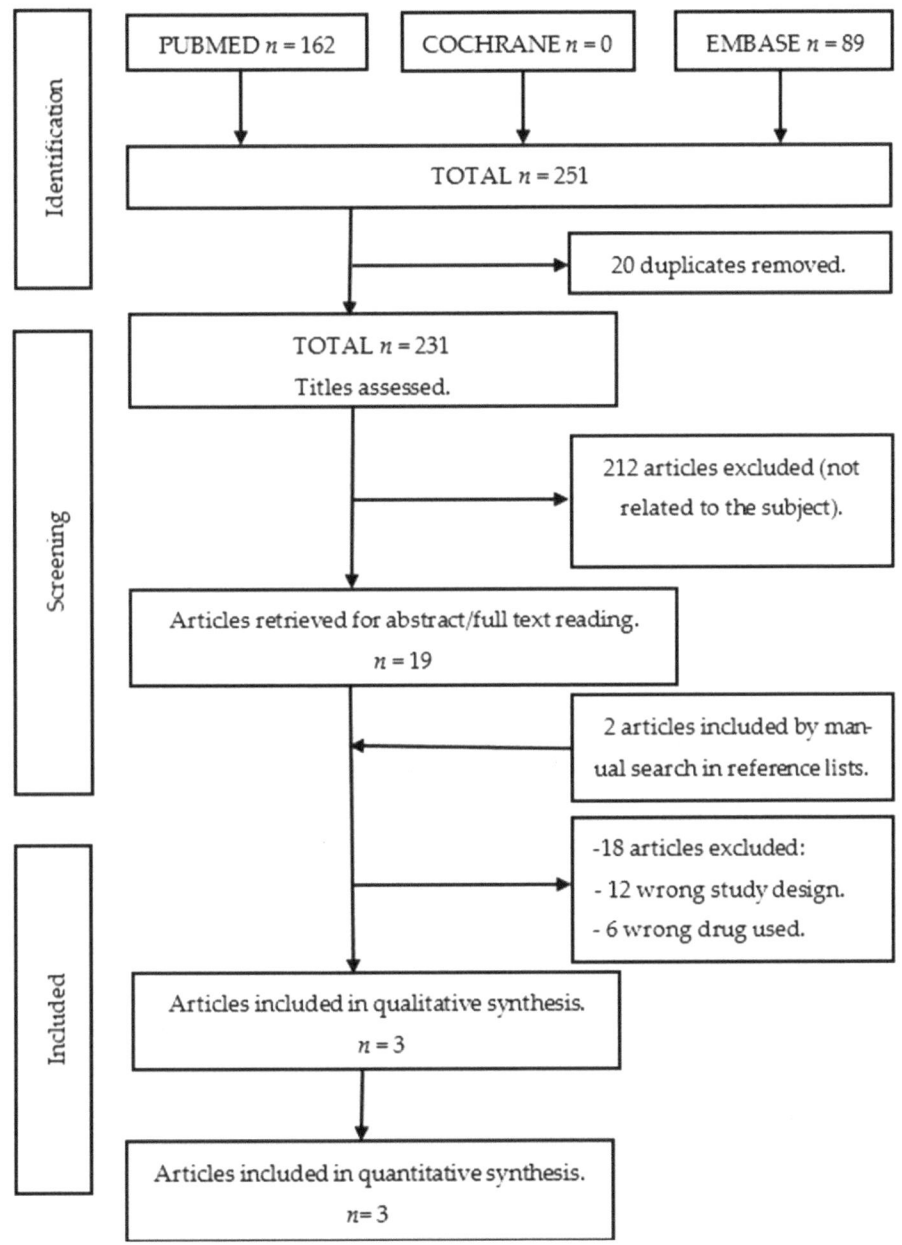

Figure 1. Flowchart of study selection according to PRISMA guidelines.

3.2. Characteristics of Articles

3.2.1. Description of the Articles

Three studies of an intervention named "ROCKET" (Rho kinase-Elevated IOP Treatment) were found. They were phase III RCTs, all conducted in the US by Serle et al. in 2018 (ROCKET 1) [24], Kahook et al. in 2019 (ROCKET 2) [25], and Khouri et al. (ROCKET 4) in 2019 [26]. These studies compared the efficacy of IOP reduction in open-angle glaucomatous patients treated with twice-daily administration of a beta-blocker (timolol 0.5%)

and a daily administration of a Rho kinase inhibitor (netarsudil 0.02%). IOP was measured on three occasions: at 8 a.m., 10 a.m. and 4 p.m. To ensure blinding control, patients belonging to the group on once daily netarsudil were given a placebo in the morning and an active drug in the evening. The ROCKET 2 study also compared efficacy after twice-daily administration of netarsudil. These data were not included in the present meta-analysis, as only the ROCKET 2 study obtained those results. As the follow-up period ranged from 3 to 12 months in the ROCKET studies, for the sake of uniformity this meta-analysis was performed on measurements obtained after a 3-month treatment period.

3.2.2. Demographic Characteristics

The mean age of participants in the included studies ranged between 63 ± 11.8 and 65 ± 11.5 years. The sample sizes ranged from 411 to 756, with a female predominance in each treatment group (59–66% women). Randomization was good, as the groups were comparable in terms of sex and age.

3.2.3. Intraocular Pressure

The articles examined individually concluded that netarsudil was not significantly inferior (non-inferior) to timolol after a 3-month treatment regime.

Appendix A, Tables A1 and A2 show additional information regarding the demographic characteristics and results of the articles included in this systematic review and meta-analysis.

3.2.4. Risk of Bias

Table 1 shows the results of the evaluation of the risk of bias of the included articles using the ROB-2 tools. Overall, the risk of bias was low in the included studies except for ROCKET 2, which had a high risk of bias in terms of missing data.

Table 1. Risk of bias assessment of the included studies according to the ROB-2 tool.

Study	Randomization Process	Deviations from Interventions	Missing Data	Outcome Measurement	Reported Results Selection	Overall Bias
ROCKET 1	Low	Low	Low	Low	Low	Low
ROCKET 2	Low	Low	High	Low	Low	Low
ROCKET 4	Low	Low	Low	Low	Low	Low

ROCKET: Rho kinase-Elevated IOP Treatment.

3.3. Assessment of Efficacy

3.3.1. Comparison of IOP Reduction at 8 a.m.

The overall mean difference in IOP reduction at 8 a.m. was 1.73 mmHg (95% CI, 1.19 to 2.27). This means that the timolol reduces the IOP of 1.73 mmHg significantly more than netarsudil after a 3-month therapy regime. A significantly high heterogeneity between studies was found ($I^2 = 92.2\%$) (Figure 2); the weight of each study was comparable. The sensitivity analysis did not reveal any significant changes in the overall effect size when individual studies were excluded, suggesting that the observed heterogeneity may not be solely driven by a specific study (Figure 2).

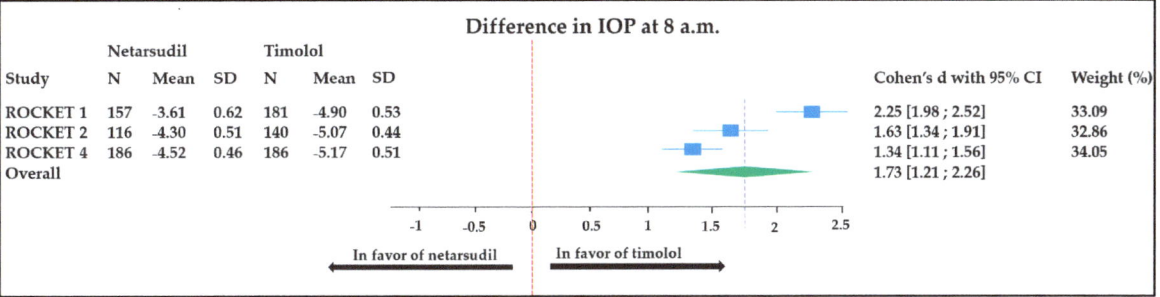

Figure 2. Forest plot representing the difference in IOP (measured at 8 a.m.) between patients treated with timolol vs. netarsudil. Heterogeneity: $T^2 = 0.20$, $I^2 = 91.96\%$, $H^2 = 12.43$; test of $\theta i = \theta j$: $Q(2) = 25.71$, $p < 0.001$; test of $\theta = 0$: $z = 6.44$, $p < 0.001$. ROCKET: Rho kinase-Elevated IOP Treatment; SD: standard deviation; CI: confidence interval; IOP: intra ocular pressure.

3.3.2. Comparison of IOP Reduction at 10 a.m.

At 10 a.m., there was an overall mean difference in IOP reduction of 0.67 mmHg (95% CI, 0.16 to 1.17). This means that timolol reduces the IOP of 0.67 mmHg significantly more than netarsudil after a 3-month therapy regime. The weight of each study was comparable. There was a significantly high heterogeneity between studies ($I^2 = 92\%$) (Figure 3).

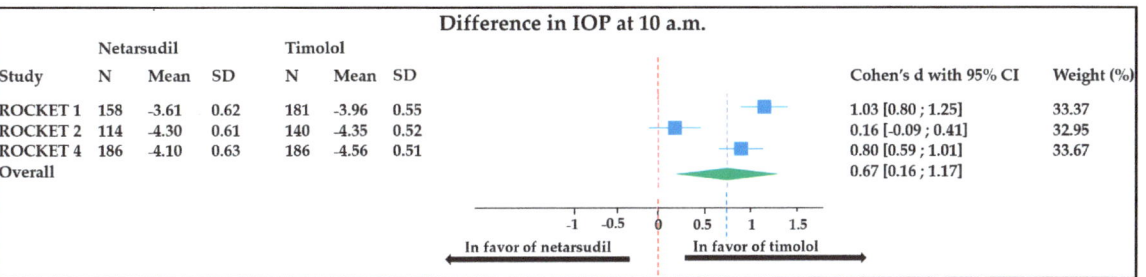

Figure 3. Forest plot representing the difference in IOP (measured at 10 a.m.) between patients treated with timolol vs. netarsudil. Heterogeneity: $T^2 = 0.19$, $I^2 = 93.23\%$, $H^2 = 14.77$; test of $\theta i = \theta j$: $Q(2) = 27.18$, $p < 0.001$; test of $\theta = 0$: $z = 2.58$, $p = 0.01$. ROCKET: Rho kinase-Elevated IOP Treatment; SD: standard deviation; CI: confidence interval; IOP: intra ocular pressure.

3.3.3. Comparison of IOP Reduction at 4 p.m.

At 4 p.m., there was an overall mean difference in IOP reduction of 0.49 mmHg (95% CI, 0.02 to 0.96). This means that the timolol reduces the IOP of 0.49 mmHg significantly more than netarsudil after 3 months of therapy. The weight of each study was comparable, although a significantly high heterogeneity between studies was found ($I^2 = 93\%$) (Figure 4).

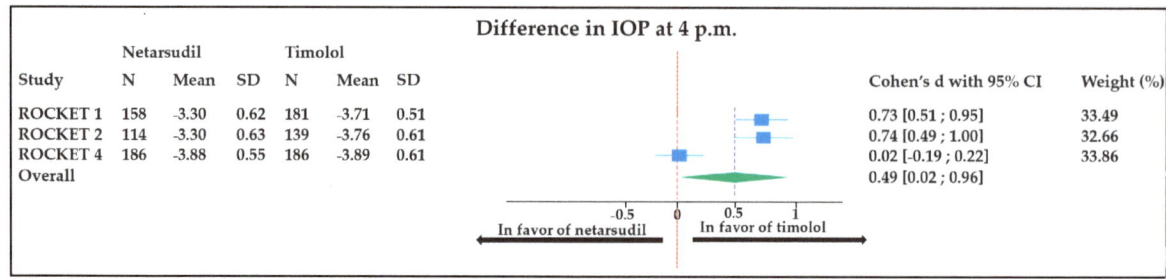

Figure 4. Forest plot representing the difference in IOP (measured at 4 p.m.) between patients treated with timolol vs. netarsudil. Heterogeneity: $T^2 = 0.16$, $I^2 = 92.41\%$, $H^2 = 13.17$; test of $\theta i = \theta j$: $Q(2) = 28.52$, $p < 0.001$; test of $\theta = 0$: $z = 2.04$, $p = 0.04$. ROCKET: Rho kinase-Elevated IOP Treatment; SD: standard deviation; CI: confidence interval; IOP: intra ocular pressure.

3.4. Assessment of Safety

3.4.1. Topical Adverse Effects

Topical side effects were significantly more common in the netarsudil-treated group in all studies. The most common side effects were conjunctival hyperemia, cornea verticillata, and subconjunctival hemorrhage (Table 2).

Table 2. Main local adverse effects in patients treated with netarsudil vs. timolol in each study.

	Local Adverse Effects											
	Conjunctival Hyperemia			Cornea Verticillata			Subconjunctival Hemorrhage			Blurred Vision		
	Netarsudil	Timolol		Netarsudil	Timolol		Netarsudil	Timolol		Netarsudil	Timolol	
Study	n (%)	n (%)	p	n (%)	n (%)	p	n (%)	n (%)	p	n (%)	n (%)	p
ROCKET 1	105 (51.7)	17 (8.1)	<0.001	11 (5.4)	NA		27 (13.3)	1 (0.5)	<0.001	NA	NA	
ROCKET 2	152 (60.5)	35 (13.9)	<0.001	64 (25.5)	2 (0.8)	<0.001	49 (19.5)	2 (0.8)	<0.001	27 (10.7)	7 (2.8)	<0.001
ROCKET 4	168 (47.9)	33 (9.2)	<0.001	86 (24.5)	0 (0)	<0.001	56 (16.0)	11 (3.1)	<0.001	22 (6.3)	4 (1.1)	0.05

NA: Not available. ROCKET: Rho kinase-Elevated IOP Treatment.

The meta-analyses comparing conjunctival hyperemia and subconjunctival hemorrhage occurrence between groups (the side effects for which all data were available) are displayed in Figures 5 and 6, respectively.

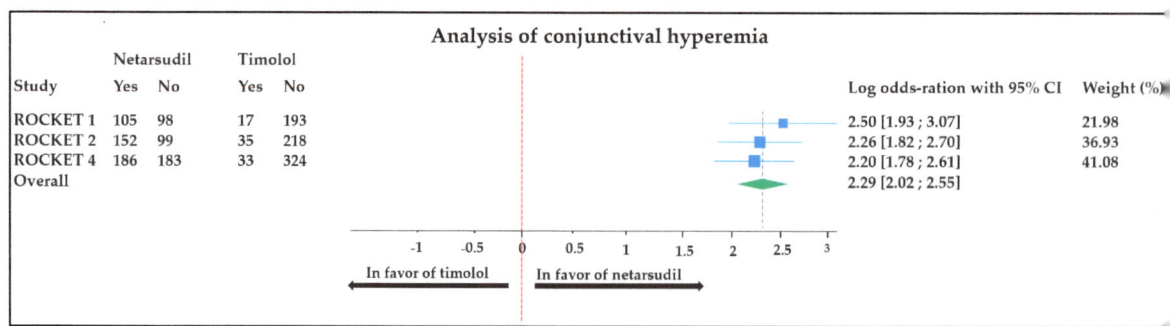

Figure 5. Comparison of conjunctival hyperemia occurrence in patients treated with netarsudil vs timolol. Heterogeneity: $T^2 = 0.00$, $I^2 = 0.00\%$, $H^2 = 1.00$; test of $\theta i = \theta j$: $Q(2) = 0.72$, $p = 0.70$; test of $\theta = 0$: $z = 16.85$, $p < 0.001$. ROCKET: Rho kinase-Elevated IOP Treatment; CI: confidence interval.

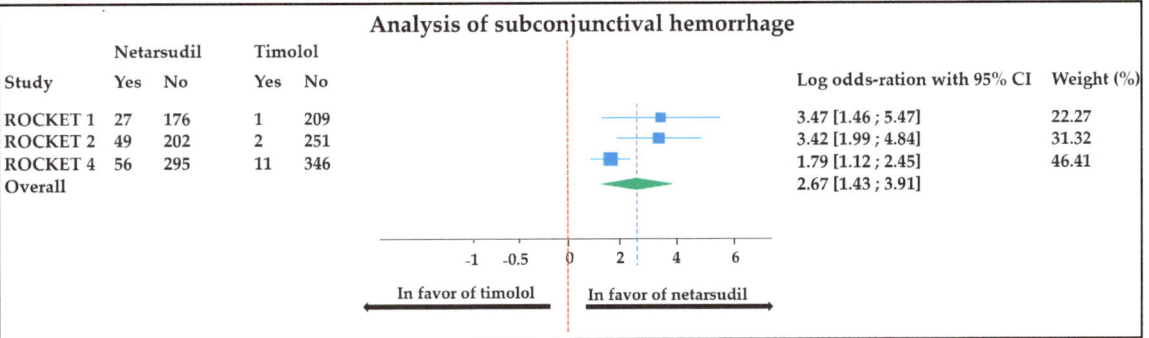

Figure 6. Comparison of subconjunctival hemorrhage occurrence in patients treated with netarsudil vs. timolol. Heterogeneity: $T^2 = 0.75$, $I^2 = 63.15\%$, $H^2 = 2.71$; test of $\theta i = \theta j$: $Q(2) = 5.81$, $p = 0.05$; test of $\theta = 0$: 4.23, $p < 0.001$. ROCKET: Rh kinase-Elevated IOP Treatment; CI: confidence interval.

Conjunctival hyperemia: the meta-analysis carried out on conjunctival hyperemia revealed a minor heterogeneity ($I^2 = 0\%$) between studies, with an overall odds ratio (OR) of 2.29 [2.02;2.55]. This means that there was significantly more (2.29 times more) conjunctival hyperemia in patients treated with netarsudil than in those treated with timolol (Figure 5).

Subconjunctival hemorrhage: the meta-analysis carried out on subconjunctival hemorrhage revealed high heterogeneity ($I^2 = 63.15\%$) between studies, with an overall OR of 2.67 [1.43;3.91]. This means there were significantly more (2.67 times more) subconjunctival hemorrhages in patients treated with netarsudil than in patients treated with timolol (Figure 6).

3.4.2. Systemic Adverse Effects

In the ROCKET 1 study, the systemic side effects were not listed. In the ROCKET 2 study, there was a significant reduction in heart rate of −2.1 beat/min with timolol therapy, while the heart rate was not changed significantly in the group receiving netarsudil therapy. The exact data were not included in the study. There was a significantly higher proportion of adverse musculoskeletal effects in patients treated with timolol ($p = 0.01$) (Table 3).

Table 3. Main systemic adverse effects in patients treated with netarsudil vs. timolol in each study.

	Systemic Adverse Effects												
	Heart Rate (beat/min)				Respiratory/Thoracic			Musculoskeletal			Gastrointestinal		
	Netarsudil		Timolol		Netarsudil	Timolol		Netarsudil	Timolol		Netarsudil	Timolol	
Study	MD ± SD	p	MD ± SD	p	n (%)	n (%)	p	n (%)	n (%)	p	n (%)	n (%)	p
ROCKET 1	NA	NA	NA	NA	NA	NA	NA	NA	NA	NA	NA	NA	NA
ROCKET 2	NA	NS	−2.1 ± 0.6	p < 0.001	10 (3.9)	14 (5.6)	0.5	3 (1.2)	17 (6.8)	0.01	2 (0.8)	9 (3.6)	0.06
ROCKET 4	0.8 ± 1.0	NS	−2 ± 1.0	p < 0.001	NA	NA	NA	NA	NA	NA	NA	NA	NA

NA: Not available; NS: non-significant: the exact p value was not specified in the study; MD = mean difference; SD: standard deviation; CI: confidence interval; ROCKET: Rho kinase-Elevated IOP Treatment.

In the ROCKET 4 study, the systemic side effects were not listed according to the body systems affected as in ROCKET 2, except for heart rate. There was a significant reduction in heart rate of −2 beat/min with timolol therapy, meanwhile the heart rate was not changed significantly in the group receiving netarsudil therapy (Table 3). Moreover, the overall systemic side effects were more frequent in the timolol group $n = 91$ (25.5%) than in the netarsudil group $n = 82$ (23.4%). This difference was not statistically significant ($p = 0.9$).

A meta-analysis of systemic side effects could not be performed because the data needed for the calculation were not provided by the studies.

4. Discussion

Efficacy: In the present study, the efficacy and safety of Rho kinase inhibitors versus beta-blockers in reducing IOP in glaucomatous patients were compared through a meta-analysis. The studies included were RCTs with a low overall risk of bias. Individually, the studies concluded that there was a non-inferiority of netarsudil compared to timolol in reducing IOP. But, once the effects were combined, a statistically significant superiority of timolol was observed. This could be because the authors chose a non-inferiority cut-off point of 10%, i.e., if the mean difference in IOP reduction between the two molecules was less than 10%, then they concluded that the efficacy was the same.

Furthermore, these studies involved only a single Rho kinase inhibitor, netarsudil. Yet, other Rho kinase inhibitors such as ripasudil have been proven to be genuinely effective in reducing IOP [27]. There was no study comparing the efficacy of ripasudil with a beta-blocker used alone.

Finally, the difference in IOP reduction between the two treatments, ranging from 0.49 to 1.73 mmHg in favor of timolol, although statistically significant, is not clinically relevant, as intra-operator variability in IOP measurements with an applanation tonometer varies from ± 2 to ± 3 mmHg [28].

The non-inferiority of Rho kinase inhibitors compared to beta-blockers is a key point for positioning Rho kinase inhibitors in the therapeutic arsenal against glaucoma.

Safety: Topical side effects were significantly more common in the netarsudil-treated groups. These included conjunctival hyperemia, which was the most common, followed by subconjunctival hemorrhage and cornea verticillata. Nevertheless, they were minor and were consistent with those reported in other Rho kinase studies [15,17]. Conversely, systemic side effects were significantly more frequent in patients treated with timolol, notably bradycardia, and musculoskeletal and gastrointestinal disorders. It is well known that beta-blocker eye drops can induce serious complications which can be life threatening, especially in the elderly or those with pre-existing comorbidities [19–21]. Overall, the better systemic safety profile of Rho kinase inhibitors is critical, as the choice of which IOP-reducing medication to use is dictated by the compatibility between the patient's comorbidity state and the sides effects of the target molecule.

Clinical setting: This meta-analysis shows that netarsudil is not inferior to timolol and that, in addition, it has a better systemic safety profile. Netarsudil appears, therefore, to be a good option for first-line treatment. It is also a valuable alternative when the patient does not tolerate other treatments, or when beta-blockers are contra-indicated.

Guidelines for the treatment of glaucoma recommend combining molecules with different mechanisms of actions for greater effectiveness [29]. While the mechanism of action of beta-blockers is through the reduction of aqueous humor production, and that of prostaglandin analogs is through the enhancement of the uveoscleral pathway, Rho kinase inhibitors provide an alternative mechanism. They reduce IOP by improving the conventional aqueous outflow pathway via cytoskeletal redistribution and changes in cell–cell interactions in the endothelial cells of the trabecular meshwork and Schlemm's canal. This alternative mechanism of IOP reduction, compared to other classes of IOP medications, therefore offers the potential for additive IOP reduction as a combination treatment [30].

Rho kinase inhibitors can thus be combined with other medications for greater effectiveness, especially when a high IOP reduction is expected. In this regard, Tanihara et al., in 2015, found significant additive IOP reduction ranging from 0.9 mmHg (95% CI, 0.4–1.3 mmHg; $p < 0.001$) to 1.6 mmHg (95% CI, 1.1–2.1 mmHg; $p < 0.001$) with combined therapy of ripasudil with timolol, compared to timolol alone [30]. Likewise, Lee et al., in 2022, found a reduction of -2.41 mmHg (95% confidence interval [CI], -2.95 to -1.87) with combined therapy of netarsudil with latanoprost, compared to -1.77 mmHg (95% CI, -2.31 to -1.87) with latanoprost alone [31].

It is interesting to note that the difference in efficacy between netarsudil and timolol decreased from the morning (10 a.m. measurements) to the evening (4 p.m. measurements). Starting at 8 a.m., the mean difference in IOP between the two groups varied from 1.29 mmHg to 0.65 mmHg, depending on the study. As the day progressed, this difference narrowed between the two groups, to the point where at 4 p.m., in the Rocket 4 study, the difference was almost zero (0.01 mmHg) (Appendix A, Figure A1). This suggests that the IOP lowering effect of netarsudil may be more constant than that of timolol. This is consistent with the longer half-life of netarsudil previously reported [32]. Therefore, netarsudil has the potential to better protect visual function in the long term As one risk factor of glaucoma progression is IOP fluctuations, this warrants further studies.

Furthermore, in the included studies, the IOP measurements were taken during the time slots when timolol was at its peak activity, while netarsudil's peak activity had passed. The peak activity of timolol occurs 2 h after instillation [33], and that of netarsudil 4 to 8 h after instillation [34]. Therefore, based on a single evening dose of netarsudil and a morning dose of timolol, IOP measurements taken between 8 a.m. and 4 p.m. would fall within the period of peak activity of timolol and low activity of netarsudil.

Moreover, as out-of-office hours were not evaluated in these studies, it is possible that during these hours netarsudil is more potent than timolol, because timolol is less effective at night [35], while netarsudil would be at its highest activity after instillation in the evening.

Finally, the authors did not perform IOP measurements after 4 p.m. It would be interesting to take IOP measurements just before the evening dose, as the persistent efficacy of a drop is protective against non-compliance in real life.

Limitations and recommendations: The limitations encountered in this study lie mainly in the paucity of clinical trials on the efficacy of Rho kinase inhibitors compared to beta-blockers. Second, the selected studies were essentially all carried out in the USA by the same team. The results could therefore not be extrapolated to Europe. Hence the need for pilot studies on European populations. Third, the selected studies did not discuss the long-term safety and efficacy of netarsudil in the management of glaucoma, which is a chronic condition. This may be related to the fact that Rho kinase inhibitors have only recently been used in the treatment of glaucoma. Long-term follow-up studies would therefore be worthwhile. Further studies analyzing evening measurements before instillation of the next dose of drops would provide information on whether Rho kinase inhibitors have a sustained 24 h IOP-lowering effect compared to beta-blockers. Also, assessing long-term functional and structural evolution would help determine whether Rho kinase inhibitors better reduce the progression of glaucoma. Finally, there was an absence of useful data, such as means and standard deviations, in the results of the selected studies. Attempts to contact the authors to obtain further information were not successful. It is therefore recommended that researchers provide readers (in their appendices at least) with as much information as possible about their study, especially in the case of pilot research.

5. Conclusions

In the current study, it was shown that Rho kinase inhibitors, specifically netarsudil, are clinically non-inferior to beta-blockers in reducing IOP. Moreover, Rho kinase inhibitors offer added benefits in the management of glaucoma as alternatives to other drug classes, mainly beta-blockers, because their side effects are essentially localized and harmless. It is suggested to carry out more RCTs on Rho kinase inhibitors, with a longer follow-up period and including European populations, and assessing Rho kinase inhibitors other than netarsudil. Finally, it is suggested to measure the IOP-lowering effect of Rho kinase inhibitors shortly before and after the evening dose administration.

Author Contributions: Conceptualization, B.N.W., A.E. and N.B.; methodology, B.N.W., A.E. and N.B.; software, B.N.W.; validation, B.N.W., A.E. and N.B.; formal analysis, B.N.W.; investigation, B.N.W., A.E. and N.B.; data curation, B.N.W.; writing—original draft preparation, B.N.W. and A.E.; writing—review and editing, B.N.W., A.E. and N.B.; visualization, B.N.W., A.E. and N.B.; supervision, A.E. All authors have read and agreed to the published version of the manuscript.

Funding: This research received no external funding.

Data Availability Statement: Data sharing is not applicable as no new data was generated and the article describes entirely theoretical research.

Acknowledgments: Many thanks to Katia Castetbon, Ecole de Santé Publique, Université Libre de Bruxelles, for the suggestions and comments on this work.

Conflicts of Interest: The authors declare no conflicts of interest.

Appendix A

Table A1. Characteristics of studies included in the meta-analysis.

Study	Authors Year	Sample Size (n)	Age (Years) Mean ± SD	Diagnosis	Follow Up. Duration
ROCKET 1	SERLE et al., 2018 [24]	411	65.1 ± 11.5	OAG or OHT >17 and <27 mmHg	Week 2 and 6, Month 3
	Netarsudil q.d	202	65.2 ± 11.3		
	Timolol b.i.d	209	NA		
ROCKET 2	KAHOOK et al. 2019 [25]	756	65.3 ± 11.48	OAG or OHT IOP < 25 mmHg	Week 2 and 6 Month 3, 6, 9 and 12
	Netarsudil q.d	251	NA		
	Timolol b.i.d	251	63 ± 11.81		
	Netarsudil b.i.d *	254	64.1 ± 12.46	OAG or OHT IOP < 25 mmHg	Week 2 and 6 Month 3, 6, 9 and 12
ROCKET 4	KHOURI et al. 2019 [26]	708	NA	OAG or OHT IOP > 20 and <30 mmHg	Week 2 and 6, Month 3 and 6
	Netarsudil q.d	351	64.1 ± 11.6		
	Timolol b.i.d	357	64.5 ± 11.0		

All studies compared the efficacy of netarsudil 0.02% once-daily with timolol 0.5% twice-daily. Abbreviations: q.d (quaque die) = once a day; b.i.d: (bis in die) = two times a day; ROCKET: Rho kinase-Elevated IOP Treatment; SD: standard deviation; OAG: Open Angle Glaucoma; OHT: Ocular Hypertension; IOP: Intra Ocular Pressure NA = not available. * Data non included in the meta-analysis.

Table A2. Mean difference of IOP after 3 month-treatment in each group.

	8 a.m.				10 a.m.				4 p.m.			
	Netarsudil Group		Timolol Group		Netarsudil Group		Timolol Group		Netarsudil Group		Timolol Group	
Study	Mean	SD	Mean	SD	Mean	SD	Mean	SD	Mean	SD	Mean	SD
ROCKET 1	−3.61	0.62	−4.9	0.51	−3.36	0.62	−3.96	0.55	−3.3	0.62	−3.71	0.51
ROCKET 2	−4.3	0.55	−5.07	0.42	−4.26	0.61	−4.35	0.52	−3.3	0.63	−3.76	0.61
ROCKET 4	−4.52	41	−5.17	0.55	−4.1	0.63	−4.56	0.51	−3.88	0.55	−3.89	0.61

ROCKET: Rho kinase-Elevated IOP Treatment; SD: Standard Deviation; IOP: intra ocular pressure.

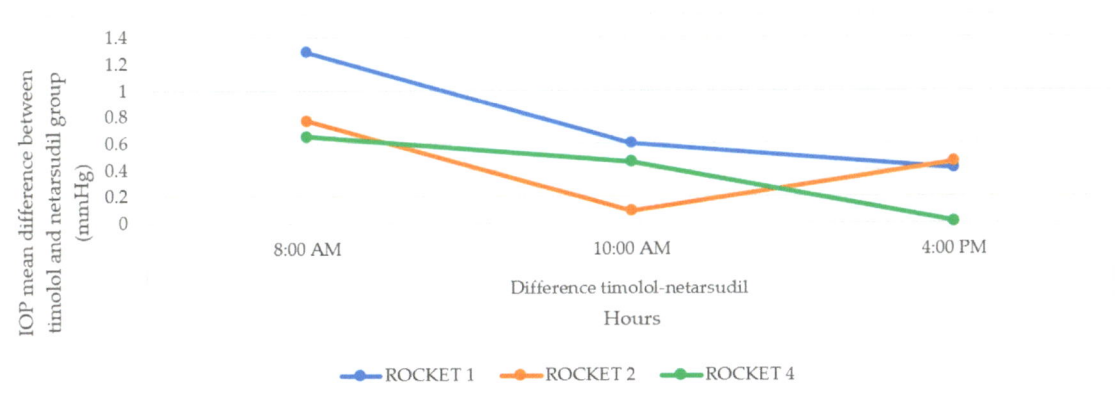

Figure A1. Hourly variation in mean IOP difference between netarsudil and timolol groups. ROCKET: Rho kinase-Elevated IOP Treatment; IOP: intra ocular pressure.

References

1. Weinreb, R.N.; Khaw, P.T. Primary open-angle glaucoma. *Lancet* **2004**, *363*, 1711–1720. [CrossRef] [PubMed]
2. Kang, J.M.; Tanna, A.P. Glaucoma. *Med. Clin. N. Am.* **2021**, *105*, 493–510. [CrossRef] [PubMed]
3. Allison, K.; Patel, D.; Alabi, O. Epidemiology of Glaucoma: The Past, Present, and Predictions for the Future. *Cureus* **2020**, *12*, e11686. [CrossRef] [PubMed]
4. Flaxman, S.R.; Bourne, R.R.A.; Resnikoff, S.; Ackland, P.; Braithwaite, T.; Cicinelli, M.V.; Das, A.; Jonas, J.B.; Keeffe, J.; Kempen, J.H.; et al. Global causes of blindness and distance vision impairment 1990–2020: A systematic review and meta-analysis. *Lancet Glob. Health* **2017**, *5*, e1221–e1234. [CrossRef] [PubMed]
5. Tham, Y.-C.; Li, X.; Wong, T.Y.; Quigley, H.A.; Aung, T.; Cheng, C.-Y. Global prevalence of glaucoma and projections of glaucoma burden through 2040: A systematic review and meta-analysis. *Ophthalmology* **2014**, *121*, 2081–2090. [CrossRef] [PubMed]
6. Gallo Afflitto, G.; Aiello, F.; Cesareo, M.; Nucci, C. Primary Open Angle Glaucoma Prevalence in Europe: A Systematic Review and Meta-Analysis. *J. Glaucoma* **2022**, *31*, 783–788. [CrossRef] [PubMed]
7. Heijl, A.; Leske, M.C.; Bengtsson, B.; Hyman, L.; Bengtsson, B.; Hussein, M.; Early Manifest Glaucoma Trial Group. Reduction of intraocular pressure and glaucoma progression: Results from the Early Manifest Glaucoma Trial. *Arch. Ophthalmol.* **2002**, *120*, 1268–1279. [CrossRef]
8. Weinreb, R.N.; Aung, T.; Medeiros, F.A. The pathophysiology and treatment of glaucoma: A review. *JAMA* **2014**, *311*, 1901–1911. [CrossRef]
9. Lusthaus, J.; Goldberg, I. Current management of glaucoma. *Med. J. Aust.* **2019**, *210*, 180–187. [CrossRef]
10. Diamond, J.P. Systemic adverse effects of topical ophthalmic agents. Implications for older patients. *Drugs Aging* **1997**, *11*, 352–360. [CrossRef]
11. Filimonova, E.E.; Sorokin, E.L.; Kogan, M.P.; Pashentsev, Y.E. Development of additive systemic effects when taking β-blockers in patients with glaucoma and concurrent chronic diseases. *Vestn. Oftalmol.* **2020**, *136*, 155–164. [CrossRef]
12. Arai, R.; Fukamachi, D.; Monden, M.; Akutsu, N.; Murata, N.; Okumura, Y. Bradycardia Shock Caused by the Combined Use of Carteolol Eye Drops and Verapamil in an Elderly Patient with Atrial Fibrillation and Chronic Kidney Disease. *Intern. Med.* **2021**, *60*, 79–83. [CrossRef]
13. Clement Freiberg, J.; von Spreckelsen, A.; Kolko, M.; Azuara-Blanco, A.; Virgili, G. Rho kinase inhibitor for primary open-angle glaucoma and ocular hypertension. *Cochrane Database Syst. Rev.* **2022**, *6*, CD013817. [PubMed]
14. Abbhi, V.; Piplani, P. Rho-kinase (ROCK) Inhibitors—A Neuroprotective Therapeutic Paradigm with a Focus on Ocular Utility. *Curr. Med. Chem.* **2020**, *27*, 2222–2256. [CrossRef] [PubMed]
15. Wu, J.-H.; Chang, S.-N.; Nishida, T.; Kuo, B.-I.; Lin, J.-W. Intraocular pressure-lowering efficacy and ocular safety of Rho-kinase inhibitor in glaucoma: A meta-analysis and systematic review of prospective randomized trials. *Graefe Arch. Clin. Exp. Ophthalmol.* **2022**, *260*, 937–948. [CrossRef]
16. Sturdivant, J.M.; Royalty, S.M.; Lin, C.-W.; Moore, L.A.; Yingling, J.D.; Laethem, C.L.; Sherman, B.; Heintzelman, G.R.; Kopczynski, C.C.; deLong, M.A. Discovery of the ROCK inhibitor netarsudil for the treatment of open-angle glaucoma. *Bioorg. Med. Chem. Lett.* **2016**, *26*, 2475–2480. [CrossRef] [PubMed]
17. Erb, C.; Konieczka, K. Rho kinase inhibitors as new local therapy option in primary open angle glaucoma. *Ophthalmologe* **2021**, *118*, 449–460. [CrossRef] [PubMed]
18. Naik, M.; Kapur, M.; Gupta, V.; Sethi, H.; Srivastava, K. Ripasudil Endgame: Role of Rho-Kinase Inhibitor as a Last-Ditch-Stand Towards Maximally Tolerated Medical Therapy to a Patient of Advanced Glaucoma. *Clin. Ophthalmol.* **2021**, *15*, 2683–2692. [CrossRef] [PubMed]

19. Morales, D.R.; Dreischulte, T.; Lipworth, B.J.; Donnan, P.T.; Jackson, C.; Guthrie, B. Respiratory effect of beta-blocker eye drops in asthma: Population-based study and meta-analysis of clinical trials. *Br. J. Clin. Pharmacol.* **2016**, *82*, 814–822. [CrossRef] [PubMed]
20. Jolobe, O.M.P. Cardiac and extracardiac side effects of eye drops. *Am. J. Emerg. Med.* **2021**, *46*, 731. [CrossRef]
21. Rains, J.; Kesterson, J. Ocular timolol as the causative agent for symptomatic bradycardia in an 89-year-old female. *Am. J. Emerg. Med.* **2021**, *42*, 263.e5–263.e6. [CrossRef] [PubMed]
22. Page, M.J.; McKenzie, J.E.; Bossuyt, P.M.; Boutron, I.; Hoffmann, T.C.; Mulrow, C.D.; Shamseer, L.; Tetzlaff, J.M.; Akl, E.A.; Brennan, S.E.; et al. The PRISMA 2020 statement: An updated guideline for reporting systematic reviews. *BMJ* **2021**, *372*, n71. [CrossRef] [PubMed]
23. Sterne, J.A.C.; Savović, J.; Page, M.J.; Elbers, R.G.; Blencowe, N.S.; Boutron, I.; Cates, C.J.; Cheng, H.-Y.; Corbett, M.S.; Eldridge, S.M.; et al. RoB 2: A revised tool for assessing risk of bias in randomised trials. *BMJ* **2019**, *366*, l4898. [CrossRef] [PubMed]
24. Serle, J.B.; Katz, L.J.; McLaurin, E.; Heah, T.; Ramirez-Davis, N.; Usner, D.W.; Novack, G.D.; Kopczynski, C.C.; ROCKET-1 and ROCKET-2 Study Groups. Two Phase 3 Clinical Trials Comparing the Safety and Efficacy of Netarsudil to Timolol in Patients with Elevated Intraocular Pressure: Rho Kinase Elevated IOP Treatment Trial 1 and 2 (ROCKET-1 and ROCKET-2). *Am. J. Ophthalmol.* **2018**, *186*, 116–127. [CrossRef] [PubMed]
25. Kahook, M.Y.; Serle, J.B.; Mah, F.S.; Kim, T.; Raizman, M.B.; Heah, T.; Ramirez-Davis, N.; Kopczynski, C.C.; Usner, D.W.; Novack, G.D.; et al. Long-term Safety and Ocular Hypotensive Efficacy Evaluation of Netarsudil Ophthalmic Solution: Rho Kinase Elevated IOP Treatment Trial (ROCKET-2). *Am. J. Ophthalmol.* **2019**, *200*, 130–137. [CrossRef] [PubMed]
26. Khouri, A.S.; Serle, J.B.; Bacharach, J.; Usner, D.W.; Lewis, R.A.; Braswell, P.; Kopczynski, C.C.; Heah, T.; Rocket-4 Study Group. Once-Daily Netarsudil Versus Twice-Daily Timolol in Patients with Elevated Intraocular Pressure: The Randomized Phase 3 ROCKET-4 Study. *Am. J. Ophthalmol.* **2019**, *204*, 97–104. [CrossRef]
27. Testa, V.; Ferro Desideri, L.; Della Giustina, P.; Traverso, C.E.; Iester, M. An update on ripasudil for the treatment of glaucoma and ocular hypertension. *Drugs Today Barc. Spain 1998* **2020**, *56*, 599–608.
28. Ottobelli, L.; Fogagnolo, P.; Frezzotti, P.; De Cillà, S.; Vallenzasca, E.; Digiuni, M.; Paderni, R.; Motolese, I.; Bagaglia, S.A.; Motolese, E.; et al. Repeatability and reproducibility of applanation resonance tonometry: A cross-sectional study. *BMC Ophthalmol.* **2015**, *15*, 36. [CrossRef]
29. Spaeth, G.L. European Glaucoma Society Terminology and Guidelines for Glaucoma, 5th Edition. *Br. J. Ophthalmol.* **2021**, *105*, 138–139.
30. Tanihara, H.; Inoue, T.; Yamamoto, T.; Kuwayama, Y.; Abe, H.; Suganami, H.; Araie, M. Additive Intraocular Pressure-Lowering Effects of the Rho Kinase Inhibitor Ripasudil (K-115) Combined with Timolol or Latanoprost: A Report of 2 Randomized Clinical Trials. *JAMA Ophthalmol.* **2015**, *133*, 755–761. [CrossRef]
31. Lee, J.-W.; Ahn, H.-S.; Chang, J.; Kang, H.-Y.; Chang, D.-J.; Suh, J.K.; Lee, H. Comparison of Netarsudil/Latanoprost Therapy with Latanoprost Monotherapy for Lowering Intraocular Pressure: A Systematic Review and Meta-analysis. *Korean J. Ophthalmol. KJO* **2022**, *36*, 423–434. [CrossRef] [PubMed]
32. Hoy, S.M. Netarsudil Ophthalmic Solution 0.02%: First Global Approval. *Drugs* **2018**, *78*, 389–396. [CrossRef] [PubMed]
33. Van der Valk, R.; Webers, C.A.B.; Schouten, J.S.A.G.; Zeegers, M.P.; Hendrikse, F.; Prins, M.H. Intraocular pressure-lowering effects of all commonly used glaucoma drugs: A meta-analysis of randomized clinical trials. *Ophthalmology* **2005**, *112*, 1177–1185. [CrossRef] [PubMed]
34. Lin, C.-W.; Sherman, B.; Moore, L.A.; Laethem, C.L.; Lu, D.-W.; Pattabiraman, P.P.; Rao, P.V.; deLong, M.A.; Kopczynski, C.C. Discovery and Preclinical Development of Netarsudil, a Novel Ocular Hypotensive Agent for the Treatment of Glaucoma. *J. Ocul. Pharmacol. Ther.* **2018**, *34*, 40–51. [CrossRef]
35. Ong, L.B.; Liza-Sharmini, A.T.; Chieng, L.L.; Cheong, M.T.; Vengadasalam, S.R.; Shin, H.C.; Balaravi, P. The Efficacy of Timolol in Gel-Forming Solution After Morning or Evening Dosing in Asian Glaucomatous Patients. *J. Ocul. Pharmacol. Ther.* **2005**, *21*, 388–394. [CrossRef]

Disclaimer/Publisher's Note: The statements, opinions and data contained in all publications are solely those of the individual author(s) and contributor(s) and not of MDPI and/or the editor(s). MDPI and/or the editor(s) disclaim responsibility for any injury to people or property resulting from any ideas, methods, instructions or products referred to in the content.

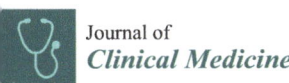 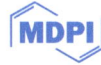

Article

Safety and Efficacy of the Rho-Kinase Inhibitor (Ripasudil) in Bleb Needling after Trabeculectomy: A Prospective Multicenter Study

Yu Mizuno [1,*], Kaori Komatsu [1], Kana Tokumo [1], Naoki Okada [1], Hiromitsu Onoe [1], Hideaki Okumichi [1], Kazuyuki Hirooka [1], Gaku Aoki [2], Yukiko Miura [3] and Yoshiaki Kiuchi [1]

1. Department of Ophthalmology and Visual Science, Hiroshima University, 1-2-3 Kasumi Minamiku, Hiroshima 734-8551, Japan
2. Department of Biostatistics, Clinical Research Center, Hiroshima University Hospital, 1-2-3 Kasumi Minamiku, Hiroshima 734-8551, Japan
3. Hiroshima Eye Clinic, 13-4, Noborimachi Nakaku, Hiroshima 730-0016, Japan
* Correspondence: ymizuno@hiroshima-u.ac.jp

Abstract: Ripasudil, a rho-associated protein kinase inhibitor ophthalmic solution, shows a protective effect in preventing excessive scarring in vitro. This study aims to evaluate the safety and efficacy of ripasudil for glaucoma patients submitted to the needling procedure. In this prospective, multicenter, single-arm study, we included 20 eyes of 20 patients with glaucoma who underwent the needling procedure without antimetabolites. All patients administered ripasudil after needling for three months. The primary endpoint of this study was the safety of ripasudil in patients, and the secondary endpoint was the change in IOP at 12 weeks after the needling procedure. No serious complications were found in the patients. One eye experienced pruritus and conjunctival follicle, while another eye had conjunctival follicle. These complications were transient and resolved quickly after discontinuation of ripasudil. The mean preoperative IOP was 14.6 ± 4.6 mmHg, which decreased to 11.0 ± 4.7 mmHg ($p = 0.0062$) at 1 week postoperatively. The IOP reduction effect continued to 12 weeks (11.8 ± 3.1 mmHg; $p = 0.0448$). The administration of the ROCK inhibitor, ripasudil, after the needling procedure is safe and effective in maintaining IOP for 12 weeks.

Keywords: glaucoma; trabeculectomy; needling; a rho-associated protein kinase inhibitor; ripasudil

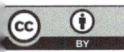

1. Introduction

Glaucoma is an optic neuropathy characterized by gradual, progressive morphological changes in the optic disc and visual field loss [1]. Trabeculectomy (TLE) is a traditional surgical technique for lowering intraocular pressure (IOP) with long-term efficacy in slowing the advancement of visual field loss among patients with glaucoma [2]. However, over time, we often experience a loss of IOP control. When filtration fails after the initial success of trabeculectomy, the most common cause is fibrosis, a natural part of the wound healing process.

The transconjunctival bleb needling procedure is designed to address the inadequacies of failing blebs thorough the mechanical removal of adhesions. Failed blebs often require multiple needling procedures due to fibrosis.

Ripasudil (Glanatec®, ophthalmic solution 0.4%, Kowa Company, Ltd., Tokyo, Japan) is an approved ophthalmic solution in Japan for managing glaucoma or ocular hypertension, which received approval in 2014. Several reports indicate that topical instillation treatment with the ROCK inhibitors Y-27632 [3,4] and ripasudil [5] can mitigate excessive scarring in vitro and following glaucoma filtration surgery in mouse or rabbit models. In our previous study, we reported that administration of ripasudil following the needling procedure with mitomycin C (MMC) did not show a more significant reduction in IOP when compared to the MMC needling procedure alone. However, this study suggests that ripasudil might reduce the number of IOP-lowering agents required after the needling procedure [6]. It is worth noting that this study was retrospective, and all subjects had received MMC just before needling. The antifibrosis effect of MMC might mask the effect of ripasudil.

In the present study, we conducted a prospective assessment of the safety profile in glaucoma patients who underwent needling without MMC and subsequently received ripasudil following the procedure. The study also thoroughly investigated the effectiveness of ripasudil administration in preventing bleb failure by suppressing fibrosis within the bleb.

2. Materials and Methods

In this prospective, multicenter, open-label, single-arm, phase II study, we evaluated patients at Hiroshima University Hospital and Hiroshima Eye Clinic in Japan. The study was conducted in accordance with the Declaration of Helsinki and received approval from the Hiroshima University Certified Review Board (Approval No. CRB210008, 26 May 2022). We analyzed 20 eyes of 20 glaucoma patients who underwent the needling procedure without the use of antimetabolites. Clinical signs of scarring determined by glaucoma specialists, including increased IOP following TLE and vascularization of the bleb, were the main indicators for the needling procedure. During the needling procedure, none of the patients encountered intraoperative complications. Our study specifically enrolled patients who underwent the needling procedure at least three months after TLE and excluded individuals with a previous history of conjunctival surgery (except for TLE).

All patients underwent comprehensive ophthalmic examination, and the following data were collected: sex, age, type of glaucoma, IOPs (Goldmann Applanation Tonometer, Haag-Streit, Köniz, Switzerland), lens status, the time interval since the most recent TLE, number of antiglaucoma medications, and corneal endothelial cell density. To categorize the morphological appearance observed through slit lamp examination, we assessed the characteristics of the blebs utilizing the Indiana Bleb Appearance Grading Scale. The scale takes into account the parameters of height, extent, vascularity, and leakage, which is graded through the Seidel test [7].

The primary endpoint of this study was to evaluate the safety profile of ripasudil administrated promptly in patients who underwent the needling procedure. Ophthalmic and systemic evaluations were conducted to scrutinize the occurrence of local and systemic adverse events (AEs) as well as adverse drug reactions (ADRs). AEs were documented irrespective of whether abnormalities occurred in the contralateral eye to which the ripasudil ophthalmic solution was administered.

We also assessed the treatment's efficacy as the secondary endpoint. We characterized absolute success as achieving a >20% reduction in IOP from the preneedling baseline without the use of antihypertensive medications (excluding the instillation of ripasudil). If the IOP exceeded the predefined criteria in two consecutive measurements, failure was deemed to have occurred at the initial time point when the IOP first exceeded the criteria. The necessity for repeat needling or an alternative glaucoma surgical intervention was categorized as a failure. We further characterized relative success as achieving an IOP within the ranges (A) 4 mmHg or higher but less than 22 mmHg, (B) 4 mmHg or higher but less than 19 mmHg, (C) 4 mmHg or higher but less than 16 mmHg, or (D) 4 mmHg or higher but less than 13 mmHg, in an attempt to adhere to the outcome criteria outlined by the World Glaucoma Association guidelines. If the IOP exceeded the defined criteria in two consecutive measurements, failure was deemed to have occurred at the initial time point when the IOP first exceeded the above criteria. The necessity for repeat needling or another glaucoma surgical intervention was classified as a treatment failure.

2.1. Needling Procedure

All needling procedures were conducted in an outpatient department by glaucoma specialists listed in the protocol. Following the application of topical anesthesia (0.4%

oxybuprocaine and 0.1% adrenaline), iodine and polyvinyl alcohol (PA·IODO ophthalmic and eye-washing solution, diluted six times with saline solution) were administered to the external eye. Subsequently, a 27-gauge needle was used to inject 0.1 mL of 2% xylocaine with epinephrine approximately 10 mm distal to the bleb. The needle was introduced between the conjunctiva and sclera, and fibrotic tissues were incised and elevated. After the procedure, patients were instructed to use ripasudil twice daily for three months, in conjunction with topical antibiotics (1.5% levofloxacin) and an anti-inflammatory (0.1% fluorometholone ophthalmic suspension) ophthalmic solution three times daily for one week.

2.2. Statistical Analysis

All the original data collected were stored in the electronic data capture (EDC) system (REDCap 12.0.33, Vanderbilt University). The EDC system was digitally secured on a password-protected internet server, and the investigators from the study team entered the data directly into the EDC system.

Considering the exploratory nature of this study, the sample size was projected by referencing historical medical records, which included an assessment of the annual patient volume at both Hiroshima University Hospital and Hiroshima Eye Clinic.

The analysis sets for this study were delineated as the Full Analysis Set (FAS) and the Per-Protocol Set (PPS). The FAS encompassed all participants in the study, excluding instances that failed to meet the eligibility criteria. The PPS was derived from the FAS, with the exclusion of individuals lacking available measurements for the primary endpoints and patients with substantial deviations from the study protocol. In this investigation, the FAS and PPS were congruent.

The primary endpoint of this study, focusing on the safety of administering ripasudil immediately following the needling procedure, was evaluated by quantifying the incidence of AEs and adverse drug reactions (ADRs), expressed in both absolute numbers and percentages. The analysis population encompassed all patients who received a minimum of one dose of ripasudil, and they were categorized based on the nature of AEs or ADRs.

For the secondary endpoint, aimed at assessing the efficacy of ripasudil, the results underwent analysis utilizing either Student's t-test or Wilcoxon's rank sum test. Survival rates were estimated by employing the Kaplan–Meier method. All statistical analyses were conducted using SAS version 9.4 (SAS Institute Inc., Cary, NC, USA). Measurement data are presented as mean ± standard deviation with a 95% confidence interval. Statistical significance was considered when the p-value was <0.05.

3. Results

We conducted an analysis on 20 eyes belonging to 20 glaucoma patients who underwent bleb needling without MMC due to TLE failure with a fornix-based conjunctival flap using MMC. A summary of demographic data is provided in Table 1. All patients were Japanese. There were 12 males and 8 females, with a mean age of 70.3 ± 11.8 years old (range: 49–89 years old). The mean time from TLE to needling was 4.2 ± 6.7 years (range: 0.30–30.02 years).

Table 1. Demographic characteristics.

Total number of eyes	20
Mean preoperative IOP (mmHg)	14.6 ± 4.6
Mean number of antihypertensive medications	1.0 ± 1.3
Age (years)	70.3 ± 11.8
Gender (male/female)	12/8
Laterality (right/left)	9/11
Glaucoma classification	
POAG	18
PACG	0

Table 1. *Cont.*

Secondary glaucoma	2
Time from TLE surgery to needling (Y)	4.3 ± 6.7
Lens status	
Phakia	7
IOL	13

IOP, intraocular pressure; POAG, primary open-angle glaucoma; PACG, primary angle-closure glaucoma; TLE, trabeculectomy.

During the study period, no serious AEs or ADRs were found in the patients. We had two minor ADRs: one eye had pruritus and conjunctival follicle, and one eye had conjunctival follicle. However, the complications were transient and resolved quickly after the discontinuation of ripasudil (Table 2).

Table 2. Type of side effects.

Total number of side effects	2 (10.0%)
Type of side effects	
conjunctival follicle	2 (10.0%)
pruritus	1 (5.0%)

Note: There was one eye with pruritus and conjunctival follicle concurrently manifested in the same eye.

Figure 1 illustrates a significant reduction in the mean IOP. The mean preoperative IOP was 14.6 ± 4.6 mmHg, which decreased to 11.0 ± 4.7 mmHg (a reduction of 25.1%, $p = 0.0006$) at 1 week postoperatively. This reduction in IOP was maintained up to 12 weeks (11.8 ± 3.1 mmHg; a reduction of 19.1%, $p = 0.0012$) (Figure 1). The Kaplan–Meier survival plot for absolute success showed a 12-week survival rate of 50.0% (Figure 2). For criteria A, B, C, and D, the relative success rates were 100.0%, 100.0%, 95.0%, and 82.0%, respectively (Figure 3).

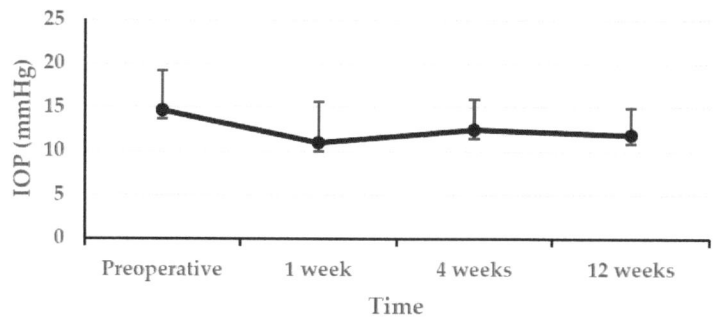

Number of eyes			
0 (preoperative)	1 week	4 weeks	12 weeks
20	19	19	16

Figure 1. Preoperative and postoperative mean IOPs (mmHg). Error bars show standard deviation. The mean preoperative IOP was lowered immediately after the needling procedure ($p = 0.0006$, Wilcoxon's rank sum test). The effect of IOP reduction was continued to 12 weeks ($p = 0.0012$, Wilcoxon's rank sum test). Error bars show the standard deviation.

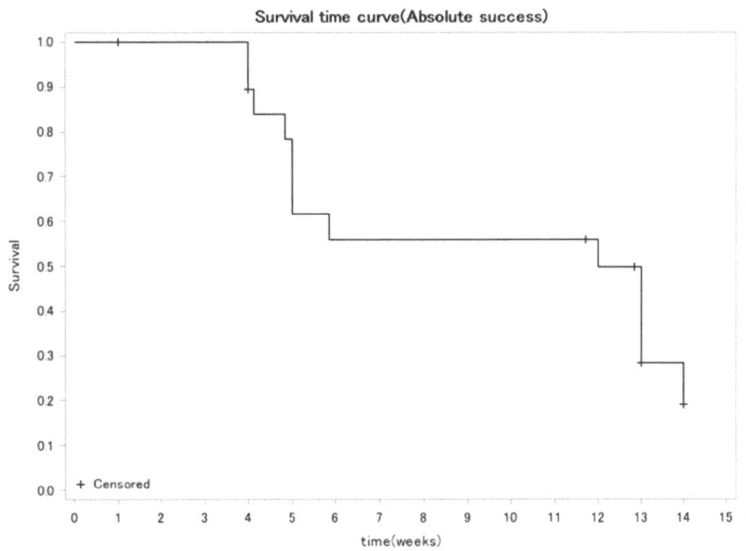

Number of eyes			
0 (preoperative)	1 week	4 weeks	12 weeks
20	19	19	16

Figure 2. Kaplan–Meier survival plot for absolute success. We characterized absolute success as achieving a >20% reduction in IOP from the preneedling baseline without the use of antihypertensive medications (excluding the instillation of ripasudil). If the IOP exceeded the predefined criteria in two consecutive measurements, failure was deemed to have occurred at the initial time point when the IOP first exceeded the criteria. The necessity for repeat needling or an alternative glaucoma surgical intervention was categorized as a failure.

There were no significant differences between the preoperative and postoperative mean numbers of antiglaucoma medications at 12 weeks ($p = 0.10$) (Table 3). The number of eyes with antiglaucoma medications before the needling procedure was nine (45%). The most utilized type of antiglaucoma medication before the needling procedure was prostaglandins (PG), followed by beta-blockers (BB). The subsequent use included carbonic anhydrase inhibitors (CAI) and alpha-2-agonists (AA) (PG: two eyes; PG + BB: two eyes; PG + CAI: one eye; PG + BB + CAI: two eyes; PG + BB + CAI + AA: one eye; BB: one eye). The number of eyes with antiglaucoma medications other than ROCK inhibitors 12 weeks after the needling procedure was two (PG: one eye; BB: one eye).

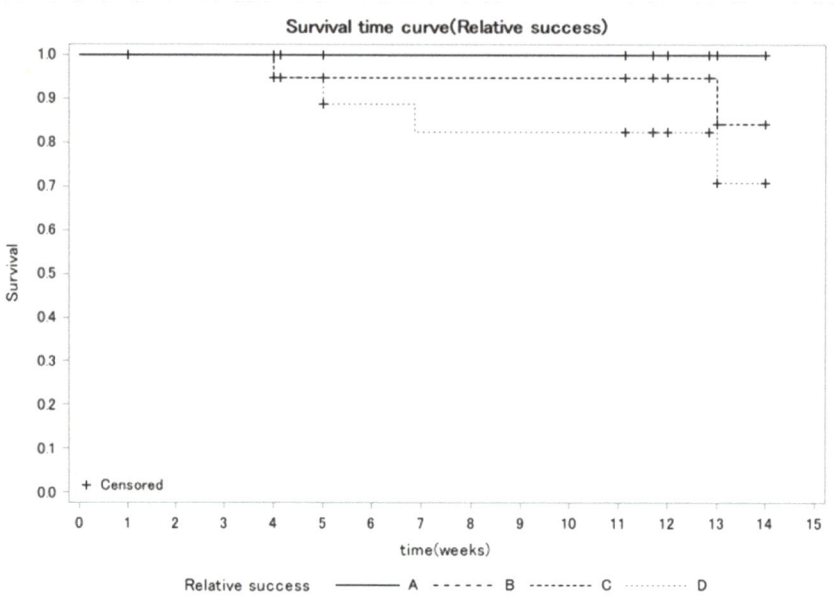

	Number of eyes			
	0 (preoperative)	1 week	4 weeks	12 weeks
(A)	19	19	19	16
(B)	17	18	18	16
(C)	14	16	16	14
(D)	6	14	12	10
total	20	19	19	16

Figure 3. Kaplan–Meier survival plot for relative success. We characterized relative success as achieving an IOP within the following ranges: (A) 4 mmHg or higher but less than 22 mmHg, (B) 4 mmHg or higher but less than 19 mmHg, (C) 4 mmHg or higher but less than 16 mmHg, or (D) 4 mmHg or higher but less than 13 mmHg. If the IOP exceeded the defined criteria in two consecutive measurements, failure was deemed to have occurred at the initial time point when the IOP first exceeded the above criteria. The necessity for repeat needling or another glaucoma surgical intervention was classified as a treatment failure. Note: Survival rate and censoring of Relative success B were equal to Relative success A.

Table 3. Number of antiglaucoma medications.

	Number of Antiglaucoma Medications	p *
preoperative	0.95 ± 1.28	
1 week	1.00 ± 0.00	0.14
4 weeks	1.05 ± 0.23	0.12
12 weeks	1.19 ± 0.54	0.10

* Wilcoxon's rank sum test.

The morphological slit lamp appearance of the blebs showed no significant difference between the preoperative and postoperative periods during the 12 weeks (Table 4).

Table 4. Changes in the morphological slit appearance of the blebs.

		Indiana Bleb Appearance Grading Scale, Height (H0–H3) **					
		Preoperative					
		H0	H1	H2	H3	Total (%)	p *
1 weeks	H0	2	0	1	0	3 (15%)	
	H1	1	3	0	0	4 (20%)	
	H2	0	5	4	0	9 (45%)	
	H3	0	0	1	2	3 (15%)	0.23
	missing values	1	0	0	0	1 (5%)	
	Total (%)	4 (20%)	8 (40%)	6 (30%)	2 (10%)	20 (100%)	
4 weeks	H0	2	0	0	9	2 (11%)	
	H1	2	3	1	0	6 (32%)	
	H2	0	3	4	1	8 (42%)	
	H3	0	1	1	1	3 (16%)	0.15
	missing values	0	0	0	0	0 (0%)	
	Total (%)	4 (21%)	7 (37%)	6 (32%)	2 (11%)	19 (100%)	
12 weeks	H0	2	0	0	0	2 (13%)	
	H1	1	2	1	0	4 (25%)	
	H2	1	4	2	1	8 (50%)	
	H3	0	1	1	0	2 (13%)	0.07
	missing values	0	0	0	0	0 (0%)	
	Total (%)	4 (25%)	7 (44%)	4 (25%)	1 (6%)	16 (100%)	
		Indiana Bleb Appearance Grading Scale, Extent (E0–E3) ***					
		Preoperative					
		E0	E1	E2	E3	Total (%)	p *
1 weeks	E0	3	0	0	0	3 (15%)	
	E1	0	7	0	0	7 (35%)	
	E2	1	3	4	0	8 (40%)	
	E3	0	0	1	0	1 (5%)	0.06
	missing values	1	0	0	0	1 (5%)	
	Total (%)	5 (25%)	10 (50%)	5 (25%)	0 (0%)	20 (100%)	
4 weeks	E0	3	0	0	0	3 (16%)	
	E1	1	7	0	0	8 (42%)	
	E2	1	2	4	0	7 (37%)	
	E3	0	0	1	0	1 (5%)	0.06
	missing values	0	0	0	0	0 (0%)	
	Total (%)	5 (26%)	9 (47%)	5 (26%)	0 (0%)	19 (100%)	
12 weeks	E0	3	0	0	0	3 (19%)	
	E1	1	5	0	0	6 (38%)	
	E2	1	3	3	0	7 (44%)	
	E3	0	0	0	0	0 (0%)	0.06
	missing values	0	0	0	0	0 (0%)	
	Total (%)	5 (31%)	8 (50%)	3 (19%)	0 (0%)	16 (100%)	

Table 4. *Cont.*

		Indiana Bleb Appearance Grading Scale, Vascularity (V0–V4) ****						
		Preoperative						
		V0	V1	V2	V3	V4	Total (%)	p *
1 weeks	V0	1	0	0	0	0	1 (5%)	0.81
	V1	0	3	0	0	0	4 (20%)	
	V2	1	0	1	2	0	7 (35%)	
	V3	1	0	4	6	0	8 (35%)	
	V4	0	0	0	0	0	0 (0%)	
	missing values	0	0	0	1	0	1 (5%)	
	Total (%)	3 (15%)	3 (15%)	5 (25%)	9 (45%)	0 (0%)	20 (100%)	
4 weeks	V0	1	0	0	0	0	1 (5%)	1.00
	V1	0	3	1	0	0	4 (21%)	
	V2	1	0	4	1	0	6 (32%)	
	V3	0	0	0	8	0	8 (42%)	
	V4	0	0	0	0	0	0 (0%)	
	missing values	0	0	0	0	0	0 (0%)	
	Total (%)	2 (11%)	3 (16%)	5 (26%)	9 (47%)	0 (0%)	19 (100%)	
12 weeks	V0	0	0	0	0	0	0 (0%)	1.00
	V1	0	2	0	0	0	2 (13%)	
	V2	1	0	4	1	0	6 (38%)	
	V3	0	0	0	8	0	8 (50%)	
	V4	0	0	0	0	0	0 (0%)	
	missing values	0	0	0	0	0	0 (0%)	
	Total (%)	1 (6%)	2 (13%)	4 (25%)	9 (56%)	0 (0%)	16 (100%)	

		Indiana Bleb Appearance Grading Scale, Leakage (S0–S2) *****				
		Preoperative				
		S0	S1	S2	Total (%)	p *
1 weeks	S0	19	0	0	19 (95%)	
	S1	0	0	0	0 (0%)	
	S2	0	0	0	0 (0%)	
	missing values	1	0	0	1 (5%)	
	Total (%)	20 (100%)	0 (0%)	0 (0%)	20 (100%)	
4 weeks	S0	19	0	0	19 (100%)	
	S1	0	0	0	0 (0%)	
	S2	0	0	0	0 (0%)	
	missing values		0	0	0 (0%)	
	Total (%)	19 (100%)	0 (0%)	0 (0%)	19 (100%)	
12 weeks	S0	19	0	0	16 (100%)	
	S1	0	0	0	0 (0%)	
	S2	0	0	0	0 (0%)	
	missing values	1	0	0	0 (0%)	
	Total (%)	16 (100%)	0 (0%)	0 (0%)	16 (100%)	

* Wilcoxon's rank sum test. ** Height: H0, flat bleb without visible elevation; H1, low bleb elevation; H2, moderate bleb elevation; and H3, high bleb. *** Extent: E0, no visible bleb extent equal to less than 1 clock hour; E1, extent equal to or greater than 1 clock hour but less than 2 clock hours; E2, extent equal to or greater than 2 clock hours but less than 4 clock hours; and E3, extent equal to or greater than 4 clock hours. **** Vascularity: V0, avascular/white (no microcysts visible on slit lamp examination); V1, avascular/cystic (microcysts of the conjunctiva visible on slit lamp examination); V2, mild vascularity; V3, moderate vascularity; and V4, extensive vascularity (vascular engorgement). ***** Leakage: S0, no bleb leak; S1, pinpoint transconjunctival leakage visible on the bleb surface (at multiple points), without streaming of fluid within 5 s of application; and S2, streaming aqueous egress visible within 5 s of application of fluorescein.

Furthermore, there was no significant difference in corneal endothelial cell density preoperatively and postoperatively at 12 weeks ($p = 0.14$) (Table 5).

Table 5. Changes in corneal endothelial cell density.

	Cells/mm^2	p *
Preoperative	2422.24 ± 479.54	
1 week	2238.34 ± 479.75	0.06
4 weeks	2375.89 ± 409.54	0.02
12 weeks	2269.53 ± 436.34	0.14

* Wilcoxon's rank sum test.

4. Discussion

This study showed that ripasudil administration after needling without any antifibrotic agents, such as MMC or 5-FU, did not result in any serious AEs or ADRs. Hidenobu T. et al. documented the results of a phase I clinical trial, elucidating that the seven-day repeated instillation of ripasudil exhibited manageable adverse events (AEs). These included mild to moderate conjunctival hyperemia observed in the healthy volunteers, and such events were resolved within 90 min following instillation [8]. The safety profile of ripasudil exhibited similarity to that observed in patients diagnosed with ocular hypertension or open-angle glaucoma [9,10]. In this study, only two eyes had temporally pruritus and conjunctival follicle, and these were resolved quickly after the discontinuation of ripasudil. These results may indicate that the safety of ripasudil after glaucoma filtration surgery was equivalent to that in patients with ocular hypertension or glaucoma who underwent filtration surgery.

The most efficacious treatment for patients with glaucoma is the reduction in IOP [11,12]. TLE is considered the gold-standard surgical technique for lowering the IOP [2]. This procedure establishes a drainage pathway connecting the anterior chamber and the sub-Tenon space, resulting in the formation of a filtrating bleb within the subconjunctival space for the aqueous humor. The success of TLE relies on the continuous passage of aqueous humor between the anterior chamber and subconjunctival space. Nevertheless, the primary factors contributing to procedure failure are commonly attributed to the proliferation of fibroblasts and the formation of scars at the conjunctival and episcleral interface of the filtrating bleb [13,14]. During glaucoma filtration surgery, the scleral flap or conjunctiva becomes exposed to cytokines and growth factors released by various types of inflammatory cells and fibroblasts [15]. These reactions elicit the activation and migration of fibroblasts and other inflammatory cells. Activated fibroblasts generate and secrete extracellular matrix, such as collagen, leading to fibrosis. ROCK inhibitors mitigate the expression of extracellular-matrix-degrading enzymes in fibroblasts, thereby reducing the secretion of extracellular matrix [16]. Ibrahim et al. revealed that the ROCK inhibitor Y-27632 has the potential to inhibit fibrosis and enhance outcomes after glaucoma filtration surgery. This is achieved by inhibiting the transdifferentiation of Tenon fibroblasts into myofibroblasts and transforming growth factor β (TGF-β) and mitogen-activated protein kinase signaling after surgery [3]. Ko et al. reported that ripasudil suppressed postoperative scar formation by altering the expression of α-SMA and vimentin after filtration surgery in a mouse model [5]. Honjyo M. et al. also reported that the topical instillation of Y-27632 inhibited wound healing and fibroproliferation after filtration surgery in a rabbit model by reducing the expression of α-SMA in the immunohistochemical staining of blebs postoperatively [4].

There are several treatment options available for addressing bleb failure after trabeculectomy, including antihypertensive medications, surgical treatments such as needling with or without antimetabolites like 5-FU or MMC [17–19], or surgical revisions with various techniques [20]. Currently, there is no universally accepted gold-standard treatment for bleb failure, and different glaucoma specialists may adapt their practices based on their individual experiences [21]. Transconjunctival bleb needling is designed to rejuvenate failing blebs by mechanically removing adhesions. To prevent fibroblast proliferation, 5-FU or MMC are commonly used in bleb needling procedures through subconjunctival injection [22–24]. The potential for achieving IOP control and reducing the need for antiglaucoma medications following needling surgery with antimetabolites is noteworthy [24]. Considering these, this study provides a prospective clinical assessment of administering the ROCK inhibitor ripasudil to clinically reduce subconjunctival scarring after the initial needling procedure without the subconjunctival injection of antifibrotic agents. This study demonstrates that ripasudil administration maintains IOP and survival rate after needling procedure for 12 weeks. Despite counting ripasudil itself as an antiglaucoma medication, there was no observed increase in the number of antiglaucoma medications from the preoperative period to 12 weeks after the needling procedure. In a prior study, we reported a reduction rate of 27.22% after the needling surgery with MMC subconjunctival injection, with IOP decreasing from 16.9 ± 4.5 mmHg to 12.3 ± 4.8 mmHg ($n = 15$) at 12 weeks post procedure [6]. A Kaplan–Meier survival plot is presented with the same definition as in this study, showing a 12-week survival rate of 60.00% after needling with MMC. While it may be challenging to make a direct comparison, ripasudil administration after needling appears to help maintain the filtration bleb through antifibrotic effects, without resulting in any serious complications.

The success of trabeculectomy or needling procedures largely depends on the formation of a filtration bleb. Bleb morphology is a crucial factor for success. Lee YS et al. identified that a smaller central bleb extension and flatter height are morphological risk factors for failure [25]. The needling procedure generally increased the spread of the bleb. In our study, although there was a tendency for improvement and maintenance of bleb extension and height after needling with the use of the ROCK inhibitor, there was no statistically significant difference in bleb extension and height before and after the needling procedure. While the study duration was too short to definitively assess the effects of the ROCK inhibitor on maintaining morphological bleb formation thorough its antifibrotic effects, it is possible that ripasudil administration after the needling procedure preserved the morphology of the bleb, potentially resulting in a reduction in IOP.

A major concern with the use of antimetabolites is their safety, as these were reported to be potentially toxic to ocular tissues. Helosa A. et al. reported that there was no significant difference in preoperative corneal endothelial cell density at 12 months [18]. However, several studies indicated that the subconjunctival injection of antimetabolites can cause severe damage to corneal endothelial cells [26–29]. While such complications are rare, they cannot be resolved through observation or treatment with ocular instillation and may require corneal transplantation. ROCK inhibitors were reported to have the potential to improve corneal endothelial diseases, such as Fuchs endothelial dystrophy or corneal edema, and to have a protective effect on corneal endothelial cells after cataract surgery [30–34]. The exact mechanism by which ROCK inhibitors improve corneal endothelial cells has not been fully elucidated, but it is possible that these promote the reactivation of cell proliferation and migration, and the restoration of the corneal endothelial pump and barrier functions, contributing to the regeneration of corneal endothelial cells [29,35]. In this study, there was no change in corneal endothelial cell density more than 12 weeks after the needling surgery. This result suggests that ripasudil may potentially preserve corneal endothelial cells after needling surgery by promoting the regeneration of corneal endothelial cells.

This study has several limitations. The first is the lack of a dose–response test including the optical frequency of ripasudil or the optical ripasudil concentration. However, ripasudil, Glanatec®, was approved in Japan as an ophthalmic solution at a concentration of 0.4% with instillation two times per day. We believe that using the approved range is an important indicator of the safety of patients. Second, this study was designed as a single-arm trial because we defined safety as the primary endpoint. Therefore, the assessment of effectiveness involves comparing patients before and after needling procedures. Specifically, the efficacy of ripasudil cannot be adequately evaluated in terms of its effect on the overall course of the disease beyond its pharmacological action, which makes it an inadequate approach compared to a placebo-controlled design. Kim JS et al. reported that bleb needling procedures without any antimetabolites resulted in an IOP reduction over 12 weeks (from 23.0 ± 6.2 mmHg to 16.4 ± 5.7 mmHg, n = 72) [36]. While it is challenging to make a direct comparison and the follow-up period was too short to calculate survival, our findings suggest that administration of ripasudil after the needling procedure may be more effective for lowering and maintaining IOP than not using any antimetabolites, even though the preneedling IOP was lower than their result (from 14.6 ± 4.6 mmHg to 11.8 ± 3.1 mmHg, n = 20). This may be attributed to the antifibrosis effect of ripasudil. Since there are no previous reports on the clinical use of ripasudil after needling without using antimetabolites such as MMC or 5-FU, it is difficult to predefine the obvious criteria of efficacy in this study. Therefore, despite the limitations in controlling bias, we plan to use the results of this study's efficacy as a reference for future studies. The study will consider success and failure criteria related to reductions in the number of preprocedure antiglaucoma medications. We also plan to incorporate a control group to assess the potential IOP-lowering effect of ripasudil due to its antifibrotic action.

5. Conclusions

In conclusion, ripasudil administration after needling is safe and effective for controlling IOP, and it seems to have a potential role in maintaining corneal endothelial cells.

Author Contributions: Y.M. (Yu Mizuno) was the principal investigator of this trial and wrote the manuscript with critical assistance from K.K., N.O., H.O. (Hiromitsu Onoe), K.T., H.O. (Hideaki Okumichi), K.H., Y.M. (Yukiko Miura) and Y.K. Authors Y.M. (Yu Mizuno) and Y.K. conceived and designed the trial protocol. Y.M. (Yu Mizuno), N.O., H.O. (Hiromitsu Onoe), K.T., H.O. (Hideaki Okumichi), K.H., Y.M. (Yukiko Miura) and Y.K. collected the clinical data. K.K. and Y.K. supported this project from a regulatory perspective. G.A. performed formal analysis. All authors contributed to multiple revisions of the trial protocol and approved the final manuscript version for publication. Y.M. (Yu Mizuno) was responsible for the statistical analyses in this study. All authors have read and agreed to the published version of the manuscript.

Funding: This research was supported by Hiroshima University Hospital.

Institutional Review Board Statement: This study was conducted in accordance with the Declaration of Helsinki and approved by the Hiroshima University Certified Review Board (approval no. CRB210008, 26 May 2022).

Informed Consent Statement: Informed consent was obtained from all subjects involved in the study. Written informed consent was obtained from the patients to publish this paper.

Data Availability Statement: Data are contained within the article.

Acknowledgments: The authors would like to thank Hiroshima University Hospital Clinical Research Center for the advice on the experimental design.

Conflicts of Interest: The authors declare no conflict of interest.

References

1. Quigley, H.A.; Addicks, E.M.; Green, W.R.; Maumenee, A.E. Optic nerve damage in human glaucoma. II. The site of injury and susceptibility to damage. *Arch. Ophthalmol.* **1981**, *99*, 635–649. [CrossRef] [PubMed]
2. Cairns, J.E. Trabeculectomy. Preliminary report of a new method. *Am. J. Ophthalmol.* **1968**, *66*, 673–679. [CrossRef]
3. Ibrahim, D.G.; Ko, J.; Iwata, W.; Okumichi, H.; Kiuchi, Y. An in vitro study of scarring formation mediated by human tenon fibroblasts: Effect of Y-27632, a Rho kinase inhibitor. *Cell Biochem. Funct.* **2019**, *37*, 113–124. [CrossRef] [PubMed]
4. Honjo, M.; Tanihara, H.; Kameda, T.; Kawaji, T.; Yoshimura, N.; Araie, M. Potential role of rho-associated protein kinase inhibitor Y-27632 in glaucoma filtration surgery. *Investig. Ophthalmol. Vis. Sci.* **2007**, *48*, 5549–5557. [CrossRef] [PubMed]
5. Ko, J.-A.; Komatsu, K.; Minamoto, A.; Kondo, S.; Okumichi, H.; Hirooka, K.; Kiuchi, Y. Effects of ripasudil, a rho-kinase inhibitor, on scar formation in a mouse model of filtration surgery. *Curr. Eye Res.* **2023**, *48*, 826–835. [CrossRef] [PubMed]
6. Mizuno, Y.; Okada, N.; Onoe, H.; Tokumo, K.; Okumichi, H.; Hirooka, K.; Kiuchi, Y. Effect of the Rho-kinase inhibitor Ripasudil in needling with Mitomycin C for the failure of filtering bleb after trabeculectomy:a cross-sectional study. *BMC Ophthalmol.* **2022**, *22*, 433. [CrossRef] [PubMed]
7. Cantor, L.B.; Mantravadi, A.; WuDunn, D.; Swamynathan, K.; Cortes, A. Morphologic classification of filtering blebs after glaucoma filtration surgery: The Indiana Bleb Appearance Grading Scale. *J. Glaucoma* **2003**, *12*, 266–271. [CrossRef]

8. Tanihara, H.; Inoue, T.; Yamamoto, T.; Kuwayama, Y.; Abe, H.; Araie, M. K-115 Clinical Study Group. Phase 1 clinical trials of a selective Rho kinase inhibitor, K-115. *JAMA Ophthalmol.* **2013**, *131*, 1288–1295. [CrossRef]
9. Tanihara, H.; Inoue, T.; Yamamoto, T.; Kuwayama, Y.; Abe, H.; Suganami, H.; Araie, M. K-115 Clinical Study Group, 2015. Intra-ocular pressure-lowering effects of a Rho kinase inhibitor, ripasudil (K-115), over 24 hours in primary open-angle glaucoma and ocular hypertension: A randomized, open-label, crossover study. *Acta Ophthalmol.* **2015**, *93*, e254–e260. [CrossRef]
10. Sakamoto, E.; Ishida, W.; Sumi, T.; Kishimoto, T.; Tada, K.; Fukuda, K.; Yoneda, T.; Kuroiwa, H.; Terao, E.; Fujisawa, Y.; et al. Evaluation of offset of conjunctival hyperemia induced by a Rho-kinase inhibitor; 0.4% Ripasudil ophthalmic solution clinical trial. *Sci. Rep.* **2019**, *9*, 3755. [CrossRef]
11. Shaarawy, T.M.; Sherwood, M.B.; Grehn, F. *Guidelines on Design and Reporting of Glaucoma Surgical Trials*; Kugler Publications: Amsterdam, The Netherlands, 2009; pp. 15–24.
12. Weinreb, R.N.; Aung, T.; Medeiros, F.A. The pathophysiology and treatment of glaucoma: A review. *JAMA* **2014**, *311*, 1901–1911. [CrossRef] [PubMed]
13. Skuta, G.L.; Parrish, R.K. Wound healing in glaucoma filtering surgery. *Surv. Ophthalmol.* **1987**, *32*, 149–170. [CrossRef] [PubMed]
14. Broadway, D.C.; Chang, L.P. Trabeculectomy, risk factors for failure and the preoperative state of the conjunctiva. *J. Glaucoma* **2001**, *10*, 237–249. [CrossRef] [PubMed]
15. Chang, L.; Crowston, J.G.; Cordeiro, M.F.; Akbar, A.N.; Khaw, P.T. The role of the immune system in conjunctival wound healing after glaucoma surgery. *Surv. Ophthalmol.* **2000**, *45*, 49–68. [CrossRef] [PubMed]
16. Akhmetshina, A.; Dees, C.; Pileckyte, M.; Szucs, G.; Spriewald, B.M.; Zwerina, J.; Distler, O.; Schett, G.; Distler, J.H. Rho-associated kinases are crucial for myofibroblast differentiation and pro-duction of extracellular matrix in scleroderma fibroblasts. *Arthritis Rheum.* **2008**, *58*, 2553–2564. [CrossRef] [PubMed]
17. Shetty, R.K.; Wartluft, L.; Moster, M.R. Slit-lamp needle revision of failed filtering blebs using high-dose Mitomycin C. *J. Glaucoma* **2005**, *14*, 52–56. [CrossRef] [PubMed]
18. Maestrini, H.A.; Cronemberger, S.; Matoso, H.D.; Reis, J.R.; Mérula, R.V.; Filho, A.D.; Sakurai, E.; Ferreira, G.A. Late needling of flat filtering blebs with adjunctive Mitomycin C: Efficacy and safety for the corneal endothelium. *Ophthalmology* **2011**, *118*, 755–762. [CrossRef]
19. Sherwood, M.B.; Spaeth, G.L.; Simmons, S.T.; Nichols, D.A.; Walsh, A.M.; Steinmann, W.C.; Wilson, R.P. Cysts of tenon's capsule following filtration surgery. Medical management. *Arch. Ophthalmol.* **1987**, *105*, 1517–1521. [CrossRef]
20. Chew, A.C.Y.; Htoon, H.M.; Perera, S.A.; Rubio, C.J.S.; Ho, C.L. Outcomes of surgical bleb revision at a tertiary Singapore eye hospital. *Int. Ophthalmol.* **2022**, *42*, 443–453. [CrossRef]
21. Mercieca, K.; Drury, B.; Bhargava, A.; Fenerty, C. Trabeculectomy bleb needling and antimetabolite administration practices in the UK: A glaucoma specialist national survey. *Br. J. Ophthalmol.* **2018**, *102*, 1244–1247. [CrossRef]
22. Ewing, R.H.; Stamper, R.L. Needle revision with and without 5-fluorouracil for the treatment of failed filtering blebs. *Am. J. Ophthalmol.* **1990**, *110*, 254–259. [CrossRef] [PubMed]
23. Mardelli, P.G.; Lederer, C.M.; Murray, P.L.; Pastor, S.A.; Hassanein, K.M. Slit-lamp needle revision of failed filtering blebs using Mitomycin C. *Ophthalmology* **1996**, *103*, 1946–1955. [CrossRef]
24. Chen, X.; Suo, L.; Hong, Y.; Zhang, C. Safety and efficacy of bleb needling with antimetabolite after trabeculectomy failure in glaucoma patients: A systemic review and meta-analysis. *J. Ophthalmol.* **2020**, *30*, 4310258. [CrossRef] [PubMed]
25. Lee, Y.S.; Wu, S.C.; Tseng, H.; Wu, W.C.; Chang, S.H.L. The relationship of bleb morphology and the outcome of needle revision with 5-fluorouracil in failing filtering bleb. *Medicine* **2016**, *95*, e4546. [CrossRef] [PubMed]
26. Anand, N.; Khan, A. Long-term outcomes of needle revision of trabeculectomy blebs with Mitomycin C and 5-fluorouracil: A comparative safety and efficacy report. *J. Glaucoma* **2009**, *18*, 513–520. [CrossRef] [PubMed]
27. Wu, K.Y.; Wang, H.Z.; Hong, S.J. Mechanism of mitomycin-induced apoptosis in cultured corneal endothelial cells. *Mol. Vis.* **2008**, *14*, 1705–1712. [PubMed]
28. Pathak-Ray, V.; Choudhari, N. Rescue of failing or failed trabeculectomy blebs with slit-lamp needling and adjunctive Mitomycin C in Indian eyes. *Indian J. Ophthalmol.* **2018**, *66*, 71–76. [CrossRef]
29. Rabiolo, A.; Marchese, A.; Bettin, P.; Monteduro, D.; Galasso, M.; Dolci, M.P.; Di Matteo, F.; Fiori, M.; Ciampi, C.; Bandello, F. Needle revision outcomes after glaucoma filtering surgery: Survival analysis and predictive factors. *Eur. J. Ophthalmol.* **2020**, *30*, 350–359. [CrossRef]
30. Schlötzer-Schrehardt, U.; Zenkel, M.; Strunz, M.; Gießl, A.; Schondorf, H.; da Silva, H.; Schmidt, G.A.; Greiner, M.A.; Okumura, N.; Koizumi, N.; et al. Potential functional restoration of corneal endothelial cells in Fuchs endothelial corneal dystrophy by ROCK inhibitor (ripasudil). *Am. J. Ophthalmol.* **2021**, *224*, 185–199. [CrossRef]
31. Syed, Z.A.; Rapuano, C.J. Rho kinase (ROCK) inhibitors in the management of corneal endothelial disease. *Curr. Opin. Ophthalmol.* **2021**, *32*, 268–274. [CrossRef]
32. Okumura, N.; Koizumi, N.; Kay, E.P.; Ueno, M.; Sakamoto, Y.; Nakamura, S.; Hamuro, J.; Kinoshita, S. The ROCK inhibitor eye drop accelerates corneal endothelium wound healing. *Investig. Ophthalmol. Vis. Sci.* **2013**, *54*, 2493–2502. [CrossRef] [PubMed]
33. Okumura, N.; Inoue, R.; Okazaki, Y.; Nakano, S.; Nakagawa, H.; Kinoshita, S.; Koizumi, N. Effect of the Rho kinase inhibitor Y-27632 on corneal endothelial wound healing. *Investig. Ophthalmol. Vis. Sci.* **2015**, *56*, 6067–6074. [CrossRef] [PubMed]
34. Fujimoto, H.; Setoguchi, Y.; Kiryu, J. The ROCK inhibitor ripasudil shows an endothelial protective effect in patients with low corneal endothelial cell density after cataract surgery. *Transl. Vis. Sci. Technol.* **2021**, *10*, 18. [CrossRef] [PubMed]

35. Okumura, N.; Koizumi, N.; Ueno, M.; Sakamoto, Y.; Takahashi, H.; Tsuchiya, H.; Hamuro, J.; Kinoshita, S. ROCK inhibitor converts corneal endothelial cells into a phenotype capable of regenerating in vivo endothelial tissue. *Am. J. Pathol.* **2012**, *181*, 268–277. [CrossRef]
36. Kim, J.S.; Kim, H.J.; Na, K.I.; Kim, Y.K.; Park, K.H.; Jeoung, J.W. Comparison of efficacy and safety of bleb needle revision with and without 5-fluorouracil for failing trabeculectomy bleb. *J. Glaucoma* **2019**, *28*, 386–391. [CrossRef]

Disclaimer/Publisher's Note: The statements, opinions and data contained in all publications are solely those of the individual author(s) and contributor(s) and not of MDPI and/or the editor(s). MDPI and/or the editor(s) disclaim responsibility for any injury to people or property resulting from any ideas, methods, instructions or products referred to in the content.

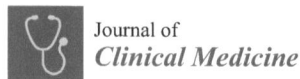 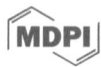

Article

Ocular Distribution of Brimonidine and Brinzolamide after Topical Instillation of a 0.1% Brimonidine Tartrate and 1% Brinzolamide Fixed-Combination Ophthalmic Suspension: An Interventional Study

Yusuke Orii [1], Eriko Kunikane [2], Yutaka Yamada [1], Masakazu Morioka [1], Kentaro Iwasaki [1], Shogo Arimura [1], Akemi Mizuno [2] and Masaru Inatani [1,*]

1 Department of Ophthalmology, Faculty of Medical Sciences, University of Fukui, Fukui 910-1193, Japan
2 Senju Pharmaceutical Co., Ltd., Osaka 541-0048, Japan
* Correspondence: inatani@u-fukui.ac.jp

Abstract: Purpose: To evaluate the concentrations of brimonidine and brinzolamide in the vitreous and aqueous humor after instillation of a 0.1% brimonidine tartrate and 1% brinzolamide fixed-combination ophthalmic suspension. Methods: The present investigation involved patients with macular holes or idiopathic epiretinal membranes who were planning to undergo vitrectomy. One week prior to surgery, the patients received twice-daily topical treatment with 0.1% brimonidine tartrate and 1% brinzolamide fixed-combination ophthalmic suspension. Before vitrectomy, vitreous and aqueous humor samples were collected, and the mean concentrations of brimonidine and brinzolamide were determined through liquid chromatography-tandem spectrometry. Results: Ten eyes (nine phakic and one pseudophakic eyes; 10 patients) were examined. The concentration of brimonidine in vitreous and aqueous humor samples was 5.02 ± 2.24 and 559 ± 670 nM, respectively. The concentration of brimonidine in the vitreous humor, which is needed to activate α2 receptors, was >2 nM in all patients. The concentration of brinzolamide was 8.96 ± 4.65 and 1100 ± 813 nM, respectively. However, there was no significant correlation between the concentrations of brimonidine in the vitreous and aqueous humor samples. Conclusions: Sufficient concentrations of brimonidine were detected in all vitreous samples. The dissociated correlation of the drug concentrations between aqueous and vitreous humors implies the possibility of another pathway to vitreous humor, different from the pathway to aqueous humor.

Keywords: brimonidine; brinzolamide; fixed-combination ophthalmic suspension; vitreous humors; aqueous humors

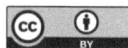

1. Introduction

Glaucoma is the most common cause of irreversible visual loss in developed countries Lowering intraocular pressure (IOP) is the most critical strategy for preventing optic nerve damage in glaucoma patients. Various randomized controlled clinical trials and related studies support the strategy that IOP lowering reduces both the onset and progression of glaucoma [1–3]. IOP-lowering treatments are classified into three procedures: medical treatment, laser therapy, and surgery. Among the three procedures, medical treatment is commonly used to lower IOP in patients with open-angle glaucoma. Although medical treatments consist of eye drops and oral medications, eye drops are the major medical treatment for glaucoma patients because of their efficiency and tolerance. Currently, various types of IOP-lowering antiglaucoma ophthalmic solutions are available [4,5]. These IOP-lowering antiglaucoma ophthalmic solutions were classified into eight categories: prostanoid receptor-related drugs [6], ß-blockers [7], carbonic anhydrase inhibitors [8], α2 adrenergic agonists [9], rho-kinase inhibitors [10], parasympathomimetic drugs [11], α1 blockers [12], and ion channel openers [13,14]. Among these categories, prostanoid receptor-related drug monotherapy is most commonly administered for the initial treatment of chronic open-angle glaucoma [15]. A randomized clinical trial using latanoprost, a prostanoid receptor-related drug, and the placebo has shown that once-daily latanoprost instillation attenuates visual field progression for glaucomatous eyes in 2 years via its IOP-lowering effect [16]. If further IOP reduction is required to prevent optic nerve damage, an additional eye drop is used for patients with glaucoma previously treated with monotherapy. A recent clinical trial reported that the combination of multiple IOP-lowering drugs with laser treatment was more effective in attenuating the progression of visual field loss than drug monotherapy [17,18]. In developed countries, most patients with glaucoma are treated with multiple types of antiglaucoma ophthalmic solutions [19]. However, half of the patients with glaucoma receiving topical antiglaucoma medications have ocular surface disease [20]. Because of increased exposure to preservatives, multidose topical instillations are associated with a high incidence of corneal epithelial damage in patients with glaucoma [21,22]. The use of multiple topical instillations results in the deterioration of adherence to medical treatment in patients with glaucoma [23]. Thus, despite the intent of further IOP reduction, this therapeutic approach is frequently associated with negative effects on the quality of vision in patients.

Medical treatment with a fixed-combination ophthalmic solution improves adherence and prevents ocular surface disease versus separate instillations of ophthalmic solutions [24]. In Japan, a fixed-combination ophthalmic suspension containing 0.1% brimonidine tartrate and 1% brinzolamide (Ailamide®; Senju Pharmaceutical Co., Ltd., Osaka, Japan) recently became available for the treatment of glaucoma and ocular hypertension. The fixed-combination suspension containing 0.2% brimonidine tartrate and 1% brinzolamide (Simbrinza®, Allergan, Dublin, Ireland) in the USA and countries in the European Union was the first fixed-combination drug to not contain a ß-blocker [25]. These combination drugs include brimonidine, a highly selective α2 adrenergic agonist that reduces IOP by suppressing the production of aqueous humor and promoting uveoscleral outflow [26,27]. Numerous in vivo and in vitro studies demonstrated that, apart from its IOP-lowering effects, brimonidine exerts potential neuroprotective effects on retinal ganglion cells (RGCs) [28–30]. In randomized clinical trials involving patients with open-angle glaucoma, 0.2% and 0.1% brimonidine tartrate ophthalmic solutions reduced the progression of visual field loss versus 0.5% timolol malate ophthalmic solution [31,32]. To perform its neuroprotective function in the RGCs of patients with glaucoma, an adequate amount of brimonidine in the ophthalmic solution should be present in the vitreous humor. Several studies have investigated the concentration of brimonidine in human vitreous samples after topical treatment with 0.1%, 0.15%, or 0.2% brimonidine tartrate ophthalmic solutions [33–35]. Following these instillations, most vitreous samples contained a concentration of brimonidine > 2 nM, which is required for the activation of α2 adrenergic receptors in neuronal cells [36].

The efficiency of drug delivery into ocular tissues is influenced by differences in the preservatives used, pH, and viscosity between the fixed-combination and single agents, as well as interactions between components. Our previous study using a 0.1% brimonidine tartrate and 0.5% timolol fixed-combination ophthalmic solution revealed that 63% of vitreous samples contained a concentration of brimonidine > 2 nM [37]. The brimonidine tartrate ophthalmic solution was homogenous. However, the brimonidine tartrate and brinzolamide fixed-combination drug is a suspension due to the composition of brinzolamide [38]. However, the effects of differences in formulations on the pharmacokinetics of brimonidine in the human vitreous remain unknown. Therefore, we examined the concentration of brimonidine in human vitreous humor following the instillation of a 0.1% brimonidine tartrate and 1% brinzolamide fixed-combination ophthalmic suspension.

2. Materials and Methods

2.1. Patient Selection

The University of Fukui Certified Review Board approved this single-arm open-label interventional trial (approval code: CRB5180014, approval date: 19 October 2020) and adhered to the principles of the Declaration of Helsinki. All participants were informed of the protocol and any potential risks and advantages of the therapies prior to enrolment. All patients provided written informed consent. The Japan Registry of Clinical Trials received registration for this study (jRCT, ID jRCTs051200089; date of access and registration, 25 November 2020).

This investigation involved adult patients (age: $\geq$20 years) who planned to undergo pars plana vitrectomy for the treatment of macular holes or idiopathic epiretinal membranes between November 2020 and June 2021. The exclusion criteria were as follows: (1) uveitis; (2) vitreous hemorrhage; (3) proliferative diabetic retinopathy; (4) corneal epithelial disorder; (5) a history of allergic reaction to an α2 stimulant or carbonic anhydrase inhibitor; and (6) difficulty in the instillation of ophthalmic solutions.

2.2. Sample Collection

Patient characteristics such as sex, lens status (phakia/pseudophakia), age, slit lamp examinations of the ocular surface including palpebral and bulbar conjunctivas and cornea, fundus retinoscopy, and optical coherence tomography for macular holes or idiopathic epiretinal membranes were examined when they were recruited in this study.

The samples were collected as previously described [33]. Briefly, the patients received twice-daily topical instillation of Ailamide® (Senju Pharmaceutical Co., Ltd.), a fixed-combination ophthalmic suspension containing 0.1% brimonidine tartrate, and 1% brinzolamide for 1 week before surgery. On the day of pars plana vitrectomy, ophthalmic suspension was applied at 8:00 a.m. within 2 h prior to surgery. The patients were requested to record their treatment adherence for 1 week using self-check sheets. Patients with an adherence rate of <75% were excluded from the analysis.

As a preoperative medication to prevent postoperative infection, levofloxacin ophthalmic solution 1.5% (Rohto-nitten Co., Ltd. Nagoya, Japan) was also administered for 3 days before surgery. We instructed the patients to allow at least a 10 min interval between multiple instillations.

Standard four-port vitrectomy was performed under retrobulbar anesthesia. Collection of vitreous humor (500 µL) and aqueous humor (100 µL) samples was performed from the anterior chamber and vitreous cavity, respectively. For the avoidance of sample dilution, the infusion line was transiently blocked until the completion of sample collection from the vitreous fluid. A 25 G vitreous cutter pointed toward the optic disc was used for the collection of vitreous humor samples from the area of the retina and optic disc. The samples were placed in Eppendorf tubes and stored at -80 °C.

2.3. Sample Size

In our previous investigation of a 0.1% brimonidine tartrate and 0.5% timolol fixed-combination ophthalmic solution (Aibeta®; Senju Pharmaceutical Co., Ltd.), the sample size was 8 patients [37]. The University of Fukui Certified Review Board approved the study design to minimize the risk of adverse events to patients because the instillation of Ailamide® (Senju Pharmaceutical Co., Ltd.) had no indication for the treatment of patients with macular holes or idiopathic epiretinal membranes planning to undergo vitrectomy. The sample size of this study was also limited to 10 patients. The sample size was applied to the present trial, including those who withdrew from the study or did not follow the study protocol.

2.4. Drug Concentration Measurement

Within 1 month after surgery, the concentrations of brimonidine and brinzolamide in the samples were quantitatively assessed in an independent bioanalytical facility through liquid chromatography and tandem mass spectrometry (CMIC Pharma Science Co., Ltd., Hokuto, Japan). The analysis was performed using a Triple Quad5500 (AB Sciex Pte. Ltd., Framingham, MA, USA) and a Nexera Ultra High-Performance Liquid Chromatography system (Shimadzu Corporation, Kyoto, Japan). Gradient chromatography was carried out using a Kinetex EVO C18 column (inner diameter: 2.1 mm, length: 150 mm, and particle size: 5 μm; Phenomenex Inc., Torrance, CA, USA). 5-Chloro-6-(2-imidazolidinylideneamino) quinoxaline was utilized as the internal standard. The mobile phase consisted of 10 mM ammonium hydrogencarbonate buffer (pH 10.0) and methanol at a flow rate of 0.5 mL/min. Brimonidine, brinzolamide, and the internal standard were examined in the positive ionization mode based on the following multiple reaction monitoring transitions: 292/212 (brimonidine); 384/136 (brinzolamide); and 248/205 (internal standard).

2.5. Primary Outcomes

The primary outcomes were as follows: (1) average concentration of brimonidine in the vitreous and aqueous humor samples; (2) percentage of patients with a concentration of brimonidine in the vitreous humor > 2 nM; and (3) correlation between the concentrations of brimonidine in vitreous and aqueous humor samples.

2.6. Secondary Outcomes

The secondary outcomes were as follows: (1) concentrations of brinzolamide in vitreous and aqueous humor samples; (2) relationship between the concentrations of brimonidine and brinzolamide in vitreous and aqueous humor samples; (3) changes in IOP after drug instillation; and (4) best-corrected visual acuity (BCVA) prior to and following surgery. To reduce patient distress, a non-contact tonometer (Nidek, Nagoya, Japan) was utilized for the measurement of IOPs in patients with macular holes or idiopathic epiretinal membranes without glaucoma.

The safety of the treatment was continuously monitored throughout the study. Ten to twenty percent of individuals with long-term brimonidine administration encounter allergic conjunctivitis [39]. Other ocular side effects include ocular itching and burning sensation, eye redness, dryness, and corneal opacity [40,41]. General systemic complications are central depression, somnolence, headache, dizziness, vomiting, nausea, and fatigue [42]. We checked the association with ocular side effects using a slit-lamp microscope and instructed the patients to inform our facility immediately if any systemic symptoms appeared.

2.7. Statistical Analysis

Statistical analysis was conducted using JMP 15 software (SAS Institute, Inc., Cary, NC, USA). Data are presented as the mean ± standard deviation. Ordinary least-squares regression analysis was used to assess the relationship between the concentrations of brimonidine and brinzolamide in the vitreous and aqueous humor samples. Changes in IOP after treatment were examined using a paired sample t-test. For all tests, the level of statistical significance was set at $p < 0.05$.

The patients, intervention providers, or outcome assessors were not blinded to the procedure.

3. Results

3.1. Patient Characteristics

Overall, 14 patients were enrolled in this study. Four patients withdrew their consent after agreeing to participate due to concerns regarding the increased number of eye drops and the complexity of the procedure. The usage of Ailamide® (Senju Pharmaceutical Co., Ltd.) did not result in any adverse effects in those patients. The remaining 10 patients complied with the study protocol and were included in the analysis (Figure 1).

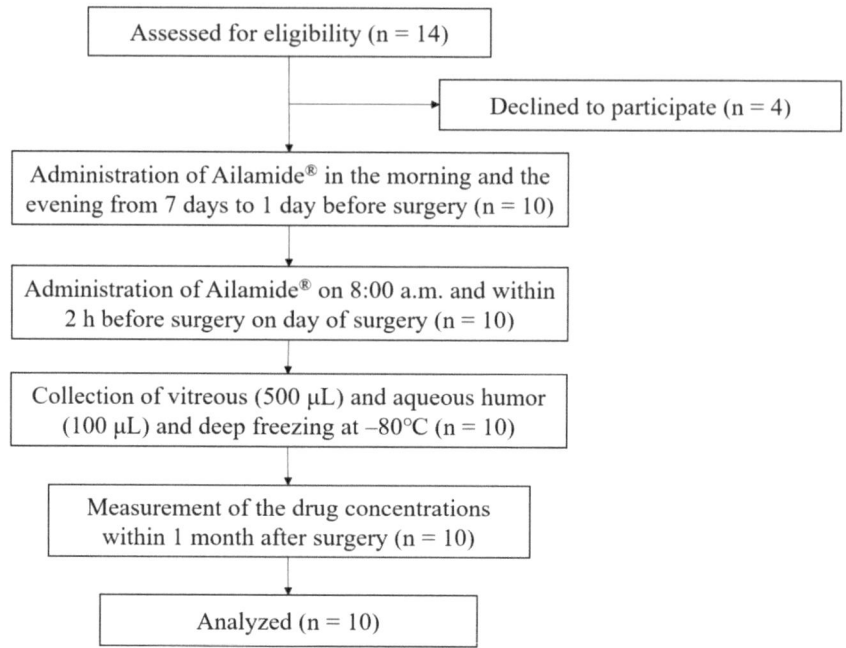

Figure 1. Study flow diagram.

All patients (five males and five females) were Japanese, with a mean age of 67.7 ± 10.0 years (Table 1). Of the 10 eyes examined, nine and one eye were phakic and pseudophakic, respectively. Of the 10 patients, nine had an idiopathic epiretinal membrane. All patient data are available in the Supplementary Materials (Table S1).

Table 1. Patient characteristics.

Characteristic	Value
Total (n)	10
Age, mean ± standard deviation (years)	67.7 ± 10.0
Sex, male/female (n)	5/5
Lens status, phakia/pseudophakia (n)	9/1
Diagnosis	
Idiopathic epiretinal membrane (n)	9
Macular hole (n)	1

All patients used levofloxacin ophthalmic solution 1.5% for 3 days preoperatively. Three patients had been using eye drops other than levofloxacin: pirenoxine ophthalmic suspension 0.005% and cyanocobalamin ophthalmic solution 0.02% (n = 1), pirenoxine ophthalmic suspension 0.005% (n = 1), and diquafosol sodium ophthalmic solution 3% (n = 1).

3.2. Primary Outcomes

The mean concentration of brimonidine in vitreous and aqueous humor samples was 5.02 ± 2.24 (95% confidence interval [CI]: 3.41–6.62) and 559 ± 670 nM (95% CI: 79.9–1040), respectively (Figure 2). In all patients, the concentration of brimonidine in the vitreous humor was >2 nM.

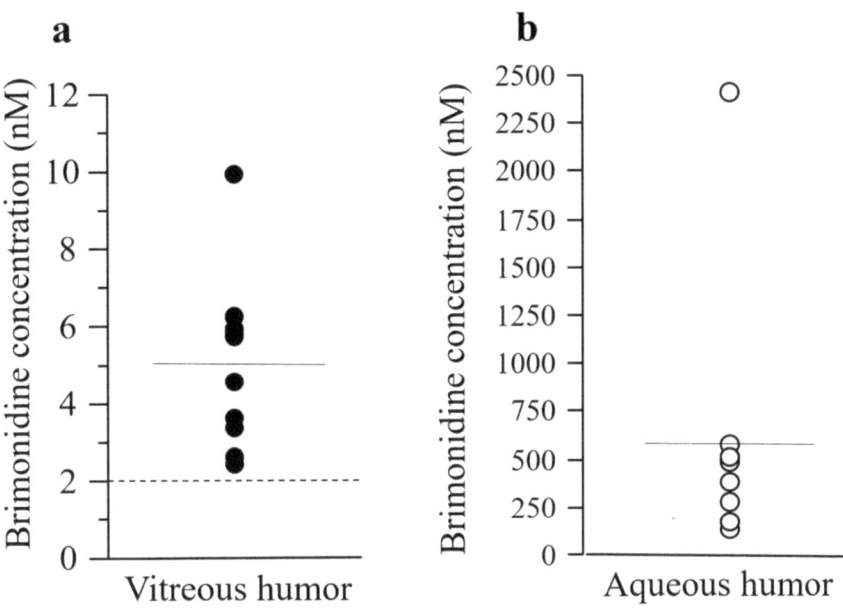

Figure 2. Concentration of brimonidine in vitreous (**a**) and aqueous (**b**) humor samples. Solid horizontal lines indicate the mean of the included data points. Dotted lines parallel to the x-axis denote the 2 nM concentration of brimonidine. Filled and open circles indicate the concentrations in vitreous and aqueous humor samples, respectively.

There was no statistically significant correlation observed between the concentrations of brimonidine in the aqueous and vitreous humor samples ($p = 0.6567$, $R^2 = 0.0259$) (Figure 3a).

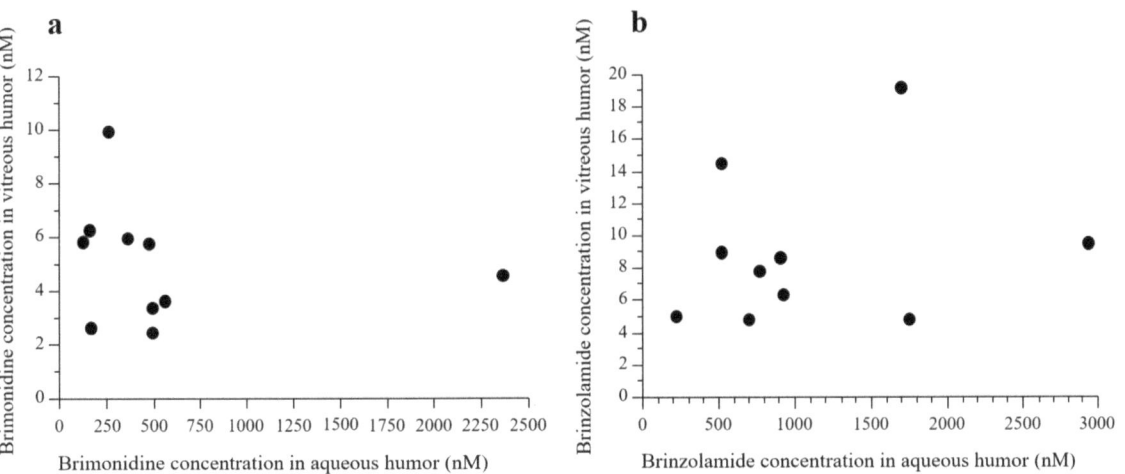

Figure 3. Correlations between the concentrations of drugs in aqueous and vitreous humor samples. There was no statistically significant correlation between the concentrations of brimonidine (**a**) and brinzolamide (**b**) in the aqueous and vitreous humor samples.

3.3. Secondary Outcomes

There was no statistically significant correlation between the concentrations of brinzolamide in the aqueous and vitreous humor samples ($p = 0.5479$, $R^2 = 0.0469$) (Figure 3b). The mean concentration of brinzolamide in vitreous and aqueous humor samples was 8.96 ± 4.65 (95% CI: 5.63–12.3) and 1100 ± 813 nM (95% CI: 513–1680), respectively (Figure 4).

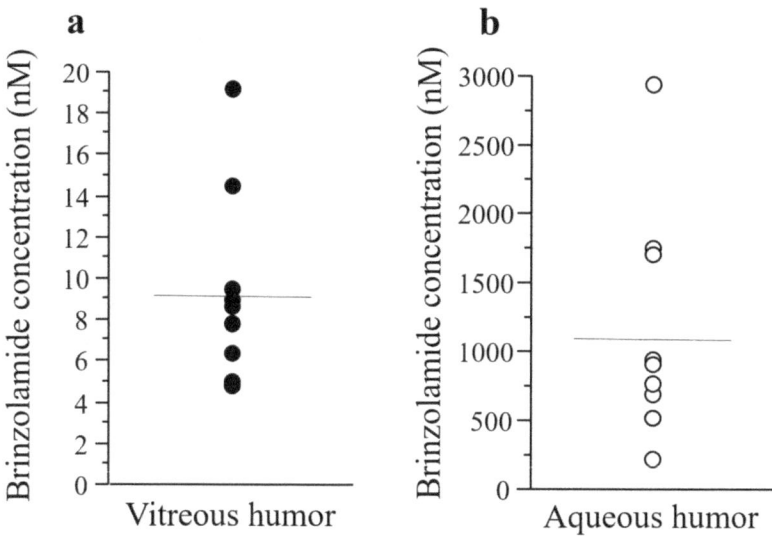

Figure 4. Concentration of brinzolamide in vitreous (**a**) and aqueous (**b**) humor samples. Solid horizontal lines indicate the mean of included data points. Filled and open circles indicate concentrations in the vitreous and aqueous humor samples, respectively.

There was no statistically significant correlation detected between the concentrations of brimonidine and brinzolamide in the vitreous humor samples ($p = 0.0789$, $R^2 = 0.336$) (Figure 5a). Nevertheless, a significant positive correlation was recorded in the aqueous humor samples ($p = 0.0006$, $R^2 = 0.792$) (Figure 5b).

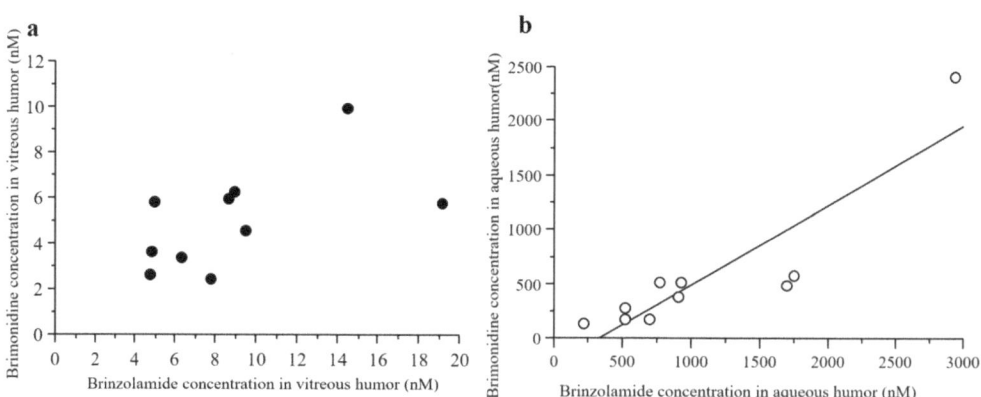

Figure 5. Linear correlations between the concentrations of brimonidine and brinzolamide in vitreous and aqueous humor samples. There were no significant correlations between the concentrations of brimonidine and brinzolamide in the vitreous humor samples (**a**). However, a significant positive correlation was noted in the aqueous humor samples (**b**). Filled and open circles indicate drug concentrations in the vitreous and aqueous humor samples, respectively.

Prior to the instillation, the mean IOP was 14.3 ± 1.9 mm Hg. The mean IOP prior to the operation was 11.2 ± 2.0 mm Hg, indicating a significant IOP reduction after the instillation ($p = 0.0008$; −3.1 ± 2.0 mmHg; 95% CI: −4.5–−1.7). Throughout the course of the study, there were no systemic or ocular side effects related to drug administration in any of the patients. Moreover, postoperative complications (e.g., infectious endophthalmitis, vitreous hemorrhage, and retinal detachment) did not occur in any of the patients.

The mean BCVA in logMAR prior to and 1 month following the operation were 0.41 ± 0.24 and 0.17 ± 0.25, respectively. The BCVA was significantly improved after surgery ($p = 0.0009$).

4. Discussion

Drugs must enter the vitreous cavity to exert their neuroprotective effects on RGCs [43]. Moreover, a concentration of brimonidine of >2 nM is needed in the animal retina for the activation of α2 adrenergic receptors in neuronal cells [36]. Therefore, the objective of this investigation was to determine whether the twice-daily topical administration of 0.1% brimonidine tartrate and 1% brinzolamide fixed-combination ophthalmic suspension (Ailamide®; Senju Pharmaceutical Co., Ltd.) for 1 week would result in a concentration of brimonidine > 2 nM. Following treatment, the concentration of brimonidine was >2 nM (mean concentration: 5.02 ± 2.24 nM; 95% CI: 3.41–6.62) in all vitreous samples.

Previous studies investigated the concentration of brimonidine in vitreous humor after the topical administration of 0.1% (Aifagan®, Senju Pharmaceutical Co., Ltd.) [33], 0.15% (Alphagan®; Allergan, Dublin, Ireland) [34] and 0.2% (Alphagan®; Allergan) [35] brimonidine tartrate ophthalmic solutions, and 0.1% brimonidine tartrate and 0.5% timolol fixed-combination ophthalmic solution (Aibeta®; Senju Pharmaceutical Co., Ltd.) [37]. Ailamide® (Senju Pharmaceutical Co., Ltd.) is an ophthalmic suspension containing brinzolamide. The liquid properties of this formulation differ from those of other brimonidine tartrate-containing ophthalmic solutions. The present study is unique because the concentration of brimonidine in the vitreous humor was evaluated following the topical administration of an ophthalmic suspension.

Previous studies quantified the concentration of brimonidine in the vitreous humor following the instillation of ophthalmic solutions, including brimonidine tartrate. The investigators reported that the concentration of brimonidine in some samples was <2 nM. However, in the present study, the concentration of brimonidine was >2 nM in all vitreous humor samples. An experimental animal study also revealed that the concentration of brimonidine after the instillation of Ailamide® (Senju Pharmaceutical Co., Ltd.) was equal to or higher than that of 0.1% brimonidine tartrate ophthalmic solution [44]. Differences in the composition of these formulations (e.g., viscosity) might contribute to the efficient penetration of brimonidine into the vitreous humor.

A significant positive correlation was detected between the concentrations of brimonidine and brinzolamide in the aqueous humor. Nevertheless, there was no significant correlation observed in the vitreous humor samples. Interestingly, in our previous study using Aibeta® (Senju Pharmaceutical Co., Ltd.), we revealed significant positive correlations between the concentrations of brimonidine and timolol in vitreous and aqueous humor samples [37]. As brimonidine tartrate and timolol are clear solutions, they may have a similar ability to penetrate the vitreous humor. Furthermore, the suspension properties may affect the penetration of brinzolamide into the vitreous humor.

Consistent with previous studies [33,37], we did not find a statistically significant correlation between the concentrations of brimonidine in vitreous and aqueous humor samples. There results suggest that the routes of entry of brimonidine into the vitreous and anterior chambers differ. The results of experimental studies using rabbit [45] and monkey eyes [46] after topical instillation of radiolabeled nipradiol ophthalmic solution indicate that nipradiol is distributed in the posterior retina from the posterior periocular tissues across the posterior sclera. A previous study using rabbits investigated ocular drug delivery after topical instillation of brimonidine. The images obtained using matrix-assisted laser desorption/ionization imaging mass spectrometry suggest that the distribution of brimonidine to the posterior ocular region is distributed through the uveal-scleral pathway [47]. Additionally, we previously demonstrated that the use of 0.1% brimonidine ophthalmic solution did not result in a significant difference in the concentrations of brimonidine between phakic and pseudophakic vitreous samples [33]. These results support the hypothesis that brimonidine diffusion from the posterior periocular tissues to the vitreous chamber contributes to the neuroprotective effect of brimonidine ophthalmic solution in clinical trials [31]. Patients had been using eye drops other than Ailamide® (Senju Pharmaceutical Co., Ltd.) The 10 min or longer interval between Ailamide® (Senju Pharmaceutical Co., Ltd.) and another eye drop instillations was designed in the present study. Therefore, the possibility that brimonidine distribution in ocular tissues might be affected by another eye drop seemed to be minimized in this study.

To be deemed neuroprotective for retinal ganglion cells, the drug must meet the following four criteria: (1) receptors on its target tissues, such as the optic nerve or retina, (2) adequate penetration into the vitreous or retina at pharmacologic levels, (3) induction of intracellular changes that enhance neuronal resistance to insult or interrupt apoptosis in animal models, and (4) demonstration of similar efficacy in clinical trials [43]. As for the distribution of α2 receptors to which brimonidine binds, several studies using animal and human tissues showed the presence of α2 receptors in the retina and optic nerve head [48,49]. As for induction of intracellular changes, in vitro and in vivo experiments demonstrated that activation of α2 receptors by brimonidine upregulates the intrinsic cell survival signaling pathway and antiapoptotic genes including Bcl-2 and BCL-X_L [30]. Furthermore, many animal experimental models have shown that brimonidine offers neuroprotection in several types of ocular injuries, including retinal ischemia [50–54], optic nerve crush [29,55], photoreceptor degeneration [56], and ocular hypertension and glaucoma [57,58]. As for the demonstration of similar efficacy in clinical trials, clinical trials using brimonidine ophthalmic solution for patients with open-angle glaucoma [31,32] have shown that brimonidine attenuates the further progression of visual field loss rather than ß-blocker, as described above. Because our present study has shown that topical administration of Ailamide® (Senju Pharmaceutical Co., Ltd.) delivered a concentration of brimonidine > 2 nM into the vitreous, it is possible that the fixed-combination ophthalmic suspension might also meet the four neuroprotective criteria.

The present study had several limitations. Firstly, we could not conclude whether brinzolamide in the vitreous humor following topical treatment with Ailamide® (Senju Pharmaceutical Co., Ltd.) affects the posterior retina. Brinzolamide inhibits the carbonic anhydrase type II isozyme (CA-II) in the ciliary body, thereby reducing the production of aqueous humor [38]. Moreover, some clinical studies have reported that topical instillation of brinzolamide improves cystoid macular edema in uveitic eyes [59] and retinal blood circulation [60]. In the present study, the mean concentration of brinzolamide in vitreous humor was 8.96 nM; of note, this concentration was higher than the IC_{50} (3.2 nM) required for the inhibition of CA-II in the ciliary body [38]. Further in vitro and in vivo experimental studies are required to determine the optimal concentration of brinzolamide for inhibiting CA-II in the retina. Secondly, one patient had extremely high concentrations of brimonidine and brinzolamide in the aqueous humor, although the concentrations of these drugs in the vitreous humor were low. Corneal epithelial defects affect the penetration of ophthalmic solutions into the cornea [61]. However, underlying ocular disorders were not identified in these patients. Moreover, as the adherence in this study was self-reported, the high concentrations detected in the aqueous humor might have been related to overdose. Multicenter clinical study would be required to obtain further samples to evaluate drug concentrations of glaucoma vitreous.

5. Conclusions

Twice-daily topical instillation of a fixed-combination ophthalmic suspension containing 0.1% brimonidine tartrate and 1% brinzolamide for 7 days resulted in a concentration of brimonidine > 2 nM in all vitreous samples. However, there was no significant correlation observed between the concentrations of brimonidine in the vitreous and aqueous humor samples. Thus, another pathway to the vitreous chamber, different from the pathway to the aqueous humor, may be involved in the neuroprotective effects of brimonidine.

Supplementary Materials: The following supporting information can be downloaded at: https://www.mdpi.com/article/10.3390/jcm12134175/s1, Table S1: Patient data.

Author Contributions: Formal analysis, M.I. and Y.O.; data curation, M.I. and Y.O.; writing—original draft, Y.O. and M.I.; writing—review & editing, E.K., Y.Y., M.M., K.I., S.A. and A.M. All authors have read and agreed to the published version of the manuscript.

Funding: This study was supported by a grant from Senju Pharmaceutical Co., Ltd., Osaka, Japan.

Institutional Review Board Statement: The University of Fukui Certified Review Board approved this single-arm open-label interventional trial (approval code: CRB5180014, approval date: 19 October 2020) and adhered to the principles of the Declaration of Helsinki. All participants were informed of the protocol and any potential risks and advantages of the therapies prior to enrolment. All patients provided written informed consent. The Japan Registry of Clinical Trials received registration for this study (jRCT, ID jRCTs051200089; date of access and registration, 25 November 2020).

Informed Consent Statement: All patients involved in the study provided written informed consent for their participation and publication of this article.

Data Availability Statement: The data presented in this study are available in the Supplementary Materials (Table S1).

Acknowledgments: Senju Pharmaceutical Co., Ltd. conceived the study protocol, contributed to the measurement of drug concentration and the data analysis and interpretation.

Conflicts of Interest: E.K. and A.M. are employees of Senju Pharmaceutical Co., Ltd., Osaka, Japan. M.I. received financial support from Senju Pharmaceutical Co., Ltd., Osaka, Japan. The other authors declare that they have no conflict of interest.

References

1. Collaborative Normal-Tension Glaucoma Study Group. Comparison of glaucomatous progression between untreated patients with normal-tension glaucoma and patients with therapeutically reduced intraocular pressures. *Am. J. Ophthalmol.* **1998**, *126*, 487–497. [CrossRef] [PubMed]
2. Kass, M.A.; Heuer, D.K.; Higginbotham, E.J. The Ocular Hypertension Treatment Study: A randomized trial determines that topical ocular hypotensive medication delays or prevents the onset of primary open-angle glaucoma. *Arch. Ophthalmol.* **2002**, *120*, 701–713. [CrossRef] [PubMed]
3. Heiji, A.; Leske, M.C.; Bengtsson, B. Reduction of intraocular pressure and glaucoma progression: Results from the Early Manifest Glaucoma Trial. *Arch. Ophthalmol.* **2002**, *120*, 1268–1279.
4. Lusthaus, J.; Goldberg, I. Current management of glaucoma. *Med. J. Aust.* **2019**, *210*, 180–187. [CrossRef]
5. MacIver, S.; Stout, N.; Ricci, O. New considerations for the clinical efficacy of old and new topical glaucoma medications. *Clin. Exp. Optom.* **2021**, *104*, 350–366. [CrossRef]
6. Aihara, M. Prostanoid receptor agonists for glaucoma treatment. *Jpn. J. Ophthalmol.* **2021**, *65*, 581–590. [CrossRef]
7. Gandolfi, S.; Cimino, L. Beta-adrenergic antagonists in the treatment of glaucoma. *Eur. J. Ophthalmol.* **2001**, *11* (Suppl. S2), 63–66. [CrossRef]
8. Stoner, A.; Harris, A.; Oddone, F.; Belamkar, A.; Verçellin, A.C.V.; Shin, J.; Januleviciene, I.; Siesky, B. Topical carbonic anhydrase inhibitors and glaucoma in 2021: Where do we stand? *Br. J. Ophthalmol.* **2022**, *106*, 1332–1337. [CrossRef]
9. Oh, D.J.; Chen, J.L.; Vajaranant, T.S. Brimonidine tartrate for the treatment of glaucoma. *Expert Opin. Pharmacother.* **2019**, *20*, 115–122. [CrossRef]
10. Tanna, A.P.; Johnson, M. Rho Kinase Inhibitors as a Novel Treatment for Glaucoma and Ocular Hypertension. *Ophthalmology* **2018**, *125*, 1741–1756. [CrossRef]
11. Yen, C.-Y.; Chen, C.-C.M.; Tseng, P.-C. Role of pilocarpine use following laser peripheral iridotomy in eyes with refractory acute angle closure glaucoma: A case report and literature review. *Medicine* **2022**, *101*, e29245. [CrossRef] [PubMed]
12. Hara, H.; Ichikawa, M.; Oku, H.; Shimazawa, M.; Araie, M. Bunazosin, a Selective α1-Adrenoceptor Antagonist, as an Anti-glaucoma Drug: Effects on Ocular Circulation and Retinal Neuronal Damage. *Cardiovasc. Drug Rev.* **2005**, *23*, 43–56. [CrossRef] [PubMed]
13. Haria, M.; Spencer, C.M. Unoprostone (Isopropyl Unoprostone). *Drugs Aging* **1996**, *9*, 213–218, discussion 219–220. [CrossRef] [PubMed]

14. Kiuchi, Y.; Inoue, T.; Shoji, N.; Nakamura, M.; Tanito, M.; Inoue, K.; Ishida, K.; Kurimoto, Y.; Suzuki, Y.; Chin, S.; et al. The Japan Glaucoma Society guidelines for glaucoma 5th edition. *Jpn. J. Ophthalmol.* **2023**, *67*, 189–254. [CrossRef] [PubMed]
15. Li, T.; Lindsley, K.; Rouse, B.; Hong, H.; Shi, Q.; Friedman, D.S.; Wormald, R.; Dickersin, K. Comparative effectiveness of firstline medications for primary open-angle glaucoma: A systematic review and network meta-analysis. *Ophthalmology* **2016**, *123*, 129–140. [CrossRef]
16. Garway-Heath, D.F.; Crabb, D.P.; Bunce, C. Latanoprost for open-angle glaucoma (UKGTS): A randomised, multicentre, placebo-controlled trial. *Lancet* **2015**, *385*, 1295–1304. [CrossRef]
17. Bengtsson, B.; Heijl, A.; Johannesson, G.; Andersson-Geimer, S.; Aspberg, J.; Lindén, C. The Glaucoma Intensive Treatment Study (GITS), a randomized clinical trial: Design, methodology and baseline data. *Acta Ophthalmol.* **2018**, *96*, 557–566. [CrossRef]
18. Bengtsson, B.; Lindén, C.; Heijl, A.; Andersson-Geimer, S.; Aspberg, J.; Jóhannesson, G. The glaucoma intensive treatment study: Interim results from an ongoing longitudinal randomized clinical trial. *Acta Ophthalmol.* **2022**, *100*, e455–e462. [CrossRef]
19. Gray, T.A.; Orton, L.C.; Henson, D.; Harper, R.; Waterman, H. Interventions for improving adherence to ocular hypotensive therapy. *Cochrane Database Syst. Rev.* **2009**, *2*, CD006132. [CrossRef]
20. Fechtner, R.D.; Godfrey, D.G.; Budenz, D.; Stewart, J.A.; Stewart, W.C.; Jasek, M.C. Prevalence of Ocular Surface Complaints in Patients with Glaucoma Using Topical Intraocular Pressure-Lowering Medications. *Cornea* **2010**, *29*, 618–621. [CrossRef]
21. Fukuchi, T.; Wakai, K.; Suda, K.; Nakatsue, T.; Sawada, H.; Hara, J.; Ueda, J.; Tanaka, T.; Yamada, A.; Abe, H. Incidence, severity and factors related to drug-induced keratoepitheliopathy with glaucoma medications. *Clin. Ophthalmol.* **2010**, *4*, 203–209. [CrossRef] [PubMed]
22. Skalicky, S.E.; Goldberg, I.; McCluskey, P. Ocular Surface Disease and Quality of Life in Patients with Glaucoma. *Am. J. Ophthalmol.* **2012**, *153*, 1–9.e2. [CrossRef] [PubMed]
23. Djafari, F.; Lesk, M.R.; Harasymowycz, P.J.; Desjardins, D.; Lachaine, J. Determinants of Adherence to Glaucoma Medical Therapy in a Long-term Patient Population. *Eur. J. Gastroenterol. Hepatol.* **2009**, *18*, 238–243. [CrossRef] [PubMed]
24. Razeghinejad, M.R.; Sawchyn, A.K.; Katz, L.J. Fixed combinations of dorzolamide-timolol and brimonidine-timolol in the management of glaucoma. *Expert Opin. Pharmacother.* **2010**, *11*, 959–968. [CrossRef]
25. Seibold, L.K.; DeWitt, P.E.; Kroehl, M.E.; Kahook, M.Y. The 24-Hour Effects of Brinzolamide/Brimonidine Fixed Combination and Timolol on Intraocular Pressure and Ocular Perfusion Pressure. *J. Ocul. Pharmacol. Ther.* **2017**, *33*, 161–169. [CrossRef]
26. Burke, J.A.; Potter, D.E. Ocular effects of a relatively selective alpha 2 agonist (UK-14, 304–318) in cats, rabbits and monkeys. *Curr. Eye Res.* **1986**, *5*, 665–676. [CrossRef]
27. Lee, P.-Y.; Serle, J.B.; Podos, S.M.; Severin, C. Time course of the effect of UK 14304-18 (Brimonidine tartrate) on rabbit uveoscleral outflow. *Investig. Ophthalmol. Vis. Sci.* **1992**, *33*, 1118.
28. Lambert, W.S.; Ruiz, L.; Crish, S.D.; Wheeler, L.A.; Calkins, D.J. Brimonidine prevents axonal and somatic degeneration of retinal ganglion cell neurons. *Mol. Neurodegen.* **2011**, *6*, 4. [CrossRef]
29. Yoles, E.; Wheeler, L.A.; Schwartz, M. Alpha2-adrenoreceptor agonists are neuroprotective in a rat model of optic nerve degeneration. *Investig. Opthalmol. Vis. Sci.* **1999**, *40*, 65–73.
30. Wheeler, L.; WoldeMussie, E.; Lai, R. Role of Alpha-2 Agonists in Neuroprotection. *Surv. Ophthalmol.* **2003**, *48* (Suppl. S1), S47–S51. [CrossRef]
31. Krupin, T.; Liebmann, J.M.; Greenfield, D.S.; Ritch, R.; Gardiner, S. A Randomized Trial of Brimonidine Versus Timolol in Preserving Visual Function: Results From the Low-pressure Glaucoma Treatment Study. *Am. J. Ophthalmol.* **2011**, *151*, 671–681. [CrossRef] [PubMed]
32. Yokoyama, Y.; Kawasaki, R.; Takahashi, H.; Maekawa, S.; Tsuda, S.; Omodaka, K.; Nakazawa, T. Effects of Brimonidine and Timolol on the Progression of Visual Field Defects in Open-angle Glaucoma: A Single-center Randomized Trial. *J. Glaucoma* **2019**, *28*, 575–583. [CrossRef] [PubMed]
33. Takamura, Y.; Tomomatsu, T.; Matsumura, T.; Takihara, Y.; Kozai, S.; Arimura, S.; Yokota, S.; Inatani, M. Vitreous and aqueous concentrations of brimonidine following topical application of brimonidine tartrate 0.1% ophthalmic solution in humans. *J. Ocul. Pharmacol. Ther.* **2015**, *31*, 282–285. [CrossRef] [PubMed]
34. Kent, A.R.; King, L.; Bartholomew, L.R. Vitreous Concentration of Topically Applied Brimonidine-Purite 0.15%. *J. Ocul. Pharmacol. Ther.* **2006**, *22*, 242–246. [CrossRef] [PubMed]
35. Kent, A.R.; Nussdorf, J.D.; David, R.; Tyson, F.; Small, D.; Fellows, D. Vitreous concentration of topically applied brimonidine tartrate 0.2%. *Ophthalmology* **2001**, *108*, 784–787. [CrossRef] [PubMed]
36. Burke, J.; Schwartz, M. Preclinical evaluation of brimonidine. *Surv. Ophthalmol.* **1996**, *41* (Suppl. S1), S9–S18. [CrossRef]
37. Orii, Y.; Kunikane, E.; Yamada, Y.; Morioka, M.; Iwasaki, K.; Arimura, S.; Mizuno, A.; Inatani, M. Brimonidine and timolol concentrations in the human vitreous and aqueous humors after topical instillation of a 0.1% brimonidine tartrate and 0.5% timolol fixed-combination ophthalmic solution: An interventional study. *PLoS ONE* **2022**, *17*, e0277313. [CrossRef]
38. DeSantis, L. Preclinical Overview of Brinzolamide. *Surv. Ophthalmol.* **2000**, *44* (Suppl. S2), S119–S129. [CrossRef]
39. Katz, L.J. Twelve-Month Evaluation of Brimonidine-Purite Versus Brimonidine in Patients with Glaucoma or Ocular Hypertension. *Eur. J. Gastroenterol. Hepatol.* **2002**, *11*, 119–126. [CrossRef]
40. Adkins, J.C.; Balfour, J.A. Brimonidine. A review of its pharmacological properties and clinical potential in the management of open-angle glaucoma and ocular hypertension. *Drugs Aging* **1998**, *12*, 225–241. [CrossRef]

41. Maruyama, Y.; Ikeda, Y.; Yokoi, N.; Mori, K.; Kato, H.; Ueno, M.; Kinoshita, S.; Sotozono, C. Severe Corneal Disorders Developed After Brimonidine Tartrate Ophthalmic Solution Use. *Cornea* **2017**, *36*, 1567–1569. [CrossRef] [PubMed]
42. Cimolai, N. A review of neuropsychiatric adverse events from topical ophthalmic brimonidine. *Hum. Exp. Toxicol.* **2020**, *39*, 1279–1290. [CrossRef] [PubMed]
43. Saylor, M.; McLoon, L.K.; Harrison, A.R.; Lee, M.S. Experimental and Clinical Evidence for Brimonidine as an Optic Nerve and Retinal Neuroprotective Agent: An Evidence-Based Review. *Arch. Ophthalmol.* **2009**, *127*, 402–406. [CrossRef] [PubMed]
44. Suzuki, G.; Kunikane, E.; Shigemi, W.; Shinno, K.; Kozai, S.; Kurata, M.; Kawamura, A. Ocular and systemic pharmacokinetics of brimonidine and brinzolamide after topical administration in rabbits: Comparison between fixed-combination and single-drug formulations. *Curr. Eye Res.* **2021**, *46*, 380–386. [CrossRef]
45. Mizuno, K.; Koide, T.; Shimada, S.; Mori, J.; Sawanobori, K.; Araie, M. Route of Penetration of Topically Instilled Nipradilol into the Ipsilateral Posterior Retina. *Investig. Opthalmol. Vis. Sci.* **2009**, *50*, 2839–2847. [CrossRef] [PubMed]
46. Mizuno, K.; Koide, T.; Saito, N.; Fujii, M.; Nagahara, M.; Tomidokoro, A.; Tamaki, Y.; Araie, M. Topical nipradilol: Effects on optic nerve head circulation in humans and periocular distribution in monkeys. *Investig. Opthalmol. Vis. Sci.* **2002**, *43*, 3243–3250.
47. Grove, K.J.; Kansara, V.; Prentiss, M.; Long, D.; Mogi, M.; Kim, S.; Rudewicz, P.J. Application of Imaging Mass Spectrometry to Assess Ocular Drug Transit. *SLAS Discov. Adv. Sci. Drug Discov.* **2017**, *22*, 1239–1245. [CrossRef]
48. Kalapesi, F.B.; Coroneo, M.T.; Hill, M.A. Human ganglion cells express the alpha-2 adrenergic receptor: Relevance to neuroprotection. *Br. J. Ophthalmol.* **2005**, *89*, 758–763. [CrossRef]
49. Woldemussie, E.; Wijono, M.; Pow, D. Localization of alpha 2 receptors in ocular tissues. *Vis. Neurosci.* **2007**, *24*, 745–756. [CrossRef]
50. Aktas, Z.; Gürelik, G.; Akyürek, N. Neuroprotective effect of topically applied brimonidine tartrate 0.2% in endothelin-1-induced optic nerve ischaemia model. *Clin. Exp. Ophthalmol.* **2007**, *35*, 527–534. [CrossRef]
51. Wheeler, L.; Lai, R.; WoldeMussie, E. From the Lab to the Clinic: Activation of an Alpha-2 agonist Pathway is Neuroprotective in Models of Retinal and Optic Nerve Injury. *Eur. J. Ophthalmol.* **1999**, *9*, S17–S21. [CrossRef] [PubMed]
52. Lafuente, M.P.; Villegas-Pérez, M.P.; Sobrado-Calvo, P.; García-Avilés, A.; De Imperial, J.M.; Vidal-Sanz, M. Neuroprotective effects of alpha(2)-selective adrenergic agonists against ischemia-induced retinal ganglion cell death. *Investig. Opthalmol. Vis. Sci.* **2001**, *42*, 2074–2084.
53. Danylkova, N.O.; Alcala, S.R.; Pomeranz, H.D. Neuroprotective effects of brimonidine treatment in a rodent model of ischemic optic neuropathy. *Exp. Eye Res.* **2007**, *84*, 293–301. [CrossRef] [PubMed]
54. Conti, F.; Romano, G.L.; Eandi, C.M.; Toro, M.D.; Rejdak, R.; Di Benedetto, G.; Lazzara, F.; Bernardini, R.; Drago, F.; Cantarella, G.; et al. Brimonidine is Neuroprotective in Animal Paradigm of Retinal Ganglion Cell Damage. *Front. Pharmacol.* **2021**, *12*, 705405. [CrossRef]
55. Levkovitch-Verbin, H.; Harris-Cerruti, C.; Groner, Y.; Wheeler, L.A.; Schwartz, M.; Yoles, E. RGC death in mice after optic nerve crush injury: Oxidative stress and neuroprotection. *Investig. Opthalmol. Vis. Sci.* **2000**, *41*, 4169–4174.
56. Wen, R.; Cheng, T.; Li, Y. Alpha 2-adrenergic agonists induce basic fibroblast growth factor expression in photoreceptors in vivo and ameliorate light damage. *J. Neurosci.* **1996**, *16*, 5986–5992. [CrossRef]
57. Hernández, M.; Urcola, J.H.; Vecino, E. Retinal ganglion cell neuroprotection in a rat model of glaucoma following brimonidine, latanoprost or combined treatments. *Exp. Eye Res.* **2008**, *86*, 798–806. [CrossRef]
58. WoldeMussie, E.; Ruiz, G.; Wijono, M.; Wheeler, L.A. Neuroprotection of retinal ganglion cells by brimonidine in rats with laser-induced chronic ocular hypertension. *Investig. Opthalmol. Vis. Sci.* **2001**, *42*, 2849–2855.
59. Bakthavatchalam, M.; Lai, F.H.; Rong, S.S.; Ng, D.S.; Brelen, M.E. Treatment of cystoid macular edema secondary to retinitis pigmentosa: A systematic review. *Surv. Ophthalmol.* **2018**, *63*, 329–339. [CrossRef]
60. Siesky, B.; Harris, A.; Brizendine, E.; Marques, C.; Loh, J.; Mackey, J.; Overton, J.; Netland, P. Literature Review and Meta-Analysis of Topical Carbonic Anhydrase Inhibitors and Ocular Blood Flow. *Surv. Ophthalmol.* **2009**, *54*, 33–46. [CrossRef]
61. Moiseev, R.V.; Morrison, P.W.J.; Steele, F.; Khutoryanskiy, V.V. Penetration Enhancers in Ocular Drug Delivery. *Pharmaceutics* **2019**, *11*, 321. [CrossRef] [PubMed]

Disclaimer/Publisher's Note: The statements, opinions and data contained in all publications are solely those of the individual author(s) and contributor(s) and not of MDPI and/or the editor(s). MDPI and/or the editor(s) disclaim responsibility for any injury to people or property resulting from any ideas, methods, instructions or products referred to in the content.

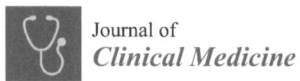

Article

Retinal Ganglion Cell Function and Perfusion following Intraocular Pressure Reduction with Preservative-Free Latanoprost in Patients with Glaucoma and Ocular Hypertension

Qëndresë Daka [1,2], Maja Sustar Habjan [2], Andrej Meglič [2], Darko Perovšek [2], Makedonka Atanasovska Velkovska [2] and Barbara Cvenkel [2,3,*]

1. Department of Pathophysiology, Medical Faculty, University of Prishtina, 10000 Prishtina, Kosovo
2. Department of Ophthalmology, University Medical Centre Ljubljana, 1000 Ljubljana, Slovenia; sustar.majchi@gmail.com (M.S.H.)
3. Faculty of Medicine, University of Ljubljana, 1000 Ljubljana, Slovenia
* Correspondence: barbara.cvenkel@gmail.com

Abstract: (1) **Background**: Given the global prevalence of glaucoma and the crucial role of intraocular pressure (IOP) reduction in the management of the disease, understanding the immediate effects on retinal structure and function is essential. (2) **Methods**: This study aimed to assess the effects of preservative-free latanoprost on morphological and functional parameters in treatment-naïve patients with ocular hypertension and open-angle glaucoma. (3) **Results**: This study showed a significant reduction in IOP by an average of 30.6% after treatment with preservative-free latanoprost. Despite the significant reduction in IOP, no statistically significant changes were observed in the electroretinogram (ERG) nor the optical coherence tomography/angiography (OCT/OCTA) parameters compared to baseline. An exploration of the correlation between IOP changes and various parameters revealed a significant association solely with the macular IPL/INL plexus vessel density (VD) measured with OCTA. (4) **Conclusions**: This finding suggests a possible association between IOP reduction and changes in the macular microcirculation and provides valuable insights into the differential effects of latanoprost. Acknowledging the study limitations, this study emphasizes the need for larger, longer-term investigations to comprehensively assess the sustained effects of preservative-free latanoprost on both IOP and retinal parameters. In addition, exploring systemic factors and conducting subgroup analyses could improve personalized approaches to glaucoma treatment.

Keywords: retinal ganglion cell; preservative-free latanoprost; electroretinogram; optical coherence tomography; optical coherence tomography angiography

Citation: Daka, Q.; Sustar Habjan, M.; Meglič, A.; Perovšek, D.; Atanasovska Velkovska, M.; Cvenkel, B. Retinal Ganglion Cell Function and Perfusion following Intraocular Pressure Reduction with Preservative-Free Latanoprost in Patients with Glaucoma and Ocular Hypertension. *J. Clin. Med.* **2024**, *13*, 1226. https://doi.org/10.3390/jcm13051226

Academic Editor: Atsushi Mizota

Received: 18 January 2024
Revised: 13 February 2024
Accepted: 19 February 2024
Published: 21 February 2024

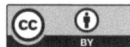

Copyright: © 2024 by the authors. Licensee MDPI, Basel, Switzerland. This article is an open access article distributed under the terms and conditions of the Creative Commons Attribution (CC BY) license (https://creativecommons.org/licenses/by/4.0/).

1. Introduction

Glaucoma, the leading cause of irreversible blindness worldwide, comprises a group of optic neuropathies characterized by the loss of retinal ganglion cells (RGCs). It is estimated that 112 million people will be affected by this disease by 2040, with open-angle glaucoma being the most common form [1–5].

The exact pathophysiology of glaucoma is still unknown as several risk factors and interacting processes have been described. However, it has been shown that only a reduction in elevated intraocular pressure (IOP) can successfully delay the onset and progression of the disease by preventing the loss of RGCs [6–13].

The clinical evaluation of glaucoma requires a thorough eye examination, but an assessment of optic nerve head (ONH) and retinal nerve fiber layer (RNFL) as well as visual field (VF) remain the cornerstone of glaucoma diagnosis and the most important parameters for monitoring disease progression and treatment efficacy [5,8,14]. However, these examinations remain largely subjective.

Optical coherence tomography angiography (OCTA), which has emerged as a non-invasive technique for imaging the microcirculation in the retina and choroid, is increasingly being used in glaucoma. It has been reported to be a useful tool for the assessment of optic disc and macular vessel density (VD) in retinal and choroidal slabs—biomarkers thought to be altered by disease [15]. Correlation of OCTA with structural and functional parameters is noted, while the quantitative data from OCTA appears to be useful for monitoring disease progression. Although OCTA has acceptable test–retest variability, it may have segmentation errors in the retinal layers as fixed boundaries are assigned to the slabs, while its parameters are associated with disease, individual, and eye-specific factors [15–18].

Electroretinography (ERG), which is not routinely used in clinical practice, provides objective information of the RGC function. Although RCGs are affected in patients with glaucoma before the appearance of subjective VF defects [19,20], they are not currently part of objective testing. Studies suggest that damaged RCGs can enter a dysfunctional state prior to apoptosis and can partially recover under certain conditions [21]. Therefore, the ERG has become an important tool to evaluate the effect of different treatments for glaucoma, as both the pattern ERG (PERG) and the photopic negative response (PhNR) are sensitive markers of RGC dysfunction, which is characteristic of glaucoma. The PERG is a measure of the electrical activity of the RGC population of the central retina (more than 40% of the total RGC population), whereas the PhNR reflects generalized activity of the RGCs and their axons [21–26].

Currently, the therapeutic goal in glaucoma is to prevent visual impairment by slowing the apoptosis of RGCs by lowering IOP. The treatment of first choice according to the guidelines is the prostaglandin analogue [14], one of the first in this class being latanoprost. Preservative-free latanoprost, which has fewer adverse effects and is thought to be tolerated better, has been introduced on the market [27,28]. However, data on the short-term effects on RGC function and perfusion are lacking.

While it is known that ERG responses vary depending on the level of IOP, the data on changes in OCTA parameters are still uncertain [23,24]. Knowledge of the effects of preservative-free latanoprost on ocular blood flow, a possible mechanism responsible for the development and progression of glaucoma, and on the RGC function may help to better understand the pathophysiology of the disease and treatment strategies. To our knowledge, this relationship has not yet been investigated, although OCTA and ERG are reasonable examinations to elucidate this relationship through an evaluation. Therefore, the aim of this study was to determine the changes and assess the relationship between the changes in macular vessel density (VD) in OCTA and the function of RGCs in ERG responses of patients with ocular hypertension (OHT) and primary open-angle glaucoma (POAG) 3 months after the initiation of IOP-lowering treatment with preservative-free latanoprost.

2. Materials and Methods

This prospective cohort intervention study was conducted in accordance with the ethical standards of the Declaration of Helsinki. The research protocol was approved by the National Ethics Committee, University Medical Centre Ljubljana, Ljubljana, Slovenia (KME 33/11/11). All patients signed a consent form after being informed about the aim of this study. This study took place from March 2022 to December 2022. The clinical examinations were performed at the Glaucoma Unit, while the electrophysiological examinations were completed at the Laboratory of Visual Electrophysiology Diagnostics, Department of Ophthalmology, University Medical Centre Ljubljana.

2.1. Population

A consecutive sample of newly diagnosed POAG and high-risk patients with OHT, as defined by the European Glaucoma Society (EGS) guidelines, were considered for inclusion. To be included in this study, the following inclusion criteria had to be met: 40 years or older; best-corrected visual acuity (BCVA) ≥ 0.8 Snellen; the spherical equivalent of <5 D; cylindrical refractive error of <2 D; clear optical media; characteristic ONH changes and/or corresponding reproducible VF defects (false-positive errors < 20%, false-negative errors < 20%); early (mean defect (MD) < 6 dB) or moderate (MD 6–12 dB) glaucoma, based on the Hodapp–Parrish–Anderson (HPA) criteria; and high untreated IOP (>21 mmHg) at baseline. The diagnosis was confirmed by two glaucoma specialists, and the MD was used as a summary measure of VF. One eye per patient was randomly selected if both eyes had the same IOP; otherwise, the eye with the higher IOP at baseline was included in the statistical analysis.

Patients with primary and secondary angle-closure glaucoma, congenital and juvenile glaucoma, and those already treated with IOP-lowering modalities were not included. In addition, patients with existing retinal, macular, or other optic nerve disorders and any type of eye surgery other than uncomplicated cataract surgery as well as patients with systemic diseases affecting retinal function were excluded.

2.2. Clinical Examination

Patients' demographic and medical history were collected, while a complete eye examination for glaucoma was performed before and three months after the start of IOP-lowering treatment including Snellen's eye chart examination for BCVA; slit lamp biomicroscopy, gonioscopy, tonometry, and fundus examination after pupil dilation with 1% tropicamide (GAT-Haag-Streit BQ900 GAT, Koeniz-Berne, Switzerland); central corneal thickness (CCT) measurement (Pachmate-DGH, Tehnology Inc., Exton, PA, USA); and standard automated perimetry (SAP) with G program, dynamic strategy for diagnosis (Octopus 900 perimeter, Haag-Streit AG, Koeniz-Berne, Switzerland). Subjects were scheduled for ERG and OCT/OCTA testing within one week.

2.3. Electroretinography

The clinical ERG testing was performed following the standards and guidelines of the International Society for Clinical Electrophysiology of Vision (ISCEV) [29,30] using the Espion visual electrophysiology testing system (Diagnosys LLC, Littleton, MA, USA). The PERG was recorded first without pupil dilation and by displaying a 0.8 checkerboard pattern with 99% contrast, reversing 4 times per second, on a $21.6° \times 27.8°$ cathode ray tube screen stimulator. Patients were positioned 70 cm from the screen stimulator with optimal refractive correction. One hundred sweeps were collected for each recording and repeated at least twice. The signals were amplified and band-pass-filtered between 0.625 and 100 Hz. The average of the two most repeatable or all three repeat recordings (from 180 to 250 sweeps) was used for further analysis. Later, the pupils were dilated with 1% tropicamide (Mydriacyl, Alcon, Geneva, Switzerland) and adapted to light for 10 min. Photopic ERGs were elicited with a Ganzfeld ColorDome flash stimulator (Diagnosys LLC, Littleton, MA, USA) using 2.5 cd s/m^2 monochromatic red stimuli (635 nm) on a 10 cd/m^2 blue background (470 nm). The rate of the stimuli was 1 Hz, and 30 sweeps were collected for each recording, repeated at least three times. The signals were amplified and band-pass-filtered between 0.17 and 300 Hz. The average of the two most repeatable or all three repeat recordings (from 50 to 80 sweeps) was used for further analysis.

2.4. OCT/OCTA

Images of the macular region were obtained using a 100 kHz scanning speed and 1050 nm Swept-Source (SS) OCT/OCTA device (DRI OCT Triton™; Topcon Inc., Tokyo, Japan) over pupils dilated with 1% tropicamide (Mydriacyl, Alcon). The device uses OCTARA™ image processing technology, which extracts the signal changes derived from vascular flow using multiple OCT B-scans acquired at the same position. The OCT/OCTA parameters were generated using the latest integrated software (IMAGEnet6), which reduces motion artefacts and improves detection sensitivity analysis and image storage.

The scanning protocols for OCT were as follows: 7×7 mm^2 area for the macula, centered on the fovea, and 6×6 mm^2 for the RNFL, centered on the ONH; while for the

OCTA, only a 6 × 6 mm² area was used for the macular area, centered on the fovea. Only scans with an image quality of >50 were accepted.

The integrated software was used to derive parameters of interest from the segmentation of the slabs and export them for analysis with the manufacturer's automatic segmentation algorithm. The algorithm used for OCTA parameters automatically segmented the superficial slab 2.6 μm below the internal limiting membrane (ILM) to 15.6 μm below the inner plexiform layer (IPL), whereas vessel density (VD) was defined as the percentage of vessel area with blood flow out of the total measured area and determined by adaptive thresholding binarization. Identification was performed using an ETDRS grid overlay.

2.5. Outcomes

The following outcomes were used for comparison: IOP change (mean, absolute); PERG—the P50 amplitude (measured from the N35 trough), the N95 amplitude (measured from the P50 peak), and the N95/P50 amplitude ratio; PhNR amplitude (measured from the baseline to the negative trough that clearly appeared after the b-wave and the i-wave); the PhNR amplitude ratio (PhNR/b-wave); OCT-average RNFL thickness from the peripapillary ONH (pRNFL) and macular (mRNFL) scans, and the ganglion cell layer (GCL)–inner plexiform layer (IPL) (GCL+) and RNFL+GCL+(GCL++) from the macular scans; OCTA-average macular VD for the RNFL/GCL plexus, the superficial vascular plexus (GCL/IPL plexus), and the IPL/INL plexus.

2.6. Statistical Analysis

All statistical analyses were performed with IBM SPSS Statistics Version 28.0 (IBM Corporation, Armonk, NY, USA). Quantitative data are described as mean (standard deviation) and percentage in continuous and numerical data. Normality of distributions for dependent variables was tested using the Shapiro–Wilk test. The two-tailed paired t-test was used to compare the changes in IOP, OCT, OCTA, and ERG measurements from baseline to month 3 post-therapy for all patients, with a p value < 0.05 considered statistically significant.

Pearson's correlation was used to determine the relationship between changes in IOP and changes in OCT/OCTA and ERG measurements 3 months after starting treatment with preservative-free latanoprost.

3. Results

Eleven eyes of eleven participants were included in this study. After baseline examinations, seven eyes were categorized as OHT, one as suspected glaucoma, one as mild POAG, and two as moderate POAG according to the HPA criteria. Six of the eleven patients (55%) were male. Mean age was 64.7 years (SD 11.2; range, 51–82 years), central corneal thickness was 580 μm (SD 30.2; range, 536–628 μm), mean baseline IOP was 24.6 mmHg (SD 3.8; range, 21–34 mmHg) with an average mean defect (MD) on Octopus perimetry of 2.8 dB (SD 3.2; range, 0–9.4 dB), and the square root of loss variance (sLV) of 4.0 dB (SD 2.2; range, 1.5–8.1 dB). The characteristics of the participants and the OCT/OCTA and ERG measurements at baseline are shown in Table 1.

Table 1. Clinical characteristics of participants at baseline.

No	Diagnosis	Eye	Age (Years)	Sex	BCVA Snellen	Systemic Diseases	CCT (μm)	IOP mmHg	VF MD (dB)	VF sLV (dB)
1	POAG	RE	59	F	1.0	AH GC	536	23	7	4.8
2	OHT	LE	59	M	1.0	DM AH HLD	620	25	2	5.6
3	OHT	LE	78	F	0.8	AH HLD OP	582	21	3.2	5.2
4	POAG	LE	71	F	0.8	BC HLD	589	21	4.4	2.8
5	OHT	RE	45	M	1.0	/	585	34	0.4	2.3
6	OHT	LE	66	M	1.0	/	588	22	0.6	3.4

Table 1. Cont.

No	Diagnosis	Eye	Age (Years)	Sex	BCVA Snellen	Systemic Diseases	CCT (μm)	IOP mmHg	VF MD (dB)	VF sLV (dB)
7	OHT	LE	76	F	1.0	OP	628	24	2.1	6.6
8	SUSPECT	RE	52	M	1.0	OSP CAT	541	27	0.4	1.5
9	OHT	RE	67	F	1.0	DM HLD COPD	584	24	0	2.2
10	POAG	RE	82	M	0.9	AH BPH DD	554	23	9.4	8.1
11	OHT	RE	45	M	1.0	/	524	25	1.9	3.0

POAG = primary open-angle glaucoma; OHT = ocular hypertension; SUSPECT = primary open-angle glaucoma suspect; RE = right eye; LE = left eye; M = male; F = female; AH = arterial hypertension; GC = gastric cancer; DM = diabetes mellitus; HLD = hyperlipidemia; OP = osteoporosis; BC = breast cancer; OSP = obstructive sleep apnea; CAT = cataract; DD = depressive disorder; BPH = benign prostatic hyperplasia; COPD = chronic obstructive pulmonary disease.

The changes in IOP, OCT/OCTA, and ERG measurements 3 months after starting IOP-lowering treatment with preservative-free latanoprost are summarized in Tables 2 and 3. Three months after starting treatment, there was a statistically significant mean reduction in IOP of 30.6% (mean 7.5 mmHg; range 5.3–9.6 mmHg; $p < 0.001$) compared to baseline IOP (Table 3).

Table 2. IOP, OCT/OCTA, and ERG measurements before (baseline) and 3 months after IOP-lowering therapy.

Case		IOP (mmHg)	OCT				OCTA			ERG				
			pRNFL	mRNFL	GCL+	GCL++	RNFL/GCL	GCL/IPL	IPL/INL	P50	N95	N95/P50	PhNR	PhNR Ratio
1	baseline	23	65	24	53	77	22.86	25.74	34.35	4.97	5.22	1.06	17.05	0.33
	3 months	16	65	29	52	81	26.57	28.12	35.52	5.15	5.20	1.01	21.8	0.36
2	baseline	25	88	30	55	85	18.97	21.86	27.43	6.57	9.27	1.41	28.68	0.42
	3 months	19	90	30	56	86	19.16	21.65	25.51	6.24	8.17	1.31	28.19	0.42
3	baseline	21	102	44	64	108	17.45	20.96	26.55	4.84	6.38	1.32	17.29	0.33
	3 months	16	104	46	65	111	15.45	18.48	22.77	8.93	11.73	1.31	17.30	0.31
4	baseline	21	93	33	60	93	33.49	37.74	50.84	4.59	6.45	1.41	28.17	0.32
	3 months	14	93	34	60	94	29.87	34.06	44.50	4.06	5.96	1.47	24.21	0.31
5	baseline	34	112	45	73	119	26.00	30.95	36.51	7.93	9.26	1.17	24.9	0.34
	3 months	18	110	44	73	116	26.73	32.02	40.32	8.68	10.95	1.26	30.72	0.37
6	baseline	22	103	36	68	105	25.13	29.74	35.33	4.78	7.25	1.52	29.25	0.35
	3 months	15	103	37	68	105	26.61	29.83	35.74	4.63	6.97	1.51	27.98	0.36
7	baseline	24	118	44	70	114	17.10	20.66	26.61	4.79	7.64	1.59	18.26	0.24
	3 months	18	117	44	70	114	16.35	18.61	21.99	5.75	8.41	1.46	20.1	0.24
8	baseline	27	95	37	56	93	24.21	27.9	30.85	4.94	6.24	1.26	30.75	0.54
	3 months	18	100	38	58	97	24.64	28.60	30.05	5.77	8.29	1.44	17.77	0.22
9	baseline	24	108	40	63	102	15.39	18.68	23.65	5.40	8.6	1.59	25.41	0.32
	3 months	19	105	41	63	104	16.83	20.32	22.98	6.14	9.35	1.52	24.92	0.25
10	baseline	23	59	18	59	78	19.52	23.42	34.08	2.79	3.09	1.11	5.55	0.18
	3 months	15	60	20	59	79	22.43	25.84	31.69	1.54	1.68	1.09	9.62	0.33
11	baseline	25	89	38	58	96	19.50	22.55	21.52	4.02	7.01	1.74	23.95	0.51
	3 months	15	89	39	58	97	18.48	22.96	28.89	4.30	6.98	1.62	25.92	0.53

IOP = intraocular pressure; OCT = optical coherence tomography; OCTA = optical coherence tomography angiography; ERG = electroretinography; pRNFL = peripapillary retinal nerve fiber layer thickness; mRNFL = macular retinal nerve fiber layer thickness; GCL = macular ganglion cell layer; GCL+ = macular ganglion cell–inner plexiform layer thickness; GCL++ = RNFL + GCL + thickness; IPL = inner plexiform layer; INL = inner nuclear layer.

There were no significant changes in mean values of the OCT and OCTA parameters compared to baseline (Table 3). Similarly, there were no statistically significant changes in the mean values of the selected ERG parameters (Table 3). However, with the comparison of values of the individual subject (Table 2), some showed an improvement of either PhNR or N95 amplitudes after 3 months of treatment (as seen for cases 3, 4, and 5), while, in some subjects, there was inconsistent worsening of one ERG parameter and an improvement of another (cases 8 and 10).

Table 3. Changes in IOP, OCT/OCTA, and ERG measurements 3 months after starting IOP-lowering treatment.

Parameters	Pre-Treatment (SD)	Post-Treatment (SD)	Mean Change: 3 Months–Baseline (SD) (95% CI)	p Value *
IOP (mmHg)	24.5 (3.6)	17.0 (1.6)	−7.5 (3.3) (−9.6 to −5.3)	<0.001
OCT				
pRNFL (μm)	97.4 (15.1)	97.6 (14.4)	0.2 (2.2) (−1.4 to 1.8)	0.78
mRNFL (μm)	37.1 (6.7)	38.2 (6.7)	1.1 (1.6) (−0.4 to 2.2)	0.06
GCL+ (μm)	62.0 (6.8)	62.3 (6.7)	0.3 (0.3) (−0.3 to 0.9)	0.23
GCL++ (μm)	99.2 (12.9)	100.5 (11.7)	1.3 (2.1) (−0.21 to 2.8)	0.08
OCTA				
RNFL/GCL (VD)	21.8 (5.2)	22.1 ((5.1)	0.3 (2.1) (−1.1 to 1.7)	0.63
GCL/IP (VD)	25.5 (5.7)	25.5 (5.4)	0.03 (2.0) (−1.3 to 1.4)	0.97
IPL/INL (VD)	31.6 (8.1)	30.9 (7.5)	−0.7 (3.9) (−2.3 to 1.9)	0.56
ERG				
P50 (μV)	5.1 (1.3)	5.6 (2.1)	0.51 (1.4) (−0.4 to 1.4)	0.25
N95 (μV)	6.9 (1.8)	7.6 (2.8)	0.7 (1.9) (−0.6 to 1.9)	0.27
N95/P50	1.4 (0.2)	1.4 (0.2)	−0.02 (0.1) (−0.1 to 0.05)	0.58
PhNR (μV)	22.7 (7.5)	22.6 (6.1)	−0.1 (5.2) (−3.5 to 3.4)	0.97
PhNR ratio	0.4 (0.1)	0.3 (0.1)	−0.02 (0.1) (−0.1 to 0.1)	0.64

* Paired t-test; IOP = intraocular pressure; OCT = optical coherence tomography; OCTA = optical coherence tomography angiography; ERG = electroretinography; pRNFL = peripapillary retinal nerve fiber layer thickness; mRNFL = macular retinal nerve fiber layer thickness; GCL = macular ganglion cell layer; GCL+ = macular ganglion cell–inner plexiform layer thickness; GCL++ = RNFL + GCL + thickness; IPL = inner plexiform layer; INL = inner nuclear layer.

The correlation between the changes in IOP and the changes in OCT/OCTA and ERG measurements 3 months after the start of treatment is shown in Table 4 and Figure 1. The correlation was significant only for the VD OCTA IPL/INL plexus ($p = 0.03$). The VD in the IPL/INL plexus increased only in four patients, an only slightly in two patients, while in another two patients—cases 5 and 11—with greater IOP-lowering treatment, the increase in VD was 3.8 and 7.4%, respectively. In seven patients with an IOP reduction between 5 and 9 mmHg, there was a decrease in VD in the IPL/INL plexus (Table 4 and Figure 1).

Table 4. Pearson's correlation between changes in IOP and changes in OCT/OCTA and ERG measurements 3 months after starting IOP-lowering treatment.

Change from Baseline Values		IOP Change from Baseline (mmHg)
OCT pRNFL (μm)	Pearson's correlation	0.10
	P	0.79
OCT mRNFL (μm)	Pearson's correlation	0.39
	P	0.26
OCT GCL+ (μm)	Pearson's correlation	0.05
	P	0.90
OCT GCL++ (μm)	Pearson's correlation	0.59
	P	0.07
OCTA RNFL/GCL (VD)	Pearson's correlation	−0.03
	P	0.92
OCTA GCL/IPL (VD)	Pearson's correlation	−0.23
	P	0.50
OCTA IPL/INL (VD)	Pearson's correlation	−0.67
	P	0.03
PERG P50 (μV)	Pearson's correlation	0.12
	P	0.97
PERG N95 (μV)	Pearson's correlation	−0.12
	P	0.73
PhNR (μV)	Pearson's correlation	−0.17
	P	0.62

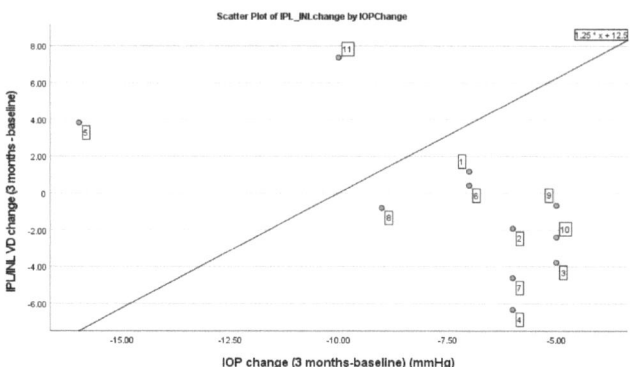

Figure 1. Scatterplot of VD change in OCTA IPL/INL by change in IOP from baseline values.

4. Discussion

In our study, we investigated the response to treatment with preservative-free latanoprost in treatment-naïve patients with POAG, suspected glaucoma, and OHT, as well as the changes associated with the reduction in IOP 3 months after the start of treatment using morphological (OCT/OCTA) and functional measurements (ERG). The efficacy of prostaglandin analogues in lowering IOP has already been emphasized in the EGS guidelines. However, with our study, we aimed to contribute to the existing evidence by focusing on the effects of prostaglandin analogues on retinal parameters, an aspect that could have broader implications for glaucoma management beyond the lowering of IOP. The significant mean reduction in IOP of 30.6% was not accompanied by statistically significant changes in ERG and OCT/OCTA parameters compared to baseline. Only the change in OCTA IPL/INL correlated significantly with the change in IOP.

Several studies have used OCTA to assess the changes in VD after lowering IOP [17,31–37]. Hollo [31] was the first to report a significant increase in peripapillary angioflow density at 2–4 weeks in six eyes of four young subjects after a large (more than 50%) decrease in IOP with topical medication. In a prospective study, an OCT/OCTA assessment was performed in 17 patients (33 eyes) with newly diagnosed early glaucoma before and 3 and 6 months after starting IOP-lowering medication [32]. Interestingly, in a subgroup of eyes with an IOP reduction of at least 20% (mean reduction 34%), a significant decrease in deep perifoveal VD was observed at 3 months compared to baseline. This was interpreted as a greater sensitivity to rapid IOP reduction with increased lability of the deep parafoveal tissue and caused a reduction in VD [32]. No changes were observed in other OCTA parameters. Gillmann and co-workers [33] measured the peripapillary and macular VD 2 and 6 months after selective laser trabeculoplasty in 21 patients with POAG. After 2 months, the mean IOP decreased by 15.4% (2.9 mmHg), with an increase in the parafoveal and perifoveal VD, which returned to near baseline after 6 months. These changes were independent of IOP, but the intensity of the signal strength had an effect on VD. After trabeculectomy, some studies [17,34–36] reported a significant increase in peripapillary and macular VD in open-angle and angle-closure glaucoma [37], which was associated with higher pre-operative IOP and greater IOP reduction [36], suggesting that ocular perfusion impairment may be improved via IOP reduction. The improvement in NFL-plexus capillary density occurred in areas with minimal RNFL thinning, in eyes with early glaucoma, which may have greater potential to restore perfusion [18], while eyes with advanced visual field loss after successful trabeculectomy had reduced peripapillary and macular VD, which may be relevant to the experience of deterioration after surgery [38,39]. Other studies found no changes in peripapillary and macular VD after a surgical reduction in IOP [40,41], while Ch'ng and co-workers [42] reported an increase in superficial foveal VD at 3 and 6 months post-operatively. A significant increase in VD was found in the deep ONH and was associated with a reduction in the curvature of the lamina cribrosa after surgically lowering IOP and not with the change in IOP [41].

In our study, two hypertensive eyes (cases 5 and 11; Figure 1) with the greatest reduction in IOP from baseline (18 and 10 mmHg, respectively) showed an increase in VD of the macular IPL/INL capillary plexus, two eyes showed a slight increase in VD, and seven eyes showed a decrease in macular VD from baseline. The reasons for the decrease in macular VD in these seven eyes despite a decrease in IOP are unclear. It would be useful to investigate the repeatability and reproducibility of our device and software in control subjects to determine whether a difference in OCTA parameter measurements in a given patient is clinically significant or within the accepted "noise" of the technology and the patient's daily physiological variation. Studies have shown good intra-session repeatability and good inter-session reproducibility of OCTA vessel parameter measurements in healthy and glaucomatous eyes using commercial software for OCTA devices [43–46]. The inter-session coefficient of repeatability is the best measure for this assessment as it represents the estimated range in which the difference between two repeated measurements for a given eye falls 95% of the time [43]. Vorperian et al. [46], using commercial software for macular VD parameters, reported the inter-session within-eye coefficient of repeatability of 1.349 (95% CI 1.173; 1.528) for non-glaucomatous eyes and 1.767 (95% CI 1.501; 2.029) for glaucomatous eyes. This means that the absolute difference between two measurements and between two sessions should not be greater than 1.349 for non-glaucomatous and 1.767 for glaucomatous eyes in 95% of cases [46]. In addition, there may be other factors that can directly affect the retinal microcirculation, such as caffeine consumption [47], nicotine [48], or level of physical activity [49]. A short-term increase in IOP of 10–15 mmHg for 1–2 h in a suspected occludable angle after laser peripheral iridotomy and dark room prone provocative test did not affect VD in the macula or ONH as examined with OCTA [50,51]. In contrast, a sudden increase in IOP of approximately 13 mmHg (50% increase from baseline) in healthy subjects using a suction cup resulted in a significant decrease in VD in the ONH and macular (superficial and deep) capillary plexus [52]. The differences in the results may be related to the amount of IOP change, the methods of lowering IOP, the age of the patients, and the extent of glaucomatous damage. The absence of changes in OCTA findings may reflect IOP-related autoregulation within a certain range of IOP change [51,53,54], which may be the case in our study with a moderate mean IOP reduction of 30.6% from baseline.

To evaluate the changes in function after lowering IOP, we used the PERG and the PhNR, which measure the integrity of the RGCs. Lowering IOP in eyes with OHT and early glaucoma was associated with an increase in PERG and PhNR amplitude, indicating an improvement in inner retinal function [55–60]. RGC dysfunction measured with PERG could be detected in suspected and mild glaucoma several years before the appearance of morphological changes measured with OCT [61]. Recently, PhNR was used to assess RGC function in patients with glaucoma and detected an improvement in inner retinal function after 12 weeks of oral nicotinamide supplementation compared to baseline [62]. Igawa and co-workers [63] showed an increase in PhNR amplitude in the first week after filtration surgery with a mean decrease in IOP of 50% from baseline, indicating rapid functional improvement. In our study, we found no significant changes in ERG parameters after lowering IOP. This could be due to the lowering of IOP too moderately and the higher variability of ERG measurements, which were found to be high compared to the morphological measurements with OCT, limiting the sensitivity of ERG in detecting changes. Inter-session variability/repeatability, calculated with a 95% limit of agreement, was within ±35.9% of the mean for PERG N95 amplitude and within 59.9% of the mean for PhNR [25], or even higher as reported by others [64,65]. In addition, the functional impairment of the RGCs must have been only very mild at baseline measurement, since in all but one patient (case 10) the baseline ERG amplitudes were within the normal range according to the laboratory reference range—so that a significant change after application of the treatment could not to be expected.

The limitations of our study should be discussed. Recognizing the limitations and addressing them in future research will contribute to a more comprehensive understanding of the effects of treatment and lead to improvements in glaucoma management strategies. This study represents a case series of 11 patients with a wide age range (51–82 years), and we recognize the need for further large studies over a longer period and with a larger sample size. The inclusion of a limited number of eyes was indeed a limitation in this initial exploration, but small sample sizes are not uncommon in preliminary studies. Our primary intention was to generate hypotheses that could be relevant to future, more comprehensive research in this area. It is known that perfusion measurements correlate significantly with age [66] and can be influenced by other diseases, such as diabetes (in 2 patients) [52]. Three patients were treated for arterial systemic hypertension and their systemic medication did not change during the study, but arterial blood pressure was not measured. Park and co-workers [67] reported that in glaucomatous eyes with an optic disc hemorrhage, high systemic blood pressure was associated with a reduction in macular VD. However, none of our patients had an optic disc hemorrhage at baseline or after 3 months of treatment with latanoprost. The wide age range in our study adds to the diversity of our patient population, but we acknowledge that a larger and more varied cohort is required for a more comprehensive understanding of the potential effects of prostaglandin analogues on retinal parameters.

The findings of this study have potential clinical implications. The significant mean reduction in IOP by 30.6% suggests that preservative-free latanoprost could be an effective treatment for lowering IOP in treatment-naïve patients with POAG, suspected glaucoma, and OHT. However, the observation that there were no statistically significant changes in ERG and OCT/OCTA parameters compared to baseline despite the reduction in IOP suggests that the reduction in IOP achieved with latanoprost may not have immediately detectable effects on retinal morphology and function.

Conducting larger and longer-term studies could help to investigate the sustained effect of preservative-free latanoprost on both IOP and retinal parameters over a longer period of time. Given the potential influence of systemic factors, future research could systematically measure and analyze systemic parameters, including arterial blood pressure, to better understand their role in ocular perfusion and treatment outcomes. Subgroup analyses based on age, presence of comorbidities, or other relevant factors could help to identify potential differences in response to treatment within specific patient groups. As the association between systemic blood pressure and macular VD has been reported in glaucomatous eyes with optic disc hemorrhages, investigating this aspect in a larger cohort could provide insight into specific subgroups that may be more susceptible to such effects.

5. Conclusions

To summarize, we investigated the change in the morphological and functional parameters 3 months after a moderate reduction in IOP in our pilot study. Objective ERG measurements of visual function (PERG, PhNR) showed no significant changes compared to baseline. Only the OCTA IPL/INL plexus showed a significant correlation with the change in IOP.

Although this study provides valuable insights, we are aware that we must be cautious when generalizing our findings. This case series serves as a starting point for investigations, and we hope to conduct future studies that build on our preliminary findings to gain a more comprehensive understanding of the potential benefits and effects of prostaglandin analogues in relation to retinal parameters.

Author Contributions: Conceptualization, Q.D. and B.C.; methodology, Q.D. and B.C.; formal analysis, Q.D. and B.C.; investigation, M.S.H., A.M. and D.P.; resources, Q.D. and M.A.V.; data curation, M.S.H., A.M. and D.P.; writing—original draft preparation, Q.D. and M.A.V.; writing—review and editing, B.C. and Q.D.; visualization, Q.D.; supervision, B.C.; project administration, B.C.; funding acquisition, B.C. All authors have read and agreed to the published version of the manuscript.

Funding: This research received no external funding.

Institutional Review Board Statement: This study was conducted in accordance with the Declaration of Helsinki and was approved on the 15 November 2011 by the National Ethics Committee, University Medical Centre Ljubljana, Ljubljana, Slovenia (KME 33/11/11).

Informed Consent Statement: Informed consent was obtained from all subjects involved in this study.

Data Availability Statement: Data are available upon reasonable request.

Conflicts of Interest: B.C. is a consultant and speaker for Thea and Santen. The other authors declare no conflicts of interest.

References

1. Tham, Y.C.; Li, X.; Wong, T.Y.; Quigley, H.A.; Aung, T.; Cheng, C.Y. Global prevalence of glaucoma and projections of glaucoma burden through 2040: A systematic review and meta-analysis. *Ophthalmology* **2014**, *121*, 2081–2090. [CrossRef]
2. Bourne, R.R.; Taylor, H.R.; Flaxman, S.R.; Keeffe, J.; Leasher, J.; Naidoo, K.; Pesudovs, K.; White, R.A.; Wong, T.Y.; Resnikoff, S.; et al. Number of People Blind or Visually Impaired by Glaucoma Worldwide and in World Regions 1990–2010: A Meta-Analysis. *PLoS ONE* **2016**, *11*, e0162229. [CrossRef]
3. Daka, Q.; Trkulja, V. Efficacy and tolerability of mono-compound topical treatments for reduction of intraocular pressure in patients with primary open angle glaucoma or ocular hypertension: An overview of reviews. *Croat. Med. J.* **2014**, *55*, 468–480. [CrossRef]
4. Quigley, H.A.; Broman, A.T. The number of people with glaucoma worldwide in 2010 and 2020. *Br. J. Ophthalmol.* **2006**, *90*, 262–267. [CrossRef]
5. Daka, Q.; Mustafa, R.; Neziri, B.; Virgili, G.; Azuara-Blanco, A. Home-Based Perimetry for Glaucoma: Where Are We Now? *J. Glaucoma* **2022**, *31*, 361–374. [CrossRef]
6. Rizzo, M.I.; Greco, A.; De Virgilio, A.; Gallo, A.; Taverniti, L.; Fusconi, M.; Conte, M.; Pagliuca, G.; Turchetta, R.; de Vincentiis, M. Glaucoma: Recent advances in the involvement of autoimmunity. *Immunol. Res.* **2017**, *65*, 207–217. [CrossRef]
7. Atanasovska Velkovska, M.; Goricar, K.; Blagus, T.; Dolzan, V.; Cvenkel, B. Association of Genetic Polymorphisms in Oxidative Stress and Inflammation Pathways with Glaucoma Risk and Phenotype. *J. Clin. Med.* **2021**, *10*, 1148. [CrossRef] [PubMed]
8. Che Hamzah, J.; Daka, Q.; Azuara-Blanco, A. Home monitoring for glaucoma. *Eye* **2020**, *34*, 155–160. [CrossRef] [PubMed]
9. Boland, M.V.; Ervin, A.M.; Friedman, D.S.; Jampel, H.D.; Hawkins, B.S.; Vollenweider, D.; Chelladurai, Y.; Ward, D.; Suarez-Cuervo, C.; Robinson, K.A. Comparative effectiveness of treatments for open-angle glaucoma: A systematic review for the U.S. Preventive Services Task Force. *Ann. Intern. Med.* **2013**, *158*, 271–279. [CrossRef] [PubMed]
10. Kass, M.A.; Heuer, D.K.; Higginbotham, E.J.; Johnson, C.A.; Keltner, J.L.; Miller, J.P.; Parrish, R.K., 2nd; Wilson, M.R.; Gordon, M.O. The Ocular Hypertension Treatment Study: A randomized trial determines that topical ocular hypotensive medication delays or prevents the onset of primary open-angle glaucoma. *Arch. Ophthalmol.* **2002**, *120*, 701–713, discussion 829–730. [CrossRef] [PubMed]
11. Heijl, A.; Leske, M.C.; Bengtsson, B.; Hyman, L.; Bengtsson, B.; Hussein, M. Reduction of intraocular pressure and glaucoma progression: Results from the Early Manifest Glaucoma Trial. *Arch. Ophthalmol.* **2002**, *120*, 1268–1279. [CrossRef]
12. The Advanced Glaucoma Intervention Study (AGIS): 7. The relationship between control of intraocular pressure and visual field deterioration.The AGIS Investigators. *Am. J. Ophthalmol.* **2000**, *130*, 429–440. [CrossRef] [PubMed]
13. Daka, Q.; Spegel, N.; Atanasovska Velkovska, M.; Steblovnik, T.; Kolko, M.; Neziri, B.; Cvenkel, B. Exploring the Relationship between Anti-VEGF Therapy and Glaucoma: Implications for Management Strategies. *J. Clin. Med.* **2023**, *12*, 4674. [CrossRef] [PubMed]
14. European Glaucoma Society. *Terminology and Guidelines for Glaucoma*, 5th ed.; GECA, Srl: Savona, Italy, 2020; p. 169.
15. Rao, H.L.; Pradhan, Z.S.; Suh, M.H.; Moghimi, S.; Mansouri, K.; Weinreb, R.N. Optical Coherence Tomography Angiography in Glaucoma. *J. Glaucoma* **2020**, *29*, 312–321. [CrossRef] [PubMed]
16. Lee, S.Y.; Son, N.H.; Bae, H.W.; Seong, G.J.; Kim, C.Y. The role of pattern electroretinograms and optical coherence tomography angiography in the diagnosis of normal-tension glaucoma. *Sci. Rep.* **2021**, *11*, 12257. [CrossRef] [PubMed]
17. Miraftabi, A.; Jafari, S.; Nilforushan, N.; Abdolalizadeh, P.; Rakhshan, R. Effect of trabeculectomy on optic nerve head and macular vessel density: An optical coherence tomography angiography study. *Int. Ophthalmol.* **2021**, *41*, 2677–2688. [CrossRef] [PubMed]
18. Liu, L.; Takusagawa, H.L.; Greenwald, M.F.; Wang, J.; Alonzo, B.; Edmunds, B.; Morrison, J.C.; Tan, O.; Jia, Y.; Huang, D. Optical coherence tomographic angiography study of perfusion recovery after surgical lowering of intraocular pressure. *Sci. Rep.* **2021**, *11*, 17251. [CrossRef] [PubMed]
19. Bach, M.; Unsoeld, A.S.; Philippin, H.; Staubach, F.; Maier, P.; Walter, H.S.; Bomer, T.G.; Funk, J. Pattern ERG as an early glaucoma indicator in ocular hypertension: A long-term, prospective study. *Investig. Ophthalmol. Vis. Sci.* **2006**, *47*, 4881–4887. [CrossRef] [PubMed]
20. Bode, S.F.; Jehle, T.; Bach, M. Pattern electroretinogram in glaucoma suspects: New findings from a longitudinal study. *Investig. Ophthalmol. Vis. Sci.* **2011**, *52*, 4300–4306. [CrossRef]

21. Tang, J.; Hui, F.; Hadoux, X.; Soares, B.; Jamieson, M.; van Wijngaarden, P.; Coote, M.; Crowston, J.G. Short-Term Changes in the Photopic Negative Response Following Intraocular Pressure Lowering in Glaucoma. *Investig. Ophthalmol. Vis. Sci.* **2020**, *61*, 16. [CrossRef]
22. Hood, D.C.; Zhang, X. Multifocal ERG and VEP responses and visual fields: Comparing disease-related changes. *Doc. Ophthalmol.* **2000**, *100*, 115–137. [CrossRef] [PubMed]
23. Chan, H.H. Detection of glaucomatous damage using multifocal ERG. *Clin. Exp. Optom.* **2005**, *88*, 410–414. [CrossRef]
24. Al-Nosairy, K.O.; Hoffmann, M.B.; Bach, M. Non-invasive electrophysiology in glaucoma, structure and function-a review. *Eye* **2021**, *35*, 2374–2385. [CrossRef]
25. Cvenkel, B.; Sustar, M.; Perovsek, D. Monitoring for glaucoma progression with SAP, electroretinography (PERG and PhNR) and OCT. *Doc. Ophthalmol.* **2022**, *144*, 17–30. [CrossRef] [PubMed]
26. Senger, C.; Moreto, R.; Watanabe, S.E.S.; Matos, A.G.; Paula, J.S. Electrophysiology in Glaucoma. *J. Glaucoma* **2020**, *29*, 147–153. [CrossRef]
27. Economou, M.A.; Laukeland, H.K.; Grabska-Liberek, I.; Rouland, J.F. Better tolerance of preservative-free latanoprost compared to preserved glaucoma eye drops: The 12-month real-life FREE study. *Clin. Ophthalmol.* **2018**, *12*, 2399–2407. [CrossRef]
28. Erb, C.; Stalmans, I.; Iliev, M.; Munoz-Negrete, F.J. Real-World Study on Patient Satisfaction and Tolerability After Switching to Preservative-Free Latanoprost. *Clin. Ophthalmol.* **2021**, *15*, 931–938. [CrossRef] [PubMed]
29. Bach, M.; Ramharter-Sereinig, A. Pattern electroretinogram to detect glaucoma: Comparing the PERGLA and the PERG Ratio protocols. *Doc. Ophthalmol.* **2013**, *127*, 227–238. [CrossRef]
30. Frishman, L.; Sustar, M.; Kremers, J.; McAnany, J.J.; Sarossy, M.; Tzekov, R.; Viswanathan, S. ISCEV extended protocol for the photopic negative response (PhNR) of the full-field electroretinogram. *Doc. Ophthalmol.* **2018**, *136*, 207–211. [CrossRef]
31. Hollo, G. Influence of Large Intraocular Pressure Reduction on Peripapillary OCT Vessel Density in Ocular Hypertensive and Glaucoma Eyes. *J. Glaucoma* **2017**, *26*, e7–e10. [CrossRef]
32. Chuang, L.H.; Li, J.H.; Huang, P.W.; Chen, H.S.L.; Liu, C.F.; Yang, J.W.; Lai, C.C. Association of Intraocular Pressure and Optical Coherence Tomography Angiography Parameters in Early Glaucoma Treatment. *Diagnostics* **2022**, *12*, 2174. [CrossRef]
33. Gillmann, K.; Rao, H.L.; Mansouri, K. Changes in peripapillary and macular vascular density after laser selective trabeculoplasty: An optical coherence tomography angiography study. *Acta Ophthalmol.* **2021**, *100*, 203–211. [CrossRef]
34. Park, H.L.; Hong, K.E.; Shin, D.Y.; Jung, Y.; Kim, E.K.; Park, C.K. Microvasculature Recovery Detected Using Optical Coherence Tomography Angiography and the Rate of Visual Field Progression After Glaucoma Surgery. *Investig. Ophthalmol. Vis. Sci.* **2021**, *62*, 17. [CrossRef]
35. Shin, J.W.; Sung, K.R.; Uhm, K.B.; Jo, J.; Moon, Y.; Song, M.K.; Song, J.Y. Peripapillary Microvascular Improvement and Lamina Cribrosa Depth Reduction After Trabeculectomy in Primary Open-Angle Glaucoma. *Investig. Ophthalmol. Vis. Sci.* **2017**, *58*, 5993–5999. [CrossRef]
36. In, J.H.; Lee, S.Y.; Cho, S.H.; Hong, Y.J. Peripapillary Vessel Density Reversal after Trabeculectomy in Glaucoma. *J. Ophthalmol.* **2018**, *2018*, 8909714. [CrossRef]
37. El-Haddad, N.; Abd Elwahab, A.; Shalaby, S.; Farag, M.M.A.; Alkassaby, M.; Ahmed, S.; Shawky, S. Comparison between open-angle glaucoma and angle-closure glaucoma regarding the short-term optic disc vessel density changes after trabeculectomy. *Lasers Med. Sci.* **2023**, *38*, 246. [CrossRef]
38. Hong, J.W.; Sung, K.R.; Shin, J.W. Optical Coherence Tomography Angiography of the Retinal Circulation Following Trabeculectomy for Glaucoma. *J. Glaucoma* **2023**, *32*, 293–300. [CrossRef]
39. Zeboulon, P.; Leveque, P.M.; Brasnu, E.; Aragno, V.; Hamard, P.; Baudouin, C.; Labbe, A. Effect of Surgical Intraocular Pressure Lowering on Peripapillary and Macular Vessel Density in Glaucoma Patients: An Optical Coherence Tomography Angiography Study. *J. Glaucoma* **2017**, *26*, 466–472. [CrossRef]
40. Lommatzsch, C.; Rothaus, K.; Koch, J.M.; Heinz, C.; Grisanti, S. Retinal perfusion 6 months after trabeculectomy as measured by optical coherence tomography angiography. *Int. Ophthalmol.* **2019**, *39*, 2583–2594. [CrossRef]
41. Kim, J.A.; Kim, T.W.; Lee, E.J.; Girard, M.J.A.; Mari, J.M. Microvascular Changes in Peripapillary and Optic Nerve Head Tissues After Trabeculectomy in Primary Open-Angle Glaucoma. *Investig. Ophthalmol. Vis. Sci.* **2018**, *59*, 4614–4621. [CrossRef]
42. Ch'ng, T.W.; Gillmann, K.; Hoskens, K.; Rao, H.L.; Mermoud, A.; Mansouri, K. Effect of surgical intraocular pressure lowering on retinal structures—Nerve fibre layer, foveal avascular zone, peripapillary and macular vessel density: 1 year results. *Eye* **2020**, *34*, 562–571. [CrossRef]
43. Lee, J.C.; Grisafe, D.J.; Burkemper, B.; Chang, B.R.; Zhou, X.; Chu, Z.; Fard, A.; Durbin, M.; Wong, B.J.; Song, B.J.; et al. Intrasession repeatability and intersession reproducibility of peripapillary OCTA vessel parameters in non-glaucomatous and glaucomatous eyes. *Br. J. Ophthalmol.* **2021**, *105*, 1534–1541. [CrossRef]
44. Venugopal, J.P.; Rao, H.L.; Weinreb, R.N.; Pradhan, Z.S.; Dasari, S.; Riyazuddin, M.; Puttiah, N.K.; Rao, D.A.S.; Devi, S.; Mansouri, K.; et al. Repeatability of vessel density measurements of optical coherence tomography angiography in normal and glaucoma eyes. *Br. J. Ophthalmol.* **2018**, *102*, 352–357. [CrossRef]
45. Shen, A.J.; Urrea, A.L.; Lee, J.C.; Burkemper, B.; LeTran, V.H.; Zhou, X.; Chu, Z.; Grisafe, D.J.; Fard, A.; Wong, B.; et al. Repeatability and Reproducibility of 4.5 by 4.5 mm Peripapillary Optical Coherence Tomography Angiography Scans in Glaucoma and Non-Glaucoma Eyes. *J. Glaucoma* **2022**, *31*, 773–782. [CrossRef]

46. Vorperian, A.; Khan, N.; Lee, J.; Burkemper, B.; Zhou, X.; Grisafe, D.; LeTran, V.; Chu, Z.; Wong, B.; Xu, B.; et al. Intrasession Repeatability and Intersession Reproducibility of Macular Vessel Parameters on Optical Coherence Tomography Angiography in Glaucomatous and Non-Glaucomatous Eyes. *Curr. Eye Res.* **2022**, *47*, 1068–1076. [CrossRef]
47. Karti, O.; Zengin, M.O.; Kerci, S.G.; Ayhan, Z.; Kusbeci, T. Acute Effect of Caffeine on Macular Microcirculation in Healthy Subjects: An Optical Coherence Tomography Angiography Study. *Retina* **2019**, *39*, 964–971. [CrossRef]
48. Ayhan, Z.; Kaya, M.; Ozturk, T.; Karti, O.; Hakan Oner, F. Evaluation of Macular Perfusion in Healthy Smokers by Using Optical Coherence Tomography Angiography. *Ophthalmic Surg. Lasers Imaging Retin.* **2017**, *48*, 617–622. [CrossRef]
49. Alnawaiseh, M.; Lahme, L.; Treder, M.; Rosentreter, A.; Eter, N. Short-Term Effects of Exercise on Optic Nerve and Macular Perfusion Measured by Optical Coherence Tomography Angiography. *Retina* **2017**, *37*, 1642–1646. [CrossRef]
50. Ma, Z.W.; Qiu, W.H.; Zhou, D.N.; Yang, W.H.; Pan, X.F.; Chen, H. Changes in vessel density of the patients with narrow antenior chamber after an acute intraocular pressure elevation observed by OCT angiography. *BMC Ophthalmol.* **2019**, *19*, 132. [CrossRef]
51. Zhang, Q.; Jonas, J.B.; Wang, Q.; Chan, S.Y.; Xu, L.; Wei, W.B.; Wang, Y.X. Optical Coherence Tomography Angiography Vessel Density Changes after Acute Intraocular Pressure Elevation. *Sci. Rep.* **2018**, *8*, 6024. [CrossRef]
52. Ashraf Khorasani, M.; Garcia, A.G.; Anvari, P.; Habibi, A.; Ghasemizadeh, S.; Ghasemi Falavarjani, K. Optical Coherence Tomography Angiography Findings after Acute Intraocular Pressure Elevation in Patients with Diabetes Mellitus versus Healthy Subjects. *J. Ophthalmic Vis. Res.* **2022**, *17*, 360–367. [CrossRef]
53. Zhi, Z.; Cepurna, W.; Johnson, E.; Jayaram, H.; Morrison, J.; Wang, R.K. Evaluation of the effect of elevated intraocular pressure and reduced ocular perfusion pressure on retinal capillary bed filling and total retinal blood flow in rats by OMAG/OCT. *Microvasc. Res.* **2015**, *101*, 86–95. [CrossRef]
54. Wang, L.; Burgoyne, C.F.; Cull, G.; Thompson, S.; Fortune, B. Static blood flow autoregulation in the optic nerve head in normal and experimental glaucoma. *Investig. Ophthalmol. Vis. Sci.* **2014**, *55*, 873–880. [CrossRef]
55. Luo, X.; Frishman, L.J. Retinal pathway origins of the pattern electroretinogram (PERG). *Investig. Ophthalmol. Vis. Sci.* **2011**, *52*, 8571–8584. [CrossRef]
56. Ventura, L.M.; Porciatti, V. Restoration of retinal ganglion cell function in early glaucoma after intraocular pressure reduction: A pilot study. *Ophthalmology* **2005**, *112*, 20–27. [CrossRef]
57. Sehi, M.; Grewal, D.S.; Goodkin, M.L.; Greenfield, D.S. Reversal of retinal ganglion cell dysfunction after surgical reduction of intraocular pressure. *Ophthalmology* **2010**, *117*, 2329–2336. [CrossRef]
58. Niyadurupola, N.; Luu, C.D.; Nguyen, D.Q.; Geddes, K.; Tan, G.X.; Wong, C.C.; Tran, T.; Coote, M.A.; Crowston, J.G. Intraocular pressure lowering is associated with an increase in the photopic negative response (PhNR) amplitude in glaucoma and ocular hypertensive eyes. *Investig. Ophthalmol. Vis. Sci.* **2013**, *54*, 1913–1919. [CrossRef]
59. Karaskiewicz, J.; Penkala, K.; Mularczyk, M.; Lubinski, W. Evaluation of retinal ganglion cell function after intraocular pressure reduction measured by pattern electroretinogram in patients with primary open-angle glaucoma. *Doc. Ophthalmol.* **2017**, *134*, 89–97. [CrossRef]
60. Ventura, L.M.; Feuer, W.J.; Porciatti, V. Progressive loss of retinal ganglion cell function is hindered with IOP-lowering treatment in early glaucoma. *Investig. Ophthalmol. Vis. Sci.* **2012**, *53*, 659–663. [CrossRef]
61. Banitt, M.R.; Ventura, L.M.; Feuer, W.J.; Savatovsky, E.; Luna, G.; Shif, O.; Bosse, B.; Porciatti, V. Progressive loss of retinal ganglion cell function precedes structural loss by several years in glaucoma suspects. *Investig. Ophthalmol. Vis. Sci.* **2013**, *54*, 2346–2352. [CrossRef]
62. Hui, F.; Tang, J.; Williams, P.A.; McGuinness, M.B.; Hadoux, X.; Casson, R.J.; Coote, M.; Trounce, I.A.; Martin, K.R.; van Wijngaarden, P.; et al. Improvement in inner retinal function in glaucoma with nicotinamide (vitamin B3) supplementation: A crossover randomized clinical trial. *Clin. Exp. Ophthalmol.* **2020**, *48*, 903–914. [CrossRef] [PubMed]
63. Igawa, Y.; Shoji, T.; Weinreb, R.; Miyake, Y.; Yoshikawa, Y.; Takano, S.; Shinoda, K. Early changes in photopic negative response in eyes with glaucoma with and without choroidal detachment after filtration surgery. *Br. J. Ophthalmol.* **2023**, *107*, 1295–1302. [CrossRef] [PubMed]
64. Mortlock, K.E.; Binns, A.M.; Aldebasi, Y.H.; North, R.V. Inter-subject, inter-ocular and inter-session repeatability of the photopic negative response of the electroretinogram recorded using DTL and skin electrodes. *Doc. Ophthalmol.* **2010**, *121*, 123–134. [CrossRef]
65. Tang, J.; Edwards, T.; Crowston, J.G.; Sarossy, M. The Test-Retest Reliability of the Photopic Negative Response (PhNR). *Transl. Vis. Sci. Technol.* **2014**, *3*, 1. [CrossRef]
66. You, Q.S.; Tan, O.; Pi, S.; Liu, L.; Wei, P.; Chen, A.; Ing, E.; Jia, Y.; Huang, D. Effect of algorithms and covariates in glaucoma diagnosis with optical coherence tomography angiography. *Br. J. Ophthalmol.* **2021**, *106*, 1703–1709. [CrossRef]
67. Park, C.K.; Lee, K.; Kim, E.W.; Kim, S.; Lee, S.Y.; Kim, C.Y.; Seong, G.J.; Bae, H.W. Effect of systemic blood pressure on optical coherence tomography angiography in glaucoma patients. *Eye* **2021**, *35*, 1967–1976. [CrossRef] [PubMed]

Disclaimer/Publisher's Note: The statements, opinions and data contained in all publications are solely those of the individual author(s) and contributor(s) and not of MDPI and/or the editor(s). MDPI and/or the editor(s) disclaim responsibility for any injury to people or property resulting from any ideas, methods, instructions or products referred to in the content.

Review

Exploring the Relationship between Anti-VEGF Therapy and Glaucoma: Implications for Management Strategies

Qëndresë Daka [1,2,3], Nina Špegel [3], Makedonka Atanasovska Velkovska [3], Tjaša Steblovnik [3], Miriam Kolko [4,5], Burim Neziri [1] and Barbara Cvenkel [3,6,*]

[1] Department of Pathophysiology, Medical Faculty, University of Prishtina, 10000 Prishtina, Kosovo; qendrese.daka@uni-pr.edu (Q.D.); burim.neziri@uni-pr.edu (B.N.)
[2] Eye Clinic, University Clinical Centre of Kosova, 10000 Prishtina, Kosovo
[3] Department of Ophthalmology, University Medical Centre Ljubljana, 1000 Ljubljana, Slovenia; spegel.nina@gmail.com (N.Š.); makedonka.atanasovskavelkovska@kclj.si (M.A.V.); tjasa.steblovnik@gmail.com (T.S.)
[4] Department of Drug Design and Pharmacology, University of Copenhagen, 2100 Copenhagen, Denmark; miriamk@sund.ku.dk
[5] Department of Ophthalmology, Copenhagen University Hospital, Rigshospitalet, 2600 Glostrup, Denmark
[6] Faculty of Medicine, University of Ljubljana, 1000 Ljubljana, Slovenia
* Correspondence: barbara.cvenkel@gmail.com

Abstract: A short-term increase in intraocular pressure (IOP) is a common side effect after intravitreal anti-VEGF therapy, but a sustained increase in IOP with the development of secondary glaucoma has also been reported in some studies after repeated intravitreal anti-VEGF injections. The aim of this review is to present and discuss the possible pathophysiological mechanisms and factors contributing to a sustained rise in IOP, as well as treatment strategies for patients at risk. Close monitoring and adjustable IOP-lowering treatment are recommended for high-risk patients, including those with glaucoma, angle-closure anomalies, ocular hypertension or family history of glaucoma; patients receiving a high number of injections or at shorter intervals; and patients with capsulotomy. Strategies are needed to identify patients at risk in a timely manner and to prevent sustained elevation of IOP.

Keywords: anti-VEGF; elevated intraocular pressure; glaucoma

1. Introduction

Overproduction of vascular endothelial growth factor (VEGF) promotes angiogenesis and induces vascular permeability, contributing to the pathogenesis of several ocular diseases in various ischemic retinal disorders and choroidal neovascularisation (CNV) in age-related macular degeneration (AMD) [1–3].

CNV is responsible for severe vision loss in these diseases. Inhibition of VEGF has been proven effective in preventing vision loss and, in some cases, improving vision [2]. However, despite the significant benefits, the use of anti-VEGF drugs is not without potential adverse effects. Over the years, several anti-VEGF drugs have been approved in the form of intravitreal injections, including pegaptanib (Macugen, Eyetech/Pfizer, Inc., Manhattan, NY, USA), a ribonucleic acid aptamer; bevacizumab (Avastin, Genentech, Inc., San Francisco, CA, USA), a recombinant humanised monoclonal antibody; ranibizumab (Lucentis, Genentech, Inc., San Francisco, CA, USA), a humanised monoclonal antibody fragment; aflibercept (Eylea, Regeneron Pharmaceuticals, Inc., Tarrytown, NY, USA), a soluble decoy receptor fusion protein; and the recently launched brolucizumab (Beovu, Novartis, Basel, Switzerland), a humanised monoclonal single-chain variable fragment, and faricimab-svoa (Vabysmo, Genentech, Inc., San Francisco, CA, USA), a bispecific monoclonal antibody that targets both VEGF and angiopoietin 2 (Ang-2) [3–5].

While RCTs have reported differences in efficacy between these drugs, real-world evidence often fails to observe such distinctions, emphasising the need to consider the limitations and confounders associated with both study types [6,7]. Furthermore, some studies demonstrated nonresponse to this therapy or a loss of efficacy over time [8,9].

The safety profile of anti-VEGF agents is generally favourable, with rare sight-threatening side effects [4,10]. Nevertheless, ocular and systemic adverse effects, such as cardiovascular and renal complications, have been reported, highlighting the importance of cautious use [11,12].

A commonly reported side effect is a transient increase in intraocular pressure (IOP), which usually normalises within 60 min without any intervention [2,13]. In recent years, several studies have reported a sustained elevation of IOP (SE-IOP) [14–19], and a few studies have reported the secondary development or progression of pre-existing glaucomatous optic neuropathy (GON) [20,21].

2. Methods

We searched the literature to examine the relationship between anti-VEGF therapy and glaucoma in terms of implications for treatment strategies.

A review was performed to summarise the relevant English-language literature on the development or progression of secondary GON development in patients treated with intravitreal anti-VEGF injections for AMD. The PubMed database was searched using the following terms: "glaucoma development*" OR "glaucoma progression" AND "anti-VEGF intravitreal injections" AND "AMD" OR "age-related macular degeneration". Articles published up to December 2022 were included in the review without any restrictions based on sex, race or geographic area. Given the different aims and designs of the included studies, a narrative review approach was adopted.

3. Literature Review

AMD and glaucoma are the most common causes of irreversible blindness worldwide [22–24]. As the prevalence of AMD increases with age, certain populations are expected to have a higher prevalence of the disease, which is estimated to affect 288 million people worldwide by 2040 [4,25]. With the increasing use of anti-VEGF injections to treat AMD, there is a possibility that the prevalence of developing secondary glaucoma and the rate of progression of pre-existing glaucoma may increase [26].

Currently, this prevalence is unknown because the data come from small, short-term and mostly retrospective studies. We found several studies with very different reports on the association of anti-VEGF treatment and other factors with IOP elevation and the development or progression of GON [3,13,26–31]. A meta-analysis of several studies on this topic concluded that the prevalence of SE-IOP was 4.7%, even after accounting for the effects of drug type, disease conditions, follow-up duration, and the exclusion of patients with pre-existing glaucoma and those using corticosteroids [32]. In contrast, the most recent network meta-analysis of eligible RCTs comparing anti-VEGF agents for different retinal diseases found no clear evidence for SE-IOP [26]. However, the authors note that the analysis was limited by imprecision, and no definitive conclusions can be drawn [26].

In addition, data from a large medical database demonstrate an increased risk of initiating IOP-lowering treatment after anti-VEGF injection, although glaucoma patients, glaucoma suspects, individuals with OHT and patients who had received an intraocular steroid injection were excluded [21]. Although data on a direct association with the development of secondary glaucoma and the rate of progression are insufficient [27], a recent retrospective study showed a significant risk [30].

The pathogenesis could be multifactorial, as many variables play a role and several theories are thought to explain the underlying mechanisms [10,17,26,27,32].

3.1. The Theory of Nitric Oxide

Nitric oxide (NO) is a crucial signalling molecule involved in various physiological and pathological processes within ocular structures, including vasodilation, neurotransmission and immune response [33]. The detrimental role of NO in GON has been confirmed in many studies that observed changes in the three isoforms of NO synthase (NOS) within ocular structures [33–35]. In eyes with normal IOP, NOS-1 was present in astrocytes, pericytes and nerve terminals in the walls of the central artery, and NOS-3 was present in the vascular endothelial cells of both large and small vessels acting as physiological vasodilators in the tissue and neuroprotecting the ONH [34–36]. In eyes with elevated IOP, no significant changes in NOS-1 or NOS-3 levels were observed, but NOS-2 appeared in astrocytes in the early stages. NOS-2 produces excessive levels of NO, which is thought to contribute to the neurodestruction of RGC axons by promoting the formation of peroxynitrite and subsequent damage to axons at the lamina cribrosa in the ONH. Furthermore, these studies have shown that inhibition of NOS-2 activity provides protection against the loss of RGCs and preserves their function [34–36].

The disruption of NO signalling pathways, particularly through endothelial NOS, by anti-VEGF agents may lead to a decrease in NO levels below physiological baseline, which is thought to be a key mechanism in the development of glaucoma and other processes [20,33,37]. Changes in NO levels may be involved in the pathogenesis of glaucoma through various mechanisms, leading to an increase in IOP, retinal vascular dysfunction and RNFL thinning [23,37]. IOP elevation may be caused by increased resistance in the outflow pathways, increased aqueous humour production in the ciliary body or increased episcleral venous pressure [33,37,38]. Retinal vascular dysfunction could result from impaired vascular autoregulation [33], while RNFL could be affected by the disruption of neuroprotective activities either directly or indirectly through changes in blood flow [38]. While the available data suggest that impaired NO signalling can contribute to glaucoma development through vascular and mechanical mechanisms, increased IOP appears to play a more significant role [33,37]. Several studies have confirmed significant RNFL thinning [38–43] and have attributed this to the underlying AMD pathology itself [38–41] rather than to the anti-VEGF injections [43]. Longitudinal studies over an 8-year period showed no difference in RNFL thickness between injected and control eyes [44], and similar findings were reported in a study involving glaucoma patients receiving anti-VEGF treatment [45]. Furthermore, the relationship between RNFL thinning and progressive visual field loss remains unknown [27].

3.2. Mechanical Effect of Elevated Intraocular Pressure

Both short- and long-term increases in IOP appear to be causative in the development and progression of glaucoma after anti-VEGF treatment [27,33,39]. The mechanisms responsible for IOP elevation have been discussed in a few studies, and the authors agree that both forms are caused by different mechanisms depending on the underlying pathophysiology and/or ocular conditions [27,33,37–39].

Anti-VEGF treatment itself may affect the endogenous expression of VEGF—a paracrine regulator of the conventional outflow pathway [46]. Many studies in humans or animal models have shown a trend towards increased levels of VEGF-A in the aqueous humour of patients with POAG, suggesting a possible neuroprotective role of VEGF in patients with POAG [47].

Brief IOP spikes following anti-VEGF treatment have been attributed to the volume of fluid injected into the eyeball, which can affect mechanical outflow pathways and transiently block axonal transport and ocular perfusion relative to IOP levels, potentially leading to RNFL damage and glaucomatous optic nerve damage [4,13,33,47].

In addition to alterations in the signalling pathways of vasodilatory modulators such as NO, mechanisms thought to be responsible for the development of SE-IOP include pharmacological blockade, damage from trauma and/or IOP spikes, drug-induced inflammation, protein aggregates/silicone oil debris and genomic profile [14–19,27,33,48–53]. Contributing factors, albeit with conflicting results, are considered to include the type of anti-VEGF agent, treatment interval, number of injections, methods of handling the agent, previous steroid use, glaucoma, angle anomalies, OHT and lens status [14–19,27,37,49–53].

SE-IOP appears to be a dominant risk factor for retinal ganglion cell death, RNFL thinning and glaucoma progression [46–50].

Anti-VEGFs can temporarily lower the IOP according to their half-life, either by decreasing aqueous humour production in the ciliary body or by mechanically dilating the outflow pathways by matrix metalloproteinase (MMP) activity. However, the IOP may increase due to rebound swelling of the cells in the outflow pathways or a renewed production of aqueous humour in the ciliary body [51].

3.3. The Role of Anti-VEGF Agents

Although results have been contradictory, studies have pointed to differences between anti-VEGF agents that may be due to either molecular properties, pharmaceutical preparation, storage or method of administration. However, it is difficult to determine which agent carries a higher risk, as patients usually receive several different agents during their treatment. The studies have mainly looked at bevacizumab, followed by ranibizumab, and less at aflibercept. Anti-VEGF agents can cause SE-IOP and, consequently, GON by different mechanisms based on their properties. Bevacizumab is considered to have a higher risk of causing SE-IOP by any mechanism.

3.3.1. Pharmacological Blockade

All molecules can accumulate in the outflow pathways and cause direct mechanical obstruction or an indirect physiological change in outflow [18,51,52]. Bevacizumab (149 kDa) is considered to have a higher risk due to its molecular weight and longer half-life, followed by aflibercept (115 kDa), ranibizumab (48 kDa), brolucizumab (26 kDa) and pegaptanib (20 kDa) [3,17,52]. However, some studies found no difference between the agents [18,53] or a higher prevalence for lower-molecular-weight ranibizumab compared to aflibercept [31,54].

3.3.2. Contamination

Outflow obstruction can result from protein aggregates and/or silicone droplets from syringes, freezing/thawing, exposure to light, mechanical shock, improper storage or administration of the anti-VEGF agent [50,55]. In addition, a number of other materials may enter the protein solution, including ions, plasticisers and other organic molecules [55]. An increase in these proportions may lead to SE-IOP due to mechanical effects, toxicity or immunity [55]. This theory is supported by the fact that in some cases, including ours, the increase in IOP could only be controlled after filtration surgery, as was the case with silicone-oil-induced glaucoma, and that SE-IOP was not observed when silicone-free syringes were used [28,50]. However, in a prospective study, silicone oil droplets were not observed in the anterior chamber [51], and no association was found between the number of injections with protein aggregates in their packaging and SE-IOP [53]. Bevacizumab is thought to have an increased risk because it is drawn from a larger vial, usually in multiple syringes not designed for protein products, and frozen for a variable time compared to single-dose vials drawn into the syringe immediately before injection [50,55]. However, the source appears to play a greater role than the drug itself, as differences in SE-IOP were found in eyes treated with repackaged bevacizumab from different suppliers [3,19,40,55].

A direct toxic effect of anti-VEGF drugs on the outflow pathways seems unlikely [3,50]. Only bevacizumab was found to be toxic to TM cells, and only when the concentration was four times higher than the clinical dose [3,40]. However, the toxic effect could be caused by impurities [55].

3.3.3. Inflammation

Inflammation can obstruct aqueous humour outflow by causing scarring and the proliferation of fibroblasts [3,52]. Theoretically, it can have different causes: subclinical inflammation after injection related to an immunological response to monomeric antibodies, especially to contaminants; chronic inflammation related to repeated injections and transient angle closure; or trabeculitis caused by the pharmacological molecule itself [15,33,49–52,55–57]. The risk of severe intraocular inflammation is increased 12-fold with bevacizumab compared with ranibizumab, probably due to the proinflammatory Fc component and the longer half-life of large antibodies [3,17,58]. Although many studies failed to demonstrate anterior chamber cells, flare, synechiae or trabeculitis [17,19,51], and some found that treatment with topical corticosteroids did not control inflammation or lower the IOP [51], the cause could still be low-grade inflammation that cannot be detected via slit-lamp examination [59,60].

3.4. The Role of the Number of Injections and Intervals between Them

The total number of injections and interval regimen may be considered as independent causal factors for the pharmacological agent, as a significant correlation of SE-IOP with the number of injections, especially if more than 20, and intervals of less than 8 weeks has been demonstrated [10,15,16,19,30,46,51,59,61]. In studies, eyes treated with more than 20 anti-VEGF injections were found to have up to a 12% reduction in aqueous humour outflow [46], while patients in whom the interval was increased were found to have a lower SE-IOP score [28] and reduced need for IOP treatment [51]. The number and interval of injections have also been associated with the risk of initiating IOP-lowering treatment for secondary glaucoma [21] and glaucoma surgery [62]. However, no significant associations were found in some studies [17,19,52,53].

3.5. The Role of Glaucoma, OHT and Angle Anomalies

An already compromised outflow system is thought to be a contributing factor for SE-IOP due to the disruption of endogenous VEGF signalling involved in outflow regulation. While a family history of glaucoma [16], compromised angles including narrow angles [20], angle synechiae, heavy trabecular pigmentation [61] and OHT [46] are associated with increased risk of SE-IOP, glaucoma itself appears to be an independent risk factor [17,27,32]. Studies found a significant decrease in tonographic outflow in OHT patients [17,46] and the development of up to 50% SE-IOP after less than 10 injections in glaucoma patients [17,52]. Studies that did not find any association pointed out their inclusion of a low number of glaucoma patients or no inclusion at all [15,16,18,19,51].

3.6. The Role of Lens Status

The relationship between lens status and the development of SE-IOP after anti-VEGF injection appears to be complex [3]. Some studies showed no association between lens status and SE-IOP [15,46], others suggested that phakic eyes or pseudophakic eyes may be risk factors after capsulotomy [16,30,52,53,61], and a few studies showed a prophylactic role of phakic lens status [18,30].

Although cataract extraction is known to lower IOP, pharmacokinetic studies of anti-VEGF agents have shown increased diffusion into the anterior chamber and increased clearance after lensectomy/vitrectomy [30,63–65]. In addition, disruption of the lens capsule, anterior hyaloid or zonules allows contaminants to enter the anterior chamber, exposing pseudophakic patients and patients undergoing laser capsulotomy to an increased risk of developing SE-IOP [3,52]. On the other hand, the increased risk of SE-IOP and glaucoma development in phakic patients is explained by the mechanical effect of pressure shifting the lens–iris diaphragm anteriorly and compressing the anterior chamber volume, leading to outflow pathway strain [30]. In pseudophakic patients, this strain can be reduced by both faster volume equilibration and faster resolution of IOP after injection due to the more open anterior chamber [30,45].

3.7. The Role of Steroid Treatment

Previous intravitreal steroid injection is listed among the risk factors for SE-IOP after anti-VEGF injection, although some studies have shown no association [3]. The association has not been studied, but it has been suggested that a common pathway is responsible [51], as the effect of steroids on extracellular matrix deposition in the TM, aqueous humour dynamics and gene expression has been demonstrated [3,60]. The same effect was also observed in patients treated with systemic and/or topical steroids who experienced a more rapid and severe increase in intraocular pressure requiring aggressive IOP-lowering treatment [3,60].

4. Conclusions and Management Strategies

Causal relationships regarding the development and/or progression of glaucoma remain very difficult to study due to glaucoma's interaction with retinal diseases [20,30]. SE-IOP associated with anti-VEGF treatment remains the main risk factor, and its mechanical effect seems to be more important for the pathogenesis of the disease [30,37]. However, the effect of elevated IOP on retinal ganglion cells and RNFL damage may be exacerbated by the ability of anti-VEGF agents to negatively affect blood flow in the retina and optic disc [33].

The pathogenesis of SE-IOP is not clear, and there have been few studies investigating genetic, molecular and protein alterations in the outflow pathways [3,60]. A reduction in aqueous humour dynamics in eyes that have received a higher number of anti-VEGF injections has been confirmed [46], but further studies are needed to clarify the pathophysiology and quantify the potential association between short- or long-term IOP elevations and the development of secondary glaucoma or progression of pre-existing glaucoma [27,51–53]. In addition, data are limited for the newer anti-VEGF agents aflibercept, brolucizumab, and faricimab.

Timely detection of SE-IOP appears to be important to delay the disease, but strategies to identify patients at risk should be explored [27]. While literature data suggest that lowering the IOP prior to treatment is beneficial in preventing IOP spikes, there is no consensus on protocols to prevent SE-IOP, while the impact on the development or progression of glaucoma is unknown [20,26,27]. The available data recommend close monitoring and prescription of medications to lower IOP in high-risk patients, including those with glaucoma, angle anomalies, family history of glaucoma or OHT; patients receiving a high number of injections or at shorter intervals; and patients with capsulotomy [3,19,39,46,57]. To prevent immediate postoperative elevation of IOP in glaucoma patients, the French Glaucoma Society suggests the instillation of 1% apraclonidine or dorzolamide/timolol a few hours before anti-VEGF injection [66], while prophylactic administration of acetazolamide 60–90 min before intravitreal ranibizumab injection showed a statistically significant but modest reduction in IOP after 30 min [67]. Currently, predicting the likelihood of a complication in the other eye is uncertain [53], and monitoring pRNFL thickness is not a standard procedure, although it seems reasonable to consider in eyes at risk of glaucoma [20,27]. Switching patients to a "pro re nata" regimen, using longer-acting agents and avoiding syringes that risk leaving particles [3,20,28,30,35,51,54,57] have been suggested as ways to avoid SE-IOP. However, it is believed that treatment with a lower frequency and higher potency is beneficial if the effect is actually related to the injection event rather than pharmacological blockade [23]. Iridotomy may be an effective preventive measure in hypermetropic eyes [30], and considerations are recommended when performing capsulotomy in patients on anti-VEGF treatment [52]. Some studies recommend modifying the injection technique [3]. Treatment of SE-IOP is required and can be performed with topical or systemic IOP-lowering drugs, laser treatment or, rarely, filtration surgery [51,57]. It is thought that better control can be achieved with NO donors as they directly target the pathophysiological decrease in NO [33]. Therefore, pharmacological neuroprotection by NOS-2 inhibition, such as the use of aminoguanidine or blocking NOS-2 induction and gene expression, may be a promising approach for the treatment of patients with glaucoma. By protecting the axons at the level of the ONH from neurodegeneration caused by chronic, moderately elevated IOP, NOS-2 inhibition has the potential to prevent the loss of retinal ganglion cells [34,35].

In some cases, IOP levels can be stabilised after switching to a "pro re nata" regimen, suggesting that a longer interval may allow for the elimination of the drug from the eye [51,57].

Further research is required to comprehensively understand and quantify the risk of developing or progressing to glaucoma associated with anti-VEGF treatment. Although a few studies have investigated the relationship between anti-VEGF treatment and the development or progression of glaucoma using visual field analysis, pRNFL thickness measurements and optic nerve analysis, the data available to date are inconclusive [21,27,62].

Author Contributions: Conceptualisation, Q.D. and B.C.; methodology, Q.D. and N.Š.; formal analysis, N.Š.; investigation, T.S. and M.A.V.; resources, N.Š., T.S. and M.A.V.; data curation, N.Š., T.S. and M.A.V.; writing—original draft preparation, Q.D. and N.Š.; writing—review and editing, B.C., M.K. and B.N.; visualisation, N.Š.; supervision, M.K. and B.C.; project administration, B.C.; funding acquisition, B.C. All authors have read and agreed to the published version of the manuscript.

Funding: This research received no external funding.

Institutional Review Board Statement: Ethical review and approval were waived for this study due to the informed consent obtained from all patients undergoing anti-VEGF treatment who agreed that data on their treatment could be further analysed, used, and published in an anonymised form.

Informed Consent Statement: Written informed consent was obtained from the patient(s) to publish this paper.

Data Availability Statement: Not applicable.

Conflicts of Interest: M.K. is a consultant and speaker for Abbvie, Santen and Thea. M.K. receives research support from Thea. B.C. is a consultant and speaker for Thea. The other authors declare no conflicts of interest.

References

1. Witmer, A.N.; Vrensen, G.F.; Van Noorden, C.J.; Schlingemann, R.O. Vascular endothelial growth factors and angiogenesis in eye disease. *Prog. Retin. Eye Res.* **2003**, *22*, 1–29. [CrossRef] [PubMed]
2. Farhood, Q.K.; Twfeeq, S.M. Short-term intraocular pressure changes after intravitreal injection of bevacizumab in diabetic retinopathy patients. *Clin. Ophthalmol.* **2014**, *8*, 599–604. [CrossRef] [PubMed]
3. Dedania, V.S.; Bakri, S.J. Sustained Elevation of Intraocular Pressure after Intravitreal Anti-Vegf Agents. *Retina* **2015**, *35*, 841–858. [CrossRef] [PubMed]
4. Solomon, S.D.; Lindsley, K.; Vedula, S.S.; Krzystolik, M.G.; Hawkins, B.S. Anti-vascular endothelial growth factor for neovascular age-related macular degeneration. *Cochrane Database Syst. Rev.* **2019**, *2019*, CD005139. [CrossRef]
5. Shirley, M. Faricimab: First Approval. *Drugs* **2022**, *82*, 825–830. [CrossRef]
6. Ricci, F.; Bandello, F.; Navarra, P.; Staurenghi, G.; Stumpp, M.; Zarbin, M. Neovascular Age-Related Macular Degeneration: Therapeutic Management and New-Upcoming Approaches. *Int. J. Mol. Sci.* **2020**, *21*, 8242. [CrossRef]
7. Rao, P.; Lum, F.; Wood, K.; Salman, C.; Burugapalli, B.; Hall, R.; Singh, S.; Parke, D.W., 2nd; Williams, G.A. Real-World Vision in Age-Related Macular Degeneration Patients Treated with Single Anti–VEGF Drug Type for 1 Year in the IRIS Registry. *Ophthalmology* **2018**, *125*, 522–528. [CrossRef]
8. Broadhead, G.K.; Hong, T.; Chang, A.A. Treating the untreatable patient: Current options for the management of treatment-resistant neovascular age-related macular degeneration. *Acta Ophthalmol.* **2014**, *92*, 713–723. [CrossRef]
9. Sun, X.; Yang, S.; Zhao, J. Resistance to anti-VEGF therapy in neovascular age-related macular degeneration: A comprehensive review. *Drug Des. Dev. Ther.* **2016**, *10*, 1857–1867. [CrossRef]
10. Kampougeris, G.; Spyropoulos, D.; Mitropoulou, A. Intraocular Pressure rise after Anti-VEGF Treatment: Prevalence, Possible Mechanisms and Correlations. *J. Curr. Glaucoma Pract.* **2013**, *7*, 19–24. [CrossRef]
11. Fogli, S.; Del Re, M.; Rofi, E.; Posarelli, C.; Figus, M.; Danesi, R. Clinical pharmacology of intravitreal anti-VEGF drugs. *Eye* **2018**, *32*, 1010–1020. [CrossRef]
12. Hanna, R.M.; Barsoum, M.; Arman, F.; Selamet, U.; Hasnain, H.; Kurtz, I. Nephrotoxicity induced by intravitreal vascular endothelial growth factor inhibitors: Emerging evidence. *Kidney Int.* **2019**, *96*, 572–580. [CrossRef] [PubMed]
13. Hollands, H.; Wong, J.; Bruen, R.; Campbell, R.J.; Sharma, S.; Gale, J. Short-term intraocular pressure changes after intravitreal injection of bevacizumab. *Can. J. Ophthalmol.* **2007**, *42*, 807–811. [CrossRef] [PubMed]
14. Bakri, S.J.; Moshfeghi, D.M.; Francom, S.; Rundle, A.C.; Reshef, D.S.; Lee, P.P.; Schaeffer, C.; Rubio, R.G.; Lai, P. Intraocular Pressure in Eyes Receiving Monthly Ranibizumab in 2 Pivotal Age-Related Macular Degeneration Clinical Trials. *Ophthalmology* **2014**, *121*, 1102–1108. [CrossRef]

15. Hoang, Q.V.; Mendonca, L.S.; Della Torre, K.E.; Jung, J.J.; Tsuang, A.J.; Freund, K.B. Effect on Intraocular Pressure in Patients Receiving Unilateral Intravitreal Anti-Vascular Endothelial Growth Factor Injections. *Ophthalmology* **2012**, *119*, 321–326. [CrossRef] [PubMed]
16. Hoang, Q.V.; Tsuang, A.J.; Gelman, R.; Mendonca, L.S.; Della Torre, K.E.; Jung, J.J.; Freund, K.B. Clinical predictors of sustained intraocular pressure elevation due to intravitreal anti–vascular endothelial growth factor therapy. *Retina* **2013**, *33*, 179–187. [CrossRef]
17. Good, T.J.; Kimura, A.E.; Mandava, N.; Kahook, M.Y. Sustained elevation of intraocular pressure after intravitreal injections of anti-VEGF agents. *Br. J. Ophthalmol.* **2010**, *95*, 1111–1114. [CrossRef]
18. Adelman, R.A.; Zheng, Q.; Mayer, H.R.; Ricca, A.M.; Morshedi, R.G.; Wirostko, B.M.; Hall, L.B.; Zebardast, N.; Huang, J.J.; Tao, Y.; et al. Persistent Ocular Hypertension Following Intravitreal Bevacizumab and Ranibizumab Injections. *J. Ocul. Pharmacol. Ther.* **2010**, *26*, 105–110. [CrossRef]
19. Mathalone, N.; Arodi-Golan, A.; Sar, S.; Wolfson, Y.; Shalem, M.; Lavi, I.; Geyer, O. Sustained elevation of intraocular pressure after intravitreal injections of bevacizumab in eyes with neovascular age-related macular degeneration. *Graefe's Arch. Clin. Exp. Ophthalmol.* **2012**, *250*, 1435–1440. [CrossRef]
20. Levin, A.M.; Chaya, C.J.; Kahook, M.Y.; Wirostko, B.M. Intraocular Pressure Elevation Following Intravitreal Anti-VEGF Injections: Short- and Long-term Considerations. *Eur. J. Gastroenterol. Hepatol.* **2021**, *30*, 1019–1026. [CrossRef]
21. Cui, Q.N.; Gray, I.N.; Yu, Y.; VanderBeek, B.L. Repeated intravitreal injections of antivascular endothelial growth factors and risk of intraocular pressure medication use. *Graefe's Arch. Clin. Exp. Ophthalmol.* **2019**, *257*, 1931–1939. [CrossRef] [PubMed]
22. Flaxman, S.R.; Bourne, R.R.A.; Resnikoff, S.; Ackland, P.; Braithwaite, T.; Cicinelli, M.V.; Das, A.; Jonas, J.B.; Keeffe, J.; Kempen, J.H.; et al. Global causes of blindness and distance vision impairment 1990–2020: A systematic review and meta-analysis. *Lancet Glob. Health* **2017**, *5*, e1221–e1234. [CrossRef] [PubMed]
23. Tham, Y.-C.; Li, X.; Wong, T.Y.; Quigley, H.A.; Aung, T.; Cheng, C.-Y. Global Prevalence of Glaucoma and Projections of Glaucoma Burden through 2040: A systematic review and meta-analysis. *Ophthalmology* **2014**, *121*, 2081–2090. [CrossRef]
24. Daka, Q.M.; Mustafa, R.; Neziri, B.M.; Virgili, G.M.; Azuara-Blanco, A.M. Home-Based Perimetry for Glaucoma: Where Are We Now? *Eur. J. Gastroenterol. Hepatol.* **2022**, *31*, 361–374. [CrossRef] [PubMed]
25. Wong, W.L.; Su, X.; Li, X.; Cheung, C.M.G.; Klein, R.; Cheng, C.Y.; Wong, T.Y. Global prevalence of age-related macular degeneration and disease burden projection for 2020 and 2040: A systematic review and meta-analysis. *Lancet Glob. Health* **2014**, *2*, e106–e116. [CrossRef]
26. Nanji, K.; Sarohia, G.S.; Kennedy, K.; Ceyhan, T.; McKechnie, T.; Phillips, M.; Devji, T.; Thabane, L.; Kaiser, P.; Sarraf, D.; et al. The 12- and 24-Month Effects of Intravitreal Ranibizumab, Aflibercept, and Bevacizumab on Intraocular Pressure: A Network Meta-Analysis. *Ophthalmology* **2021**, *129*, 498–508. [CrossRef] [PubMed]
27. Hoguet, A.; Chen, P.P.; Junk, A.K.; Mruthyunjaya, P.; Nouri-Mahdavi, K.; Radhakrishnan, S.; Takusagawa, H.L.; Chen, T.C. The Effect of Anti-Vascular Endothelial Growth Factor Agents on Intraocular Pressure and Glaucoma: A Report by the American Academy of Ophthalmology. *Ophthalmology* **2018**, *126*, 611–622. [CrossRef]
28. Wehrli, S.J.; Tawse, K.; Levin, M.H.; Zaidi, A.; Pistilli, M.M.; Brucker, A.J. A lack of delayed intraocular pressure elevation in patients treated with intravitreal injection of bevacizumab and ranibizumab. *Retina* **2012**, *32*, 1295–1301. [CrossRef]
29. Kim, D.; Nam, W.H.; Kim, H.K.; Yi, K. Does Intravitreal Injections of Bevacizumab for Age-related Macular Degeneration Affect Long-term Intraocular Pressure? *Eur. J. Gastroenterol. Hepatol.* **2014**, *23*, 446–448. [CrossRef]
30. Wingard, J.B.; AP Delzell, D.; Houlihan, N.; Lin, J.; Gieser, J.P. Incidence of Glaucoma or Ocular Hypertension After Repeated Anti-Vascular Endothelial Growth Factor Injections for Macular Degeneration. *Clin. Ophthalmol.* **2019**, *13*, 2563–2572. [CrossRef]
31. Rusu, I.M.; Deobhakta, A.; Yoon, D.B.; Lee, M.B.; Slakter, J.S.; Klancnik, J.M.; Thompson, D.; Freund, K.B. Intraocular pressure in patients with neovascular age-related macular degeneration switched to aflibercept injection after previous anti-vascular endothelial growth factor treatments. *Retina* **2014**, *34*, 2161–2166. [CrossRef]
32. Zhou, Y.; Zhou, M.; Xia, S.; Jing, Q.; Gao, L. Sustained Elevation of Intraocular Pressure Associated with Intravitreal Administration of Anti-vascular Endothelial Growth Factor: A Systematic Review and Meta-Analysis. *Sci. Rep.* **2016**, *6*, 39301. [CrossRef]
33. Ricca, A.M.; Morshedi, R.G.; Wirostko, B.M. High Intraocular Pressure Following Anti-Vascular Endothelial Growth Factor Therapy: Proposed Pathophysiology due to Altered Nitric Oxide Metabolism. *J. Ocul. Pharmacol. Ther.* **2015**, *31*, 2–10. [CrossRef] [PubMed]
34. Neufeld, A.H.; Sawada, A.; Becker, B. Inhibition of nitric-oxide synthase 2 by aminoguanidine provides neuroprotection of retinal ganglion cells in a rat model of chronic glaucoma. *Proc. Natl. Acad. Sci. USA* **1999**, *96*, 9944–9948. [CrossRef] [PubMed]
35. Shareef, S.; Sawada, A.; Neufeld, A.H. Isoforms of nitric oxide synthase in the optic nerves of rat eyes with chronic moderately elevated intraocular pressure. *Investig. Opthalmology Vis. Sci.* **1999**, *40*, 2884–2891.
36. Husain, S.; Abdul, Y.; Singh, S.; Ahmad, A.; Husain, M. Regulation of Nitric Oxide Production by δ-Opioid Receptors during Glaucomatous Injury. *PLoS ONE* **2014**, *9*, e110397. [CrossRef]
37. Morshedi, R.G.; Ricca, A.M.; Wirostko, B.M. Ocular Hypertension Following Intravitreal Antivascular Endothelial Growth Factor Therapy: Review of the Literature and Possible Role of Nitric Oxide. *Eur. J. Gastroenterol. Hepatol.* **2016**, *25*, 291–300. [CrossRef]
38. Cavet, M.E.; Vittitow, J.L.; Impagnatiello, F.; Ongini, E.; Bastia, E. Nitric Oxide (NO): An Emerging Target for the Treatment of Glaucoma. *Investig. Opthalmology Vis. Sci.* **2014**, *55*, 5005–5015. [CrossRef]

39. de Vries, V.A.; Bassil, F.L.; Ramdas, W.D. The effects of intravitreal injections on intraocular pressure and retinal nerve fiber layer: A systematic review and meta-analysis. *Sci. Rep.* **2020**, *10*, 13248. [CrossRef]
40. Parlak, M.; Oner, F.H.; Saatci, A.O. The long-term effect of intravitreal ranibizumab on retinal nerve fiber layer thickness in exudative age-related macular degeneration. *Int. Ophthalmol.* **2014**, *35*, 473–480. [CrossRef]
41. Jo, Y.-J.; Kim, W.-J.; Shin, I.-H.; Kim, J.-Y. Longitudinal Changes in Retinal Nerve Fiber Layer Thickness after Intravitreal Anti-vascular Endothelial Growth Factor Therapy. *Korean J. Ophthalmol.* **2016**, *30*, 114–120. [CrossRef] [PubMed]
42. Entezari, M.; Ramezani, A.; Yaseri, M. Changes in retinal nerve fiber layer thickness after two intravitreal bevacizumab injections for wet type age-related macular degeneration. *J. Ophthalmic Vis. Res.* **2014**, *9*, 449–452. [CrossRef] [PubMed]
43. Martinez-De-La-Casa, J.M.; Ruiz-Calvo, A.; Saenz-Frances, F.; Reche-Frutos, J.; Calvo-Gonzalez, C.; Donate-Lopez, J.; Garcia-Feijoo, J. Retinal Nerve Fiber Layer Thickness Changes in Patients with Age-Related Macular Degeneration Treated with Intravitreal Ranibizumab. *Investig. Opthalmology Vis. Sci.* **2012**, *53*, 6214–6218. [CrossRef]
44. Valverde-Megías, A.; Ruiz-Calvo, A.; Murciano-Cespedosa, A.; Hernández-Ruiz, S.; Martínez-De-La-Casa, J.M.; García-Feijoo, J. Long-term effect of intravitreal ranibizumab therapy on retinal nerve fiber layer in eyes with exudative age-related macular degeneration. *Graefe's Arch. Clin. Exp. Ophthalmol.* **2019**, *257*, 1459–1466. [CrossRef]
45. Swaminathan, S.S.; Kunkler, A.L.; Quan, A.V.; Medert, C.M.; Vanner, E.A.; Feuer, W.; Chang, T.C. Rates of RNFL Thinning in Patients with Suspected or Confirmed Glaucoma Receiving Unilateral Intravitreal Injections for Exudative AMD. *Am. J. Ophthalmol.* **2021**, *226*, 206–216. [CrossRef]
46. Wen, J.C.; Reina-Torres, E.; Sherwood, J.M.; Challa, P.; Liu, K.C.; Li, G.; Chang, J.Y.H.; Cousins, S.W.; Schuman, S.G.; Mettu, P.S.; et al. Intravitreal Anti-VEGF Injections Reduce Aqueous Outflow Facility in Patients with Neovascular Age-Related Macular Degeneration. *Investig. Opthalmology Vis. Sci.* **2017**, *58*, 1893–1898. [CrossRef]
47. Dimtsas, G.S.; Tsiogka, A.; Moschos, M.M. VEGF levels in the aqueous humor of patients with primary open angle glaucoma: A systematic review and a meta-analysis. *Eur. J. Ophthalmol.* **2023**, 11206721231168146. [CrossRef]
48. Barash, A.; Chui, T.Y.P.; Garcia, P.; Rosen, R.B. Acute macular and peripapillary angiographic changes with intravitreal injections. *Retina* **2020**, *40*, 648–656. [CrossRef] [PubMed]
49. Sniegowski, M. Sustained Intraocular Pressure Elevation After Intravitreal Injection of Bevacizumab and Ranibizumab Associated with Trabeculitis. *Open Ophthalmol. J.* **2010**, *4*, 28–29. [CrossRef]
50. Liu, L.; Ammar, D.A.; Ross, L.A.; Mandava, N.; Kahook, M.Y.; Carpenter, J.F. Silicone Oil Microdroplets and Protein Aggregates in Repackaged Bevacizumab and Ranibizumab: Effects of Long-term Storage and Product Mishandling. *Investig. Opthalmol. Vis. Sci.* **2011**, *52*, 1023–1034. [CrossRef]
51. Tseng, J.J.; Vance, S.K.; Della Torre, K.E.; Mendonca, L.S.; Cooney, M.J.; Klancnik, J.M.; Sorenson, J.A.; Freund, K.B. Sustained Increased Intraocular Pressure Related to Intravitreal Antivascular Endothelial Growth Factor Therapy for Neovascular Age-related Macular Degeneration. *Eur. J. Gastroenterol. Hepatol.* **2012**, *21*, 241–247. [CrossRef] [PubMed]
52. Sternfeld, A.; Ehrlich, R.; Weinberger, D.; Dotan, A. Effect of different lens status on intraocular pressure elevation in patients treated with anti-vascular endothelial growth factor injections. *Int. J. Ophthalmol.* **2020**, *13*, 79–84. [CrossRef]
53. Choi, D.Y.B.; Ortube, M.C.; A Mccannel, C.; Sarraf, D.; Hubschman, J.-P.; Mccannel, T.A.; Gorin, M.B. Sustained elevated intraocular pressures after intravitreal injection of bevacizumab, ranibizumab, and pegaptanib. *Retina* **2011**, *31*, 1028–1035. [CrossRef]
54. Freund, K.B.; Hoang, Q.V.; Saroj, N.; Thompson, D. Intraocular Pressure in Patients with Neovascular Age-Related Macular Degeneration Receiving Intravitreal Aflibercept or Ranibizumab. *Ophthalmology* **2015**, *122*, 1802–1810. [CrossRef]
55. Kahook, M.Y.; Liu, L.; Ruzycki, P.B.; Mandava, N.; Carpenter, J.F.; Petrash, J.M.; Ammar, D.A. High-molecular-weight aggregates in repackaged bevacizumab. *Retina* **2010**, *30*, 887–892. [CrossRef] [PubMed]
56. Georgopoulos, M.; Polak, K.; Prager, F.; Prunte, C.; Schmidt-Erfurth, U. Characteristics of severe intraocular inflammation following intravitreal injection of bevacizumab (Avastin). *Br. J. Ophthalmol.* **2008**, *93*, 457–462. [CrossRef]
57. Leleu, I.; Penaud, B.; Blumen-Ohana, E.; Rodallec, T.; Adam, R.; Laplace, O.; Akesbi, J.; Nordmann, J.-P. Late and sustained intraocular pressure elevation related to intravitreal anti-VEGF injections: Cases requiring filtering surgery (French translation of the article). *J. Fr. Ophtalmol.* **2018**, *41*, 789–801. [CrossRef]
58. Kahook, M.Y.; Kimura, A.E.; Wong, L.J.; Ammar, D.A.; Maycotte, M.A.; Mandava, N. Sustained Elevation in Intraocular Pressure Associated with Intravitreal Bevacizumab Injections. *Ophthalmic Surg. Lasers Imaging Retin.* **2009**, *40*, 293–295. [CrossRef] [PubMed]
59. Menke, M.N.; Salam, A.; Framme, C.; Wolf, S. Long-Term Intraocular Pressure Changes in Patients with Neovascular Age-Related Macular Degeneration Treated with Ranibizumab. *Ophthalmologica* **2013**, *229*, 168–172. [CrossRef]
60. Bakri, S.J.; McCannel, C.A.; Edwards, A.O.; Moshfeghi, D.M. Persistent ocular hypertension following intravitreal ranibizumab. *Graefe's Arch. Clin. Exp. Ophthalmol.* **2008**, *246*, 955–958. [CrossRef] [PubMed]
61. Pershing, S.; Bakri, S.J.; Moshfeghi, D.M. Ocular Hypertension and Intraocular Pressure Asymmetry After Intravitreal Injection of Anti–Vascular Endothelial Growth Factor Agents. *Ophthalmic Surg. Lasers Imaging Retin.* **2013**, *44*, 460–464. [CrossRef] [PubMed]
62. Eadie, B.D.; Etminan, M.; Carleton, B.; Maberley, D.A.; Mikelberg, F.S. Association of Repeated Intravitreous Bevacizumab Injections with Risk for Glaucoma Surgery. *JAMA Ophthalmol* **2017**, *135*, 363–368. [CrossRef] [PubMed]

63. Niwa, Y.; Kakinoki, M.; Sawada, T.; Wang, X.; Ohji, M. Ranibizumab and Aflibercept: Intraocular Pharmacokinetics and Their Effects on Aqueous VEGF Level in Vitrectomized and Nonvitrectomized Macaque Eyes. *Investig. Opthalmology Vis. Sci.* **2015**, *56*, 6501–6505. [CrossRef]
64. Edington, M.; Connolly, J.; Chong, N.V. Pharmacokinetics of intravitreal anti-VEGF drugs in vitrectomized versus nonvitrectomized eyes. *Expert Opin. Drug Metab. Toxicol.* **2017**, *13*, 1217–1224. [CrossRef] [PubMed]
65. Christoforidis, J.B.; Williams, M.M.M.; Wang, J.B.; Jiang, A.; Pratt, C.D.; Abdel-Rasoul, M.; Hinkle, G.H.R.; Knopp, M.V. Anatomic and pharmacokinetic properties of intravitreal bevacizumab and ranibizumab after vitrectomy and lensectomy. *Retina* **2013**, *33*, 946–952. [CrossRef]
66. Poli, M.; Denis, P.; Dot, C.; Nordmann, J.-P. Ocular hypertension after intravitreal injection: Screening and management. *J. Fr. Ophtalmol.* **2017**, *40*, e77–e82. [CrossRef]
67. Murray, C.D.; Wood, D.; Allgar, V.; Walters, G.; Gale, R.P. Short-term intraocular pressure trends following intravitreal ranibizumab injections for neovascular age-related macular degeneration—The role of oral acetazolamide in protecting glaucoma patients. *Eye* **2014**, *28*, 1218–1222. [CrossRef]

Disclaimer/Publisher's Note: The statements, opinions and data contained in all publications are solely those of the individual author(s) and contributor(s) and not of MDPI and/or the editor(s). MDPI and/or the editor(s) disclaim responsibility for any injury to people or property resulting from any ideas, methods, instructions or products referred to in the content.

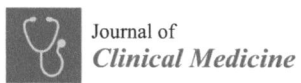 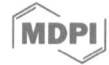

Review

Update on Diagnosis and Treatment of Uveitic Glaucoma

Ioannis Halkiadakis [1,*], Kalliroi Konstantopoulou [1], Vasilios Tzimis [1], Nikolaos Papadopoulos [1], Klio Chatzistefanou [2] and Nikolaos N. Markomichelakis [3]

[1] Ophthalmiatrion Athinon, Athens Eye Hospital, 10672 Athens, Greece; kalikonsta@yahoo.gr (K.K.); tzimisv@hotmail.com (V.T.); papadopoulosn1992@gmail.com (N.P.)
[2] First Department of Ophthalmology, National and Kapodistrian University of Athens School of Medicine, Athens General Hospital "G. Gennimatas", 11527 Athenbs, Greece; kliochat@med.uoa.gr
[3] Ocular Inflammation Institute of Athens, Sarantaporou 7 Agios Stefanos, 14565 Athens, Greece; nmarkom@otenet.gr
* Correspondence: ihalkia@gmail.com; Tel.: +30-21-0813-1378 or +30-69-4495-8013; Fax: +30-21-0779-1808

Abstract: Glaucoma is a common and potentially blinding complication of uveitis. Many mechanisms are involved alone or in combination in the pathogenesis of uveitic glaucoma (UG). In terms of diagnostic evaluation, the effects of inflammatory activity in the retinal nerve fiber layer may be a source of bias in the interpretation of optical coherence tomography measurements. For the successful treatment of UG, the control of intraocular inflammation specific to the cause or anti-inflammatory treatment, combined with IOP management, is mandatory. The early institution of specific treatment improves the prognosis of UG associated with CMV. The young age of UG patients along with increased failure rates of glaucoma surgery in this group of patients warrants a stepwise approach. Conservative and conjunctival sparing surgical approaches should be adopted. Minimally invasive surgical approaches were proved to be effective and are increasingly being used in the management of UG along with the traditionally used techniques of trabeculectomy or tubes. This review aims to summarize the progress that recently occurred in the diagnosis and treatment of UG.

Keywords: uveitic glaucoma; inflammatory glaucoma; CMV; minimally invasive glaucoma surgrery; Ahmed valve; Baerveldt tube

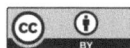

1. Introduction

Uveitis is the most common inflammatory eye disease, with an incidence of 17–52.4 cases per 100,000 population [1–7]. The incidence of secondary glaucoma caused by uveitis is reported to be 10–20% [8–11]. Daniel et al. reported that in adults with non-infectious uveitis, mean annual incidence rates for ocular hypertension (OHT) with intraocular pressure (IOP) $\geq$ 21 mmHg and IOP $\geq$ 30 mmHg were 14.4% and 5.1% per year, respectively [12]. Furthermore, OHT in uveitis, in contrast to POAG, progresses rapidly to uveitic glaucoma (UG) [13]. Uveitic glaucoma is aggressive, with a high likelihood of requiring surgical management and a high risk of central vision loss. Glaucoma is the most common cause of permanent vision loss in cases of anterior uveitis, accounting for 30.1% of cases with moderate visual loss [14,15]. Certain types of uveitis carry a higher risk of developing secondary glaucoma; namely, Posner–Schlossman syndrome (PSS), herpetic uveitis, Fuchs heterochromic iridocyclitis and juvenile idiopathic arthritis. Risk factors which increase the incidence of UG apart from etiology are race, age, duration of inflammation and steroid use [6,9,16,17].

In cases of UG, a successful clinical course implies prompt and effective treatment of uveitis, high suspicion and early identification of glaucomatous changes and aggressive control of the IOP. Management can be particularly challenging with medical therapy alone; meanwhile, the success of glaucoma surgery is lower in these patients compared to the general population, with a higher incidence of postoperative complications [13,18].

2. Pathophysiology of Uveitic Glaucoma

Several mechanisms may be responsible (alone or in combination) for the occurrence of glaucoma in uveitis patients.

1. Alteration of aqueous humor consistency and reduced permeability of trabecular meshwork: The breakdown of the blood aqueous barrier during inflammation results in higher concentrations of proteins in aqueous humor. This transudate may not in all cases of uveitis immediately affect pressure; however, over time its accumulation at the trabecular meshwork reduces drainage rate [6,19]. Trabecular precipitates in the form of circulating inflammatory cells and debris may further clog the Schlemm's canal and reduce drainage.
2. Inflammation of the trabecular meshwork (trabeculitis) resulting in thick and edematous trabecular filaments, as well as the accumulation of fibrin and inflammatory cells in the outflow channels (as shown in herpetic and cytomegalovirus trabeculitis) produces significant obstruction to drainage and extremely high IOP Figure 1 [20,21]. Granulomas in the angle in cases of granulomatous uveitis may also impair drainage.
3. Acute angle-closure pupillary block: The formation of synechiae posteriorly between the iris and the lens may lead to seclusion of the pupil, forward iris bowing with apposition to the angle and angle-closure glaucoma (Figure 2).

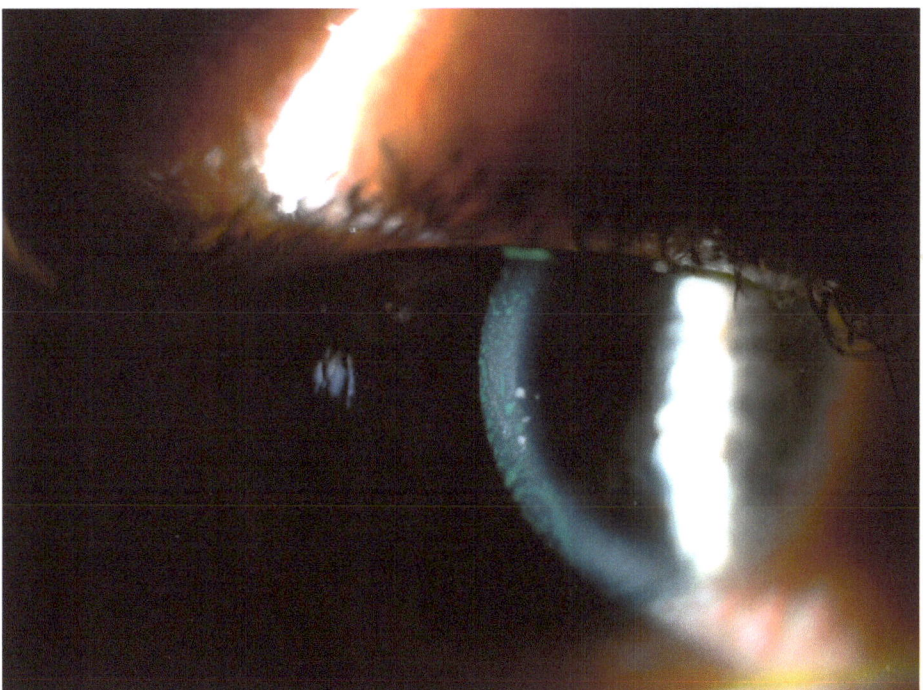

Figure 1. CMV anterior uveitis with characteristic large keratic precipates.

4. Secondary acute angle closure: swelling and anterior rotation of the ciliary body, as well as choroidal effusion, can lead to angle obstruction.
5. Chronic angle closure: Anterior synechiae formation between the iris and the angle due to the increased coagulative state of the inflamed iris may cause chronic angle closure [22]. Recently Alvarez Guzman et al. reported that the majority (80%) of cases of glaucoma associated with Vogt–Koyanagi–Harada disease were due to angle closure [23]. In the event of a uveitis that causes significant retinal or ocular ischemia,

pronounced neovascularization can affect the trabeculum, with inevitable aqueous flow obstruction and intractable glaucoma [24].

6. Special consideration should be given to the impact of corticosteroid use in glaucoma, as their use in effectively controlling the inflammation is a double-edged sword. Steroids may be the cause of UG in up to 42% of cases [10,25]. Common risk factors for steroid response in uveitis are primary open-angle glaucoma, familial history of glaucoma, rheumatoid arthritis, extremes of age (children and the elderly) and diabetes [21,26,27]. It becomes evident that in uveitis, glaucoma may present either with an open angle or with an angle-closure mechanism, or even with a combination of both.

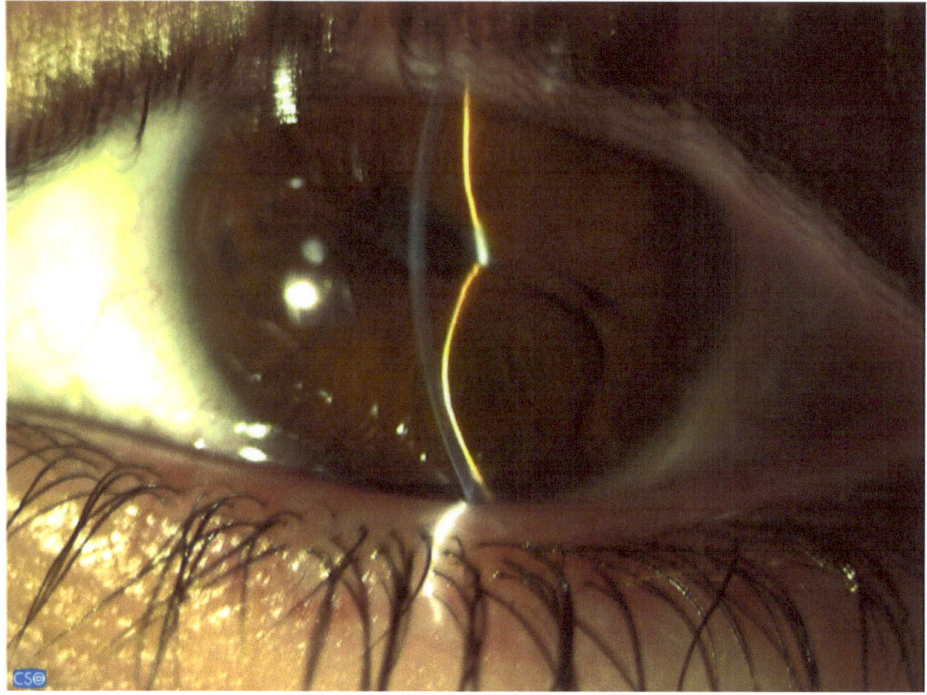

Figure 2. Angle-closure glaucoma with iris bombe.

There are also poorly studied mechanisms involved. For example, an attempt to identify a causal association between uveitis and glaucoma in the general population has disclosed a possible genetic link [28].

3. Diagnosis

High vigilance for early signs of IOP elevation and optic nerve damage in patients with uveitis is important.

Sequential visual field tests and optical coherence tomography (OCT) tests with attention to the retinal nerve fiber and ganglion cell layer thickness are mandatory. However, diagnosing glaucomatous changes during episodes of inflammation can pose a significant challenge to the ophthalmologist, as active uveitis may influence the results. Studies have revealed that in patients with active uveitis and no glaucoma, OCT displays a thickened retinal fiber layer (RNFL) compared to healthy individuals. The RNFL thickness may remain normal even in eyes with quiescent uveitis and early glaucoma. Therefore, RNFL thickness measurements should be interpreted cautiously, and screening for glaucoma is best performed when the eyes are going through periods of quiescence [29], as shown in

Figure 3. The measurement of blood flow by OCT angiography is an additional method for the detection of early glaucomatous lesions. The vessel density in the area of the optic nerve head and the macula has been shown to be reduced in primary open angle glaucoma (POAG). Several studies have indicated that the peripapillary vessel density and RNFL thickness have a similar sensitivity and specificity in diagnosing POAG [30]. In the sole study to date evaluating the use of OCT angiography in UG, Liepsech et al., reported that vessel density was reduced in the area of the optic nerve head and the macula in UG eyes in comparison to normal eyes [31]. Another case report verified the use of OCT angiography in diagnosing glaucoma in an instance of active uveitis [32].

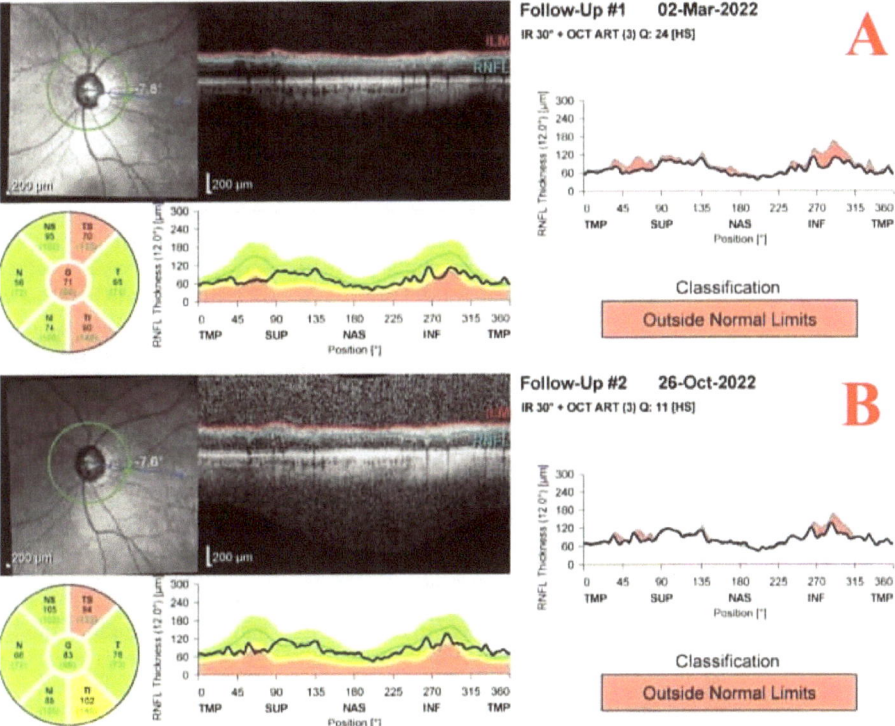

Figure 3. Retinal nerve fiber layer thickness before (**A**) and during (**B**) inflammation.

Additionally, anterior-segment OCT (AS-OCT) may assist in revealing corneal thickness, abnormal irises, the ciliary body and angle configuration; this will lead to early intervention. At the same time, if the cornea precludes visualization of the anterior segment, ultrasound biomicroscopy can offer valuable information regarding the anterior segment structures. Importantly, these ancillary tests should never negate or replace regular and meticulous clinical examination and gonioscopy; this is crucial for these patients, for whom persistent inflammation, increasing pigment deposition, granulomas, posterior or anterior synechiae and early neovascularization of the angle may be identified and treated accordingly. Gonioscopy should always be performed to identify the presence of synechiae nodules or neovascularization in the angle and to establish the extent of angle closure [22].

4. Treatment

Management of UG is multidisciplinary and involves both strict control of the inflammation and treatment of the IOP elevation. Treatment can be both medical and surgical.

4.1. Medical Treatment

Identifying the cause of uveitis is crucial, as in cases of infectious etiology, where treating the underlying infection will expedite resolution of the disease. This is best exemplified in herpetic or toxoplasmic uveitis, where antiviral and antiparasitic medication produce an immediate improvement to the clinical signs and symptoms [33,34]. It has been shown that IOP in CMV-positive PSS is more difficult to control than in CMV-negative cases. Treatment of CMV infection with valganciclovir or ganciclovir has been shown to improve PSS control [35] and contribute to withdrawal of the steroids in cases of steroid-dependent PSS [36]. Touhami et al. have found that in cases of CMV anterior uveitis, the institution of early (<700 days) antiviral treatment reduced the need for later antiglaucoma surgery [37]. This is attributable to the fact that early antiviral treatment prevented permanent damage to the trabecular meshwork.

In the event of idiopathic or immune-mediated diseases, corticosteroids (administered either locally or systematically), immunosupressants or the recently introduced monoclonal antibodies should be used accordingly. Treatment should be aggressive, aiming to achieve quiescence; furthermore, one should not choose to undertreat in order to avoid corticosteroid-induced IOP rise, as the adverse effects of chronic inflammation may further complicate the outcome [6,27]. However, great consideration should be given to the mode of implementation of steroid treatment. A recent multicenter study has shown that eyes treated with fluocinolone implant have substantially higher risk of developing glaucoma than eyes treated with systemic therapy (40% vs. 8% in 6.9 years) [38].

B-blockers, prostaglandin (PG) analogs, a-adrenergic agonists, topical and systemic carbonic anhydrase inhibitors and combined preparations may be used for the control of IOP in cases of UG. There is controversy regarding the use of prostaglandin analogues (PGAs) as first-line agents in UG due to their proinflammatory properties, the possibility of exacerbation of herpes simplex keratouveitis and the occurrence of cystoid macular oedema [39]. There are studies that support their safety for UG patients [40], and some authorities advocate the use of PGAs as first-line treatment [41,42]. Furthermore, there are indications that bimatoprost has a much lower propensity in causing uveitis or macular edema than latanoprost [43]. On the contrary, cholinergic agonists are usually avoided in uveitic patients, as they are proven to aggravate inflammation (by increasing blood aqueous barrier breakdown) and promote posterior synechiae formation.

Investigations for effective treatment are ongoing and ripasudil, a rho-kinase inhibitor that was first introduced in Japan in 2014 has demonstrated effectiveness in approximately 50% of patients suffering from glaucoma [44,45]. Recent studies suggest that ripasurdil is particularly effective in eyes with ocular inflammation that receive steroids, as it may have an anti-inflammatory effect along with its effects to the IOP [45,46].

4.2. Laser Treatment

Nd-YAG laser peripheral iridotomy (LPI) is used for anterior chamber angle closure due to posterior synechiae and iris bombe, but it is not always successful in UG. According to the sole study to date that evaluated the results of LPI in acute angle closure secondary to UG, 62% of LPIs performed did not remain functional after 85 days. Therefore, the performance of at least two iridotomies and intensive treatment with corticosteroids and cycloplegics is recommend. The performance of LPI should be avoided in eyes with severe active anterior uveitis, corneal oedema or iridocorneal touch, as a shallow anterior chamber increases the risk of endothelial damage during LPI [22,47].

Argon laser iridoplasty was successful in one case of acute angle closure associated with uveitis that did not respond to repeated LPIs and medical treatment [48].

Until recently, SLT was not considered a treatment option for UG because of the inflammation that it may induce [49]. However, recent publications tend to refute this theory. Initially Maleki et al. performed SLT in 15 eyes of 14 patients with stable uveitis who had received one fluocinolone implant that caused glaucoma. Their success rate at 1 year was 46.7%, slightly less favorable than in patients with POAG [50]. Xiao et al. performed high-energy (1.2–1.5 mJ per pulse as opposed to 0.9 mJ for regular treatment) SLT treatment in 20 patients with steroid-induced glaucoma and quiescent uveitis and reported a 65% success rate without complications. A more frequent postoperative steroid regimen was followed [51]. Recently, Zhou et al. compared the reduction of IOP and complications after SLT in UG and POAG or PEX glaucoma. They did not find a difference except at a time point 3–8 weeks after treatment [52]. At this time point, the reduction of IOP was greater in the UG group than in the PEX glaucoma group. In conclusion, even though data are limited, it seems that SLT is a promising treatment which can be applied in quiescent uveitis cases with steroid-induced glaucoma.

Cyclodestructive procedures using the 810 nm diode laser are most of the time reserved for cases in which all other methods of surgical treatment have failed. Because of the very serious complications they cause, they are a final choice in UG. Applying transcleral diode laser cyclophotocoagulation (TD-CPC) to an already inflamed and underactive ciliary body can cause severe damage. Laser cyclophotocoagulation may cause severe hypotony in 19% of patients and is likely to cause phthisis, irreversible anatomical lesions to the globe and loss of vision [53]. However, in a small series of 20 patients using a treatment mode of 10–15 applications of 2.0 W energy applied for 2 s to treat no more than 270°, Shlote et al. reported a 72.2% success rate without any serious adverse effect [54]. Voykov et al. used TD-CPC to treat 16 patients with Fuchs uveitis. In 10 of them, TD-CPC was the sole surgical treatment. After 1 year, control of IOP was achieved in 6 out of 10 patients (60%). There was no exacerbation of intraocular inflammation, no postoperative hypotony and no phthisis bulbi in the 16 patients who underwent CPC [55]. In contrast, Heinz et al. used TD-CPC to treat UG attributed to juvenile rheumatoid arthritis and reported a 32% qualified success after 9 months [56].

Recently, micropulse wave transscleral diode cyclophotocoagulation has been proposed as an alternative to TD-CPC, offering a better safety profile. Its operating principle is based on short laser pulses (ON cycles) separated by intervals corresponding to the thermal relaxation time (OFF cycles). During ON cycles, energy accumulates in the pigmented epithelium to achieve the coagulation threshold. It has been proposed that the OFF cycles allow thermal dissipation and thus reduce collateral damage and adverse effects such as inflammation and chronic hypotony. Several studies reporting favorable results with micro-pulse diode cyclophotocoagulation included a small number of eyes with UG [57,58].

4.3. Surgical Treatment

According to several studies, almost 30% of patients with UG will need surgical treatment [8,59,60]. This percentage may be significantly higher in children [8]. Surgical treatment of UG may be challenging for a variety of reasons. Persistent intraocular inflammation, extensive use of steroids and extreme IOP range are factors that need to be considered when choosing the appropriate surgical technique. Uveitis patients may have a wide variation in their IOP and there is always a possibility of ocular hypertension alternating with ocular hypotony, with devastating consequences for the eye. While reviewing the literature of more than two decades, it is generally accepted that either trabeculectomy [59] or valve [60] implantation are safe and most of the times successful procedures in the treatment of UG. However, most of studies evaluating surgical techniques in UG are retrospective in their design with a small number of participants; furthermore, they present data in various different ways, and many of them have a limited follow-up period. Given the limited lifespan thattraditional glaucoma surgery has and the fact that UG patients who present for glaucoma surgery are either in their mid-fifties or children, alternative conjuctival sparing approaches are being considered. Recently, various techniques of minimally invasive glaucoma surgery (MIGS) are being instituted in the surgical treatment of UG. Most of the instances are performed as primary procedures or along with cataract surgery, but some are tried after other methods have failed.

5. Trabeculectomy

Trabeculectomy has been the preferred surgical procedure for UG for many years [61,62]. Although studies evaluating the success rate of trabeculectomy in UG are retrospective with a small number of patients, most of them agree that the success rate of trabeculectomy with MMC is reduced in UG in comparison to POAG [63]. There are at least two reasons for this: Inflammatory activity is likely to be more pronounced in uveitic eyes following intraocular surgery, leading either to hypotony due to ciliary body impairment or to bleb failure due to subconjunctival scarring. Almarobac et al. reported that the cumulative probabilities of success were 60% and 35.7% at 36 and 60 months postoperation, respectively, whereas in the largest up-to-date series, Iwao et al. reported probabilities of success 1, 3 and 5 years after trabeculectomy in the UG group of 89.5%, 71.3% and 61.7%, respectively [63,64]. In a recent study, Kanaya et al. reported that the success rates in UG and POAG were 91.7% and 88.0% at 12 months, 82.2% and 75.6% at 36 months, and 66.5% and 61.8% at 120 months, respectively [65]. The authors attributed the increased success rate of trabeculectomy in UG (which was similar to that in POAG) to the successful control of the inflammation. Different studies evaluated risk factors for the failure of trabeculectomy in cases with UG. Iwao et al. considered cataract surgery and granulomatous uveitis as a risk factor for failure [63]. Almobarac et al. reported that in UG eyes that underwent phacoemulsification following MMC-enhanced trabeculectomy, the bleb survived but the eyes required more medication to control the IOP after the procedure [66]. In contrast to Iwao et al. [63], Kanaya et al. reported that granulomatous uveitis was significantly associated with favorable prognosis [65]. There is controversy regarding whether preoperative inflammation affects the results of surgery. On the contrary, most studies agree that postoperative inflammation is a risk factor of worsening failure rate for trabeculectomy surgery [67,68].

Kwon et al. looked specifically at the effect of the activity of inflammation on the success rate of trabeculectomies in UG and concluded that the initial activity of inflammation did not affect the success rate, but relapses of the inflammation were risk factors for failure [69]. In contrast, recently, Magliya et al. concluded that proper perioperative uveitis control in patients attending UG surgeries results in lower IOP levels and less inflammation over 2 years postoperatively [70]. Finally, Gregory et al. evaluated the effect of race on the course of UG and concluded that trabeculectomy has a higher risk of failure in black patients [71].

6. Minimally Invasive Glaucoma Surgical (MIGS) Devices in Uveitic Glaucoma

Minimally invasive glaucoma surgical (MIGS) devices have been developed as a surgical option for glaucoma, to improve surgical safety, conserve conjunctiva and maintain efficacy in terms of lowering IOP. Procedures that disrupt, ablate, or bypass the trabecular meshwork (TM) constitute MIGS. These procedures include ab interno trabeculectomy using the Trabectome® (NeoMedix, Tustin, CA, USA), goniotomy with the Kahook Dual Blade® (New World Medical, Cucamonga, CA, USA) and gonioscopy-assisted transluminal trabeculotomy (GATT). These techniques are blebless and target the TM, the primary anatomic structure responsible for aqueous outflow resistance.

Goniotomy has traditionally been used to treat pediatric UG. It has been shown that it results in a significant decrease in IOP and number of IOP-lowering medications, although multiple interventions are often needed [72,73]. Recently, Meerwijk et al. reported success rates of 100%, 93% and 80% at 1, 2 and 5 years, respectively, after performing goniotomy in children with a mean age of 7 years and non-infectious UG [74]. There were no significant changes in visual acuity and uveitis activity or its treatment, and there were no major complications.

Trabectome (Neomedix, Tustin, CA, USA) is a MIGS device that uses electrocautery, irrigation and aspiration to selectively ablate the trabecular meshwork and the inner wall of Schlemm's canal and allow aqueous free access to the canal and its collector channels. Anton et al. used Trabectome to treat 24 patients with UG and reported that there was no patient who achieved absolute success but 87.5% of the patients achieved qualified success after 1 year. Three (12.5%) patients needed further glaucoma surgery [75]. According to Swamy et al., who reported the results of the operation from 45 eyes with UG from the Trabectome Study Group database, the qualified success rate at 12 months was 91%. Six (13.4%) cases required secondary glaucoma surgery and no other serious complication were noticed [76].

The Kahook dual blade (KDB) is a disposable handpiece that employs two parallel blades to remove a strip of trabecular meshwork to improve outflow. It may be combined with phacoemulsification. Murata et al. performed ab interno trabeculotomy with KDB in 24 eyes with UG and reported that the success rate was 33% in 1 year [77]. In contrast, Chen et al. performed KDB in 24 eyes of 22 patients and reported an 86% success rate after 2 years [78]. TrabEx+ (MST, Redmond, WA, USA) consists of a handpiece with a dual blade that is also connected with an irrigation and aspiration system that adapts to each machine for phacoemulsification. Tanev et Kirkova reported 100% qualified success 18 months after performing TrabEx in 12 patients with UG [79].

Gonioscopy-assisted transluminal trabeculotomy (GATT) is a minimally invasive ab interno procedure that has evolved from traditional trabeculotomy techniques and is performed with a prolene suture or with the guidance of an illuminating micro-catheter device. The surgical procedure involves cutting through the trabecular meshwork, cannulating the Schlemm's canal 360° and unroofing the Schlemm's canal. GATT is believed to reduce IOP by fracturing the trabecular meshwork and removing the resistance to aqueous outflow. Initially, Sachdev et al. successfully used GATT in three young patients with JRA uveitis [80]. Very recently, Gunay et al. reported favorable results in two other patients [81]. Parkish et al., in a small study of 16 eyes with uncontrolled UG, reported a cumulative success rate of 81% at 12 months. Transient hyphema was seen in 44% of eyes [82]. In the largest series to date, Belkin et al. used GATT in 33 eyes of 32 patients with UG who underwent GATT with or without concomitant cataract extraction. Surgical success was achieved in 71.8% of cases in 1 year. No sight-threatening complications occurred during surgery or follow-up [83]. Sotani et al. performed microhook trabeculotomy with a straight Tanito microhook (M-2215 s, Inami & Co., Ltd., Tokyo, Japan) in 36 eyes of 30 patients and reported that after 1 year, surgical success was achieved in 67% of eyes [84]. Other MIGS used are the i-stent and Hydrous, which might have a role as primary or secondary conjunctival sparing procedures in UG [85].

Bleb-Forming Devices

Similar to traditional filtering surgery, another MIGS approach to reducing IOP is to shunt aqueous from the anterior chamber to the subconjunctival space. The Xen® gel stent (Allergan INC, Dublin, Ireland) and PreserFlo® (Santen, Osaka, Japan) microShunt utilize this approach. Because this approach results in the formation of a filtering bleb, there is debate as to whether they may truly be classified in the MIGS category.

The Xen implant stent is a hydrophilic tube that is 6 mm long with a lumen of 45 μm, and it is composed of porcine gelatine crosslinked with glutaraldehyde to prevent degradation when implanted [86]. In 2018, Sng et al. published the first results with Xen-45 in UG. They implanted Xen-45 in 24 consecutive UG patients, in the majority of whom conventional glaucoma surgery was considered inevitable. The 12-month cumulative Kaplan–Meier survival probability was 79.2% [87].

Qureshi et al. performed Xen-45 implantation in urgent basis in 37 eyes with uncontrolled glaucoma. At the end of the follow-up period (12 to 23 months; mean: 16.7 months) five eyes (13.5%) failed, needing further glaucoma surgery. The cumulative probability of absolute success was 89.2% 1 year after surgery [88].

Recently, Evers et al. reported results for Xen-45 implantation in 25 eyes with uncontrolled UG. Six eyes (24%) underwent surgical revision and were considered failures. At the final follow-up (mean: 17.7 months), 72% of eyes achieved complete success and 4% of eyes qualified success. Notably, the Xen implant did not prevent IOP spikes during uveitis activity [89].

Serar et al. reported the successful use of Xen-63 with a larger lumen in the case of a refractory neovascular glaucoma due to Fuchs heterochromic iridocyclitis and retinal vein occlusion after the failure of an Ahmed tube. After one-year, intraocular pressure was 16 mmHg without any medication and the bleb was well-formed [90].

The PreserFlo® microShunt is an 8.5-mm-long glaucoma filtration surgical device with a 350 μm outer diameter and a 70 μm lumen that is implanted through an ab externo technique. The device's proximal tip rests in the anterior chamber while the distal tip sits under the conjunctiva and Tenon's capsule, about 6 mm beyond the limbus, enabling aqueous humor to pass through the lumen to produce a posterior bleb after implantation [91]. Triolo et al. reported 36-month results of PreserFlo implants in a consecutive series of 21 patients with UG. The mean rates of success were 68%, 47% and 47% at 12, 24 and 36 months postoperation, respectively [92].

7. No Penetrating Glaucoma Procedures in Uveitic Glaucoma

In uveitic patients, non-penetrating surgery offers the advantage of minimal postoperative anterior chamber inflammation and a reduced risk of delayed complications such as hypotony and bleb-related infections, which are more common with trabeculectomy. The absence of an iridectomy and anterior chamber penetration is supposed to reduce the inflammatory response while the presence of a trabecular meshwork may act as a barrier to infectious organisms entering the eye. Satisfactory long-term results have been reported for non-penetrating glaucoma procedures (deep sclerectomy (DS) and viscocanalostomy) in the management of UG. Obeidan et al. performed DS in 33 consecutive eyes of 21 patients and after a mean follow-up of 33.2 months reported that complete success was obtained in 72.7% of eyes, whereas qualified success was obtained in 21.2% of eyes, yielding an overall success rate of 93.9% [93].

Mercieca et al. reported that after performing DS with 0.2–04 mgr/l MMC in 43 eyes of 43 patients, the probabilities of IOP < 22 mmHg and <19 mmHg were 69% and 62% at 3 years and 60% and 51% at 5 years, respectively. Most eyes (60%) had a Nd:Yag laser goniopuncture (LGP) by the fifth year. Recurrence of uveitis was observed in 16 eyes. Seven eyes (16.3%) had subsequent glaucoma procedures [94].

The limitation of deep sclerectomy is that it is technically difficult to perform manually, which has limited its popularity. CO^2 laser-assisted sclerectomy surgery (CLASS) is an improved version of DS that uses a CO^2 laser, which is precise and easily strips the deep sclera, unroofs the Schlemm's canal (SC) and leaves the trabecular meshwork thin enough for aqueous humor percolation. Xiao et al. performed CLASS in 22 eyes with UG and in 25 eyes with POAG and compared the results. After 1 year, the qualified surgical success was comparable between the UG (86.9%) and POAG (96.0%) groups, and the complete success rates were 60.9% and 64.0% in the UG group and POAG group, respectively [95].

Recently, Salloukh et al. presented long-term results after performing vicocanalostomy in 16 patients with UG. Complete and qualified success was seen in 75% and 94% of patients at year 1, 50% and 86% of patients at year 3 and 19% and 75% of patients at year 5 [96]. The long term (>2 years) outcomes of the aforementioned procedures, according to the recent literature, are presented in Table 1.

Table 1. Recent studies reporting long term (>2 years) outcomes of surgical treatment in adult uveitic glaucoma.

	Procedure	Patients/Eyes	Diagnosis (%)	F/U (Months)	Success Rate (%) *	Complications	Secondary Procedures (%)
Almobarac (2017) [64]	Trabeculectomy	50/70	VKH 38.6% Idiopathic 24.3 Fuchs 15.7	77 ± 40.9	35.7	Cataract 45.3 Hypotony 30 IOP spike 10	25.7
Kanaya (2021) [65]	Trabeculectomy	50/50	Idiopathic 42 Sarcoidosis 34 VKH 8 Bechset 8	120	66.5	Hyphema 14 Choroidals 14	16
Known (2017) [69]	Trabeculectomy	54/54	Idiopathic 42 Fuchs 14	24 ± 21	67	Late hypotony 15	
	BGI	28/28	Herpetic 8.5 Sarcoidosis 8.5	31 ± 21	75	Late hypotony 11 Corneal edema 3.6 Endophthalmitis 7.1	
Chen (2023) [78]	KDB	22/24	Idiopathic anterior 45 idiopathic posterior 17.5	24	69	Cyclodialysis cleft 8.3 Transients IOP elevation 17 Early hypotony 8	12.5
	GATT	40/33		24	80	Cyclodialysis cleft 3 Transient IOP elevation 20 Hyphema 10	7.5
Triolo (2023) [92]	Preserflo	21/21	Idiopathic 52 Possner Schlosman 10 Sarcoidosis 10		47	Button hole 4.7	57.1
Merceica (2017) [94]	Deep sclerectomy	43/43	Idiopathic 35 Fuchs 32.5 Herpes 9.3	68 ± 33	60	Transient hypotonoous maculopathy 5 Vision loss 2	16.3
Salloukh (2021) [96]	Viscocanalostomy	16		60	75	Transient IOP > 30.73	25

(*): according to the definition by the author; VKH: Vogt–Koyanagi–Harada; BGI: Baerveldt glaucoma implant; KDB: Kahook dual blade; GATT: gonioscopy-assisted transluminal trabeculotomy; JIA: juvenile idiopathic arthritis.

8. Tube Shunt Surgery in Uveitic Glaucoma

Tube shunt (aqueous shunt) surgery has traditionally been reserved for refractory glaucoma. Therefore, shunts are commonly performed as primary surgery in UG.

Ahmed Valve and UG: The Ahmed Glaucoma Valve® (AGV, New World Medical Inc., Rancho Cucamonga, CA, USA) is a glaucoma drainage device commonly used for the treatment of glaucoma. It can be used as a primary surgical procedure or after failure of a previous filtration procedure. As the AGV has an internal valve mechanism consisting of thin silicone elastomer membranes, it does not require additional restrictive mechanisms to limit aqueous humour flow from the anterior chamber to the subconjunctival space. The above valve mechanism prevents early hypotony, which is considered advantageous, especially in UG. The body plate is usually placed 8–10 mm from the limbus while the tube is inserted 2–3 mm into the anterior chamber (AC), sulcus or even the vitreous cavity, depending on AGV type. More recently, a new type of AGV was introduced (Ahmed ClearPath GDD) which lacks the internal valve mechanism. It is available in 250 mm^2 and 350 mm^2 sizes and a pre-threaded 4-0 rip cord is provided by the manufacturer to prevent hypotony during the early postoperative period.

Data for more than 20 years can give us a general idea of what to expect when using these shunts as far as outcomes and complications are concerned. Earlier studies indicated that a significant IOP reduction (at least 25% from preoperative values) was achieved in more than 70% and 50% of patients at 1 and 4 years postoperation [97–99]. A significant reduction of glaucoma medications was also detected in all cases, but up to 17% of eyes experienced complications during the follow-up period [97]. The most important complications were tube occlusion, valve exposure and corneal decompensation [97,99]. It has been proposed that sulcus placement of the tube is associated with a moderate decrease in endothelial cell count and is strongly recommended in eyes at high risk of corneal failure. Macular edema as well as ocular hypotony is still a concern even with the use of AGV. Ramdas et al. reported that 13.2% and 15.8% of UG patients developed macular edema and hypotony, respectively, after AGV and Baerveldt-350 implantation. These percentages were higher compared to non-uveitic patients, but the difference was not statistically significant. IOP reduction was comparable to that of non-uveitic glaucoma patients (44.9% vs. 42.8% decrease) [18]. When AGV performance was evaluated as the mean IOP decrease postoperatively, this was ranged from 11 mmHg to 25.2 mmHg [100–104]. A mean decrease in the number of antiglaucoma medications was also achieved (1.88) [100–104]. Combining AGV with fluocinolone implant resulted in even less need for glaucoma medications [105]. The success rate was relatively higher in eyes with pars planitis and lower in eyes with ankylosing spondylitis, suggesting that there might be differences in valve performance depending on the uveitis cause [101]. Another study indicated that aqueous suppression early after surgery, when IOP is 10–15 mmHg, was associated with lower IOP later [106].

Baerveldt Valve and UG: The Baerveldt Implant® (BGI-250/350, Johnson & Johnson Vision, Irvine, CA, USA) has been used for more than three decades in glaucoma practice worldwide. It consists of a non-valved silicone tube attached to a silicon plate of 250 mm^2 or 350 mm^2 total surface. The implant is placed under two recti muscles (usually superior and lateral) and the absence of any internal valve mechanism requires additional surgical steps to restrict aqueous flow during the early postoperative period. BGI was extensively used and evaluated in a tube vs. trabeculectomy study (TVT) and primary TVT study where surgery was performed in either glaucoma patients with previous glaucoma and/or cataract surgery (TVT) or in patients with no prior incisional surgery (PTVT). BGI surgery and trabeculectomy with MMC produced similar IOPs at 5 years postoperatively in both studies while tube shunt surgery had a higher success rate (TVT), suggesting BGI's good performance in a wide range of glaucoma patients [107,108]. Tan et al. reported results after using BGI in 47 eyes with UG. With an upper limit of 18 mmHg, the qualified success was 87% and 74% at 1 and 5 years, respectively [109]. The presence of a tube did not prevent IOP spikes during inflammation. Tan et al. reported a high rate of corneal decompensation (9%) and hypotony maculopathy (11%) as well. Chambra et al. reported a 76% qualified success rate at 5 years [110]. Casana compared the results of BGI implantation in 24 eyes with UG and 38 eyes with other forms of glaucoma. The median follow-up period was 592 days for UG and 764 days for other forms of glaucoma. At the end of follow-up time, 52.5% of UG and 32.5% of other glaucoma cases showed qualified success [111]. Manako et al. have recently reported significant IOP reductions from around 30 mmHg to 15 mmHg 1 year postoperation following BGI surgery in UG patients. This corresponded to a 1-year success rate of 88% [112]. The authors reported that the use of immunosuppressive treatment (that indicated a strong inflammatory response) was a risk factor for failure.

It is difficult to compare efficacy between different types of aqueous shunts in UG. Data from the Ahmed–Baerveldt comparison study group showed a higher vision-threatening complication rate in the BGI group at a 5-year follow up, but authors included all types of refractory glaucomas [113]. Several studies compared AGV and BGI in the management of UG. Shisha et al. compared results after performing AGV and BGI implantation in 122 eyes and concluded that after a mean follow-up of 29.6 ± 3.6 months in the AGV group and 33.1 ± 3.8 months in the BGI group, the BGI group had a greater IOP reduction (60.3% vs. 44.5%) and complete success rate (30% vs. 9%) with a higher complication rate (51.4% vs. 20.9%). The glaucoma reoperation rate was significantly higher in the AGV group (19% in the AGV group and 4% in the BGI group). Hypotony resulted in failure in 7 eyes (10%) in the BGI group and none in the AGV group [114]. The same group reported a greater incidence of corneal complications in BGI compared to AGV. Previous trabeculectomy was considered a risk factor for corneal decompensation [115].

Molteno Valve and UG: The Molteno® Implant (IOP, Inc., Costa Mesa, CA, USA/Molteno Ophthalmic Limited, Dunedin, New Zealand) is a non-valved device which consists of a silicon tube attached to a single or a double plate. The double-plate model provides more surface for aqueous humour drainage but implantation is considered surgically demanding. Molteno implants have also been used for UG patients even if this is not the most frequently inserted valve. Vuori et al. reported an 85% success rate after 4 years [116].

Recently, Garagani et al. reported the results of tube implantation (mostly Molteno) in 50 eyes of 36 children with UG. Success rates were 98% at 1 year, 87% at 5 years, and 59% at 15 years; postoperative complications occurred in 36% of patients and included hypotony (22%), tube exposure (6%), tube obstruction (4%), corneal decompensation (2%) and cystoid macular edema (2%) [117].

The question of whether UG patients lose visual acuity and/or the visual field deteriorates postoperatively needs to be addressed. Vision loss in UG patients is multifactorial and can be associated not only with IOP control but also with the level of inflammation, cataract/macula status and ciliary body function. Tan et al. reported that approximately 1/3 of BGI patients suffered significant vision loss (mean follow-up: 63.6 months) [109]. Earlier reports estimated the rate to be no more than 26% after AGV implantation but the follow-up period was shorter [97,99]. A tendency of visual field loss over the first 2 years postoperation with further stabilization has been observed in BGI patients, but contemporary literature provides insufficient data regarding visual field deterioration. The long term (>2 years) outcomes of tubes according to the recent literature are presented in Table 2.

Table 2. Recent studies reporting long term (>2 years) outcomes of tubes in adult uveitic glaucoma.

	Procedure	Patients/Eyes	Diagnosis (%)	F/U (Months)	Success Rate * (%)	Complications (%)	Secondary Procedures (%)
Kubaisi (2017) [118]	AGV + FAI	9/10	Panuveitis 44.4			RD 10	
Bao (2018) [102]	AGV	57/66	Unknown 35.8 Ankylosing spondylitis 31.3	53.3 ± 8.5	61.2	Tube erosion 7.6% RD 3%	40
Voykov (2018) [119]	AGV	17	Fuchs	36	38.4	Tube erosion 23.5 Tube obstruction 23.5 Diplopia 4	35
Yakin (2017) [120]	AGV	35/47	ABD	57.7 ± 26.1	35.9	Tube erosion 3.2 Early wound dehiscence 2.1	6.4
Sungur (2017) [101]	AGV	39/46	Idiopathic anterior uveitis 17.3 Ankylosing spondilitis 17.3 Fuchs 17.3	51.9 ± 23	63	Tube exposure 2.2	
Tan (2018) [109]	BGI	47/47	Unknown 30 Fuchs 17 Sarcoidosis 13	63.6 ± 43.1	75	Cornea decompensation 9 Hypotony maculopathy 11	17
Chambra (2019) [110]	BGI	42/34	Sarcoidosis 31 Idiopathic 21 Tuberculosis 14	58.5. ± 20.8	76	CME 5 Hypotony maculopathy 2	31
Sisha (2020) [114]	AGV	67	Anterior uveitis 86 Panuveitis 7 Posterior 6	30 ± 4	63	Tube exposure 12	45
Sisha (2020) [114]	BGI	70		33 ± 4	70	Corneal edema 6 Tube exposure 4 Endophthalmitis 1	59

(*): according to the definition by the author; AGV: Ahmed Glaucoma Valve; FAI: fluocinolone implant; BGI: Baerveldt glaucoma implant; ABD: Adamantiades–Behcet's disease; RD: retinal detachment.

9. Comparison of Tubes to Trabeculectomy

The choice of a surgical procedure for UG is not an easy task. The benefits of tube surgery over trabeculectomy remains a matter of debate. Various studies have compared the two procedures. The most reported complications have been hypotony, corneal edema and hyphema for tube implantation and aqueous leakage, macular edema and cataract progression for trabeculectomy [121]. Initially, Bettis et al., in a retrospective study of 41 eyes, reported that AGV had a higher success rate compared to trabeculectomy (100% vs. 66.7% after 1 year). Most trabeculectomies failed because of relapse of the inflammation [100]. Similar results were reported by Iverson et al., who compared BGI to trabeculectomy [122]. Later studies failed to detect a difference in the success rate [69,104]. Chow et al. [104] reported significantly worse IOP control and a higher number of antiglaucoma medications in the AGV group, compared with the trabeculectomy and BGI group. Lee et al. found that trabeculectomy had a significant benefit over AGV implantation; namely, its lower postoperative IOP values, as achieved with significantly fewer antiglaucoma medications [121].

Recently, El-Saied HMA et al. prospectively compared three surgical modalities for treatment of UG in a total of 105 patients: trabeculectomy AGV implantation and transscleral diode laser cyclophotocoagulation. They concluded that the three modalities had the same efficacy in reducing IOP and no significant difference in complications. After 2 years, complete success was achieved in 60% via trabeculectomy, 68.6% via AGV and 62.9% via TD-CPC [123].

Nevertheless, according to most experts, certain situations most clearly call for a tube as the first surgical intervention. These include patients with active inflammation at the time of surgery as well as those with other known risk factors for trabeculectomy failure: young age, black race, aphakia or pseudophakia and prior failed glaucoma surgery.

No matter which surgical approach is elected, up to 1/3 of UG will need a second or even a third operation. The activity of postoperative inflammation may be a critical factor for the longevity of the procedure [124].

10. Management Algorithm in a Patient with Uveitic Glaucoma

Initial treatment for UG should target the cause of uveitis (especially in cases of infectious uveitis), the inflammation and the IOP. PCR to detect viral DNA may be performed in cases of anterior uveitis with a PSS or Fuchs phenotype to detect CMV, as specific antiviral treatments may significantly improve the prognosis of glaucoma. In the follow-up of UG glaucoma patients' visual fields, disc photos should not be omitted along with OCT. The value of OCT angiography should be verified with further studies. Gonioscopy should define whether there is angle closure and indicate the need of laser peripheral iridotomy in cases of angle-closure glaucoma. Any class of antihypertensive medication (except cholinergic agonists) may be used for IOP control. SLT may only be considered in cases of quiescent inflammation when steroid response is suspected. Once surgical intervention for medically uncontrolled IOP is deemed necessary, glaucoma and uveitis specialists must coordinate to succeed in this task. Ocular surgery will produce a significant amount of inflammation, regardless of the adequate control that may have been achieved preoperatively. Additional perioperative suppression of the inflammatory cascade that the operation will generate is mandatory. There are no large-scale studies providing a specific algorithm; however, in our practice, the type of uveitis (anterior or posterior) and the means to achieve quiescence employed in the past (from the patient's medical records) is reviewed, in order to decide upon the best perioperative approach. A common agreement suggests that either topical, periocular or systemic steroids should be introduced a few days prior to surgery, according to the severity of previous ocular inflammation, and a slow taper should follow postoperatively. A difficult subject is the need for glaucoma surgery in eyes for which uveitis control is suboptimal; however, in real-world situations, the quiescent period may be small or even absent, or a low-grade inflammation may persist despite maximum treatment. These situations are not well described in literature and a leap of faith may be required. There is no unanimity regarding the best surgical approach, and trabeculectomy, tubes or even MIGS may be tried depending on the clinical picture and the preference of the surgeon [85].

11. Future Directions

In recent years, many advances have occurred in the diagnosis and especially the treatment of UG. However, there are various subjects that need to be clarified by further studies. The value of OCT angiography in the follow up of UG has not been adequately studied. The place of MIGS in the surgical algorithm of UG should also be assessed. The best surgical treatment of UG according to the clinical scenario (anterior vs. posterior uveitis, active vs. inactive, open angle glaucoma vs. angle-closure glaucoma) should also be defined. Finally, given that a recent prospective study regarding UG treatment indicated that TD-CPC is not inferior to surgical treatment, we should reassess its role in UG treatment, especially in the micropulse mode.

12. Conclusions

Uveitic glaucoma is a complex disease. Many pathogenic mechanisms are involved alone or in combination. The diagnostic approach is problematic as inflammatory activity may affect the interpretation of diagnostic and staging tests. In turn, the treatment poses a lot of dilemmas. Intraocular inflammation along with IOP should be controlled and the benefits of steroid treatment should be carefully balanced with the risks. The young age of glaucoma patients warrants a stepwise approach. Conservative and conjunctival sparing surgical approaches should be adopted. Minimally invasive surgical approaches have been proven effective and are increasingly being adopted in the management of UG. Whether indicated, either trabeculectomy or a tube may be equally effective depending on the condition of the patient and the preference of the doctor.

Author Contributions: All authors wrote, read, and revised the final version of the manuscript. All authors have read and agreed to the published version of the manuscript.

Funding: This research received no external funding.

Institutional Review Board Statement: Not applicable.

Informed Consent Statement: Not applicable.

Data Availability Statement: Not applicable.

Conflicts of Interest: The authors declare no conflicts of interest.

References

1. Acharya, N.R.; Tham, V.M.; Esterberg, E.; Borkar, D.S.; Parker, J.V.; Vinoya, A.C.; Uchida, A. Incidence and prevalence of uveitis: Results the Pacific ocular inflammation study. *JAMA Ophthalmol.* **2013**, *131*, 1405–1412. [CrossRef] [PubMed]
2. Gritz, D.; Wong, I.G. Incidence and prevalence of uveitis in northern California the Northern California epidemiology of uveitis study. *Ophthalmology* **2004**, *111*, 491–500. [CrossRef] [PubMed]
3. Miettinen, R. Incidence of uveitis in northern Finland. *Acta Ophthalmol.* **1997**, *55*, 252–260. [CrossRef] [PubMed]
4. Suhler, E.B.; Lloyd, M.J.; Choi, D.; Rosenbaum, J.T.; Austin, D.F. Incidence and prevalence of uveitis in Veterans Affairs medical centers of the Pacific Northwest. *Am. J. Ophthalmol.* **2008**, *146*, 890. [CrossRef]
5. Van Tran, T.; Auer, C.; Guex-Crosier, Y.; Pittet, N.; Herbort, C.P. Epidemiological characteristics of uveitis in Switzerland. *Int. Ophthalmol.* **1994**, *18*, 293–298. [CrossRef]
6. Kalogeropoulos, D.; Sung, V.C. Pathogenesis of Uveitic Glaucoma. *J. Curr. Glaucoma Pract.* **2018**, *12*, 125–138. [CrossRef]
7. Tsirouki, T.; Dastiridou, A.; Symeonidis, C.; Tounakaki, O.; Brazitikou, I.; Kalogeropoulos, C.; Androudi, S. A Focus on the Epidemiology of Uveitis. *Ocul. Immunol. Inflamm.* **2018**, *26*, 2–16. [CrossRef]
8. Heinz, C.; Koch, J.M.; Zurek-Imhoff, B.; Heiligenhaus, A. Prevalence of uveitic secondary glaucoma and success of nonsurgical treatment in adults and children in a tertiary referral center. *Ocul. Immunol. Inflamm.* **2009**, *17*, 243–248. [CrossRef]
9. Neri, P.; Azuara-Blanco, A.; Forrester, J.V. Incidence of glaucoma in patients with uveitis. *J. Glaucoma.* **2004**, *13*, 461–465. [CrossRef]
10. Kanda, T.; Shibata, M.; Taguchi, M.; Ishikawa, S.; Harimoto, K.; Takeuchi, M. Prevalence and aetiology of ocular hypertension in acute and chronic uveitis. *Br. J. Ophthalmol.* **2014**, *98*, 932–936. [CrossRef]

11. Kalogeropoulos, D.M.; Asproudis, I.; Stefaniotou, M.; Moschos, M.M.; Kozobolis, V.P.; Voulgari, P.V.; Katsanos, A.; Gartzonika, C.; Kalogeropoulos, C. The Large Hellenic Study of Uveitis: Diagnostic and Therapeutic Algorithms, Complications, and Final Outcome. *Asia Pac. J. Ophthalmol.* **2023**, *12*, 44–57. [CrossRef] [PubMed]
12. Daniel, E.; Pistilli, M.; Kothari, S.; Khachatryan, N.; Kaçmaz, R.O.; Gangaputra, S.S.; Sen, H.N.; Suhler, E.B.; Thorne, J.E.; Foster, C.S.; et al. Risk of Ocular Hypertension in Adults with Noninfectious Uveitis. *Ophthalmology* **2017**, *124*, 1196–1208. [CrossRef] [PubMed]
13. Ma, T.; Sims, J.L.; Bennett, S.; Chew, S.; Niederer, R.L. High rate of conversion from ocular hypertension to glaucoma in subjects with uveitis. *Br. J. Ophthalmol.* **2022**, *106*, 1520–1523. [CrossRef] [PubMed]
14. Tomkins-Netzer, O.; Talat, L.; Bar, A.; Lula, A.; Taylor, S.R.; Joshi, L.; Lightman, S. Long-term clinical outcome and causes of vision loss in patients with uveitis. *Ophthalmology* **2014**, *121*, 2387–2392. [CrossRef] [PubMed]
15. Al-Ani, H.H.; Sims, J.L.; Tomkins-Netzer, O.; Lightman, S.; Niederer, R.L. Vision loss in anterior uveitis. *Br. J. Ophthalmol.* **2020**, *104*, 1652–1657. [CrossRef]
16. Baneke, A.J.; Lim, K.S.; Stanford, M. The Pathogenesis of Raised Intraocular Pressure in Uveitis. *Curr. Eye Res.* **2016**, *41*, 137–149. [CrossRef]
17. Kok, H.; Barton, K. Uveitic glaucoma. *Ophthalmol. Clin. N. Am.* **2002**, *15*, 375–387. [CrossRef]
18. Ramdas, W.D.; Pals, J.; Rothova, A.; Wolfs, R.C.W. Efficacy of Glaucoma Drainage Devices in Uveitic Glaucoma and a Meta-Analysis of the Literature. *Graefes Arch. Clin. Exp. Ophthalmol. Albrecht Von. Graefes Arch. Klin. Exp. Ophthalmol.* **2019**, *257*, 143–151. [CrossRef]
19. Kesav, N.; Palestine, A.G.; Kahook, M.Y.; Pantcheva, M.B. Current management of uveitis-associated ocular hypertension and glaucoma. *Surv. Ophthalmol.* **2020**, *65*, 397–407. [CrossRef]
20. Yan, X.; Li, M.; Wang, J.; Zhang, H.; Zhou, X.; Chen, Z. Morphology of the Trabecular Meshwork and Schlemm's Canal in Posner-Schlossman Syndrome. *Investig. Ophthalmol. Vis. Sci.* **2022**, *63*, 1. [CrossRef]
21. Kalogeropoulos, D.; Kalogeropoulos, C.; Moschos, M.M.; Sung, V. The Management of Uveitic Glaucoma in Children. *Turk. J. Ophthalmol.* **2019**, *49*, 283–293. [CrossRef] [PubMed]
22. Sng, C.C.A.; Barton, K. Mechanism and Management of Angle Closure in Uveitis. *Curr. Opin. Ophthalmol.* **2015**, *26*, 121–127. [CrossRef]
23. Alvarez-Guzman, C.; Valdez-Garcia, J.E.; Ruiz-Lozano, R.E.; Rodriguez-Garcia, A.; Navas-Villar, C.F.; Hartleben-Matkin, C.; Pedroza-Seres, M. High prevalence of angle-closure glaucoma in Vogt-Koyanagi-Harada disease. *Int. Ophthalmol.* **2022**, *42*, 3913–3921. [CrossRef] [PubMed]
24. Călugăru, D.; Călugăru, M. Etiology, Pathogenesis, and Diagnosis of Neovascular Glaucoma. *Int. J. Ophthalmol.* **2022**, *15*, 1005–1010. [CrossRef] [PubMed]
25. Dibas, A.; Yorio, T. Glucocorticoid Therapy and Ocular Hypertension. *Eur. J. Pharmacol.* **2016**, *787*, 57–71. [CrossRef] [PubMed]
26. Yakin, M.; Kumar, A.; Kodati, S.; Jones, L.; Sen, H.N. Risk of Elevated Intraocular Pressure with Difluprednate in Patients with Non-Infectious Uveitis. *Am. J. Ophthalmol.* **2022**, *240*, 232–238. [CrossRef]
27. Sherman, E.R.; Cafiero-Chin, M. Overcoming Diagnostic and Treatment Challenges in Uveitic Glaucoma. *Clin. Exp. Optom.* **2019**, *102*, 109–115. [CrossRef]
28. Seo, J.H.; Lee, Y. Causal Association between Iritis or Uveitis and Glaucoma: A Two-Sample Mendelian Randomisation Study. *Genes* **2023**, *14*, 642. [CrossRef]
29. Yilmaz, H.; Koylu, M.T.; Çakır, B.A.; Küçükevcilioğlu, M.; Durukan, A.H.; Bayer, A.; Mutlu, F.M. Uveitis as a Confounding Factor in Retinal Nerve Fiber Layer Analysis Using Optical Coherence Tomography. *Ocul. Immunol. Inflamm.* **2022**, *30*, 386–391. [CrossRef]
30. Rao, H.L.; Pradhan, Z.S.F.; Suh, M.H.; Moghimi, S.; Mansouri, K.; Weinreb, R.N. Optical Coherence Tomography Angiography in Glaucoma. *J. Glaucoma* **2020**, *29*, 312–321. [CrossRef] [PubMed]
31. Lommatzsch, C.; Bauermann, P.; Heimes-Bussmann, B.; Nolte, C.; Heinz, C. Optical Coherence Tomography Angiography in Uveitic Glaucoma—A Pilot Study. *Ocul. Immunol. Inflamm.* **2021**, *29*, 1410–1416. [CrossRef]
32. Do, J.L.; Sylvester, B.; Shahidzadeh, A.; Wang, R.K.; Chu, Z.; Patel, V.; Richter, G.M. Utility of optical coherence tomography angiography in detecting glaucomatous damage in a uveitic patient with disc congestion: A case report. *Am. J. Ophthalmol. Case Rep.* **2017**, *8*, 78–83. [CrossRef] [PubMed]
33. Fan, X.; Li, Z.; Zhai, R.; Sheng, Q.; Kong, X. Clinical Characteristics of Virus-Related Uveitic Secondary Glaucoma: Focus on Cytomegalovirus and Varicella Zoster Virus. *BMC Ophthalmol.* **2022**, *22*, 130. [CrossRef] [PubMed]
34. Ahmad, F.; Deshmukh, N.; Webel, A.; Johnson, S.; Suleiman, A.; Mohan, R.R.; Fraunfelder, F.; Singh, P.K. Viral infections and pathogenesis of glaucoma: A comprehensive review. *Clin. Microbiol. Rev.* **2023**, *36*, e0005723. [CrossRef] [PubMed]
35. Su, C.-C.; Hu, F.-R.; Wang, T.-H.; Huang, J.-Y.; Yeh, P.-T.; Lin, C.-P.; Wang, I.-J. Clinical outcomes in cytomegalovirus-positive Posner-Schlossman syndrome patients treated with topical ganciclovir therapy. *Am. J. Ophthalmol.* **2014**, *15*, 1024–1031. [CrossRef]
36. Sheng, Q.; Sun, Y.; Zhai, R.; Fan, X.; Ying, Y.; Kong, X. 2% Ganciclovir Controlled Posner-Schlossman Syndrome Relapse and Reduced the Chance of Corticosteroid Dependence: A Large Cohort in East China. *Ocul. Immunol. Inflamm.* **2023**, 1–8. [CrossRef]
37. Touhami, S.; Qu, L.; Angi, M.; Bojanova, M.; Touitou, V.; Lehoang, P.; Rozenberg, F.; Bodaghi, B. Cytomegalovirus Anterior Uveitis: Clinical Characteristics and Long term Outcomes in a French Series. *Am. J. Ophthalmol.* **2018**, *194*, 134–142. [CrossRef]

38. Kempen, J.H.; Van Natta, M.L.; Friedman, D.S.; Altaweel, M.M.; Ansari, H.; Dunn, J.P.; Elner, S.G.; Holbrook, J.T.; Lim, L.L.; Sugar, E.A.; et al. Incidence and Outcome of Uveitic Glaucoma in Eyes with Intermediate, Posterior, or Panuveitis Followed up to 10 Years After Randomization to Fluocinolone Acetonide Implant or Systemic Therapy. *Am. J. Ophthalmol.* **2020**, *219*, 303–316. [CrossRef]
39. Horsley, M.B.; Chen, T.C. The use of prostaglandin analogs in the uveitic patient. *Semin. Ophthalmol.* **2011**, *26*, 285–289. [CrossRef]
40. Markomichelakis, N.N.; Kostakou, A.; Halkiadakis, I.; Chalkidou, S.; Papakonstantinou, D.; Georgopoulos, G. Efficacy and safety of latanoprost in eyes with uveitic glaucoma. *Graefes Arch. Clin. Exp. Ophthalmol.* **2009**, *247*, 775–780. [CrossRef]
41. Siddique, S.S.; Suelves, A.M.; Baheti, U.; Foster, C.S. Glaucoma and uveitis. *Surv. Ophthalmol.* **2013**, *58*, 1–10. [CrossRef]
42. Hu, J.; Vu, J.T.; Hong, B.; Gottlieb, C. Uveitis and cystoid macular oedema secondary to topical prostaglandin analogue use in ocular hypertension and open angle glaucoma. *Br. J. Ophthalmol.* **2020**, *104*, 1040–1044. [CrossRef]
43. Araie, M.; Sugiyama, K.; Aso, K.; Kanemoto, K.; Iwata, R.; Hollander, D.A.; Senchyna, M.; Kopczynski, C.C. Phase 3 Clinical Trial Comparing the Safety and Efficacy of Netarsudil to Ripasudil in Patients with Primary Open-Angle Glaucoma or Ocular Hypertension: Japan Rho Kinase Elevated Intraocular Pressure Treatment Trial (J-ROCKET). *Adv. Ther.* **2023**, *40*, 4639–4656. [CrossRef] [PubMed]
44. Kusuhara, S.; Katsuyama, A.; Matsumiya, W.; Nakamura, M. Efficacy and safety of ripasudil, a Rho-associated kinase inhibitor, in eyes with uveitic glaucoma. *Graefes Arch. Clin. Exp. Ophthalmol.* **2018**, *256*, 809–814. [CrossRef]
45. Pinnock, C.; Yip, J.L.Y.; Khawaja, A.P.; Luben, R.; Hayat, S.; Yanai, R.; Uchi, S.-H.; Kobayashi, M.; Nagai, T.; Teranishi, S.; et al. Efficacy of Ripasudil in Reducing Intraocular Pressure and Medication Score for Ocular Hypertension with Inflammation and Corticosteroid. *Int. J. Ophthalmol.* **2023**, *16*, 904–908.
46. Yasuda, M.; Takayama, K.; Kanda, T.; Taguchi, M.; Someya, H.; Takeuchi, M. Comparison of intraocular pressure-lowering effects of ripasudil hydrochloride hydrate for inflammatory and corticosteroid-induced ocular hypertension. *PLoS ONE* **2017**, *12*, e0185305. [CrossRef]
47. Spencer, N.A.; Hall, A.J.; Stawell, R.J. Nd:YAG laser iridotomy in uveitic glaucoma. *Clin. Exp. Ophthalmol.* **2001**, *29*, 217–219. [CrossRef] [PubMed]
48. Mansouri, K.; Ravinet, E. Argon-laser iridoplasty in the management of uveitis-induced acute angle-closure glaucoma. *Eur. J. Ophthalmol.* **2009**, *19*, 304–306. [CrossRef]
49. Koktekir, B.E.; Gedik, S.; Bakbak, B. Bilateral severe anterior uveitis after unilateral selective laser trabeculoplasty. *Clin. Exp. Ophthalmol.* **2013**, *41*, 305–307. [CrossRef]
50. Maleki, A.; Swan, R.T.; Lasave, A.F.; Ma, L.; Foster, C.S. Selective lasertrabeculoplasty in controlled uveitis with steroid-induced glaucoma. *Ophthalmology* **2016**, *123*, 2630–2632. [CrossRef] [PubMed]
51. Xiao, J.; Zhao, C.; Liang, A.; Zhang, M.; Cheng, G. Efficacy and Safety of High-Energy Selective Laser Trabeculoplasty for Steroid-Induced Glaucoma in Patients with Quiescent Uveitis. *Ocul. Immunol. Inflamm.* **2021**, *29*, 766–770. [CrossRef] [PubMed]
52. Zhou, Y.; Pruet, C.M.; Fang, C.; Khanna, C.L. Selective laser trabeculoplasty in steroid-induced and uveitic glaucoma. *Can. J. Ophthalmol.* **2022**, *57*, 277–283. [CrossRef] [PubMed]
53. Sung, V.C.T.; Barton, K. Management of inflammatory glaucomas. *Curr. Opin. Ophthalmol.* **2004**, *15*, 136–140. [CrossRef] [PubMed]
54. Schlote, T.; Derse, M.; Zierhut, M. Transscleral diode laser cyclophotocoagulation for the treatment of refractory glaucoma secondary to inflammatory eye diseases. *Br. J. Ophthalmol.* **2000**, *84*, 999–1003. [CrossRef]
55. Voykov, B.; Deuter, C.; Zierhut, M.; Leitritz, M.A.; Guenova, E.; Doycheva, D. Is cyclophotocoagulation an option in the management of glaucoma secondary to Fuchs' uveitis syndrome? *Graefes Arch. Clin. Exp. Ophthalmol.* **2014**, *252*, 485–489. [CrossRef]
56. Heinz, C.; Koch, J.M.; Heiligenhaus, A. Transscleral diode laser cyclophotocoagulation as primary surgical treatment for secondary glaucoma in juvenile idiopathic arthritis: High failure rate after short term follow up. *Br. J. Ophthalmol.* **2006**, *90*, 737–740. [CrossRef]
57. De Crom, R.M.P.C.; Slangen, C.G.M.M.; Kujovic-Aleksov, S.; Webers, C.A.B.; Berendschot, T.T.J.M.; Beckers, H.J.M. Micropulse Trans-scleral Cyclophotocoagulation in Patients with Glaucoma: 1- and 2-Year Treatment Outcomes. *J. Glaucoma* **2020**, *29*, 794–798. [CrossRef]
58. Souissi, S.; Baudouin, C.; Labbé, A.; Hamard, P. Micropulse transscleral cyclophotocoagulation using a standard protocol in patients with refractory glaucoma naive of cyclodestruction. *Eur. J. Ophthalmol.* **2021**, *31*, 112–119. [CrossRef]
59. Rojas-Carabali, W.; Mejía-Salgado, G.; Cifuentes-González, C.; Chacón-Zambrano, D.; Cruz-Reyes, D.L.; Delgado, M.F.; Gómez-Goyeneche, H.F.; Saad-Brahim, K.; de-la-Torre, A. Prevalence and clinical characteristics of uveitic glaucoma: Multicentric study in Bogotá, Colombia. *Eye* **2023**. [CrossRef]
60. Pillai, M.R.; Balasubramaniam, N.; Wala, N.; Mathews, A.M.; Tejeswi, B.; Krishna, H.; Ishrath, D.; Rathinam, S.R.; Sithiq Uduman, S.M. Glaucoma in Uveitic Eyes: Long-Term Clinical Course and Management Measures. *Ocul. Immunol. Inflamm.* **2023**, 1–7. [CrossRef]
61. Jampel, H.D.; Jabs, D.A.; Quigley, H.A. Trabeculectomy with 5-fluo-rouracil for adult inflammatory glaucoma. *Am. J. Ophthalmol.* **1990**, *109*, 168–173. [CrossRef]
62. Ceballos, E.M.; Beck, A.D.; Lynn, M.J. Trabeculectomy with antiproliferative agentsin uveitic glaucoma. *J. Glaucoma* **2002**, *11*, 189–196. [CrossRef]

63. Iwao, K.; Inatani, M.; Seto, T.; Takihara, Y.; Ogata-Iwao, M.; Okinami, S.; Tanihara, H. Long-term outcomes and prognostic factors for trabeculectomy with mitomycin C in eyes with uveitic glaucoma: A retrospective cohort study. *J. Glaucoma* 2014, *23*, 88–94. [CrossRef]
64. Almobarak, F.A.; Alharbi, A.H.; Morales, J.; Aljadaan, I. Intermediate and Long-term Outcomes of Mitomycin C-enhanced Trabeculectomy as a First Glaucoma Procedure in Uveitic Glaucoma. *J. Glaucoma* 2017, *26*, 478–485. [CrossRef]
65. Kanaya, R.; Kijima, R.; Shinmei, Y.; Shinkai, A.; Ohguchi, T.; Namba, K.; Chin, S.; Ishida, S. Surgical Outcomes of Trabeculectomy in Uveitic Glaucoma: A Long-Term, Single-Center, Retrospective Case-Control Study. *J. Ophthalmol.* 2021, *2021*, 5550776. [CrossRef]
66. Almobarak, F.A.; Alharbi, A.H.; Morales, J.; Aljadaan, I. The Influence of Phacoemulsification on Intraocular Pressure Control and Trabeculectomy Survival in Uveitic Glaucoma. *J. Glaucoma* 2017, *26*, 444–449. [CrossRef]
67. Shimizu, A.; Maruyama, K.; Yokoyama, Y.; Tsuda, S.; Ryu, M.; Nakazawa, T. Characteristics of uveitic glaucoma and evaluation of its surgical treatment. *Clin. Ophthalmol.* 2014, *8*, 2383–2389. [CrossRef]
68. Kaburaki, T.; Koshino, T.; Kawashima, H.; Numaga, J.; Tomidokoro, A.; Shirato, S.; Araie, M. Initial trabeculectomy with mitomycin C in eyes with uveitic glaucoma wit inactive uveitis. *Eye* 2009, *23*, 1509–1517. [CrossRef]
69. Kwon, H.J.; Kong, Y.X.G.; Tao, L.W.; Lim, L.L.; Martin, K.R.; Green, C.; Ruddle, J.; Crowston, J.G. Surgical outcomes of trabeculectomy and glaucoma drainage implant for uveitic glaucoma and relationship with uveitis activity. *Clin. Exp. Ophthalmol.* 2017, *45*, 472–480. [CrossRef]
70. Magliyah, M.S.; Badawi, A.H.; Alshamrani, A.A.; Malik, R.; Al-Dhibi, H. The Effect of Perioperative Uveitis Control on the Success of Glaucoma Surgery in Uveitic Glaucoma. *Clin. Ophthalmol.* 2021, *15*, 1465–1475. [CrossRef]
71. Gregory, A.C., 2nd; Zhang, M.M.; Rapoport, Y.; Ling, J.D.; Kuchtey, R.W. Racial Influences of Uveitic Glaucoma: Consolidation of Current Knowledge of Diagnosis and Treatment. *Semin. Ophthalmol.* 2016, *31*, 400–404. [CrossRef]
72. Bohnsack, B.L.; Freedman, S.F. Surgical Outcomes in Childhood Uveitic Glaucoma. *Am. J. Ophthalmol.* 2013, *155*, 134–142. [CrossRef]
73. Ho, C.L.; Wong, E.Y.M.; Walton, D.S. Goniosurgery for glaucoma complicating chronic childhood uveitis. *Arch. Ophthalmol.* 2004, *122*, 838–844. [CrossRef]
74. Meerwijk, C.L.L.I.V.; Edema, A.B.; Rijn, L.J.V.; Los, L.I.; Jansonius, N.M. Goniotomy for Non-Infectious Uveitic Glaucoma in Children. *J. Clin. Med.* 2023, *12*, 2200. [CrossRef]
75. Anton, A.; Heinzelmann, S.; Neß, T.; Lübke, J.; Neuburger, M.; Jordan, J.F.; Wecker, T. Trabeculectomy ab interno with the Trabectome® as a therapeutic option for uveitic secondary glaucoma. *Graefes Arch. Clin. Exp. Ophthalmol.* 2015, *253*, 1973–1978. [CrossRef]
76. Swamy, R.; Francis, B.A.; Akil, H.; Yelenskiy, A.; Francis, B.A.; Chopra, V.; Huang, A. Clinical results of ab interno trabeculotomy using the trabectome in patientswith uveitic glaucoma. *Clin. Exp. Ophthalmol.* 2020, *48*, 31–36. [CrossRef]
77. Murata, N.; Takahashi, E.; Saruwatari, J.; Kojima, S.; Inoue, T. Outcomes and risk factors for ab interno trabeculotomy with a Kahook Dual Blade. *Graefes Arch. Clin. Exp. Ophthalmol.* 2023, *261*, 503–511. [CrossRef]
78. Chen, R.I.; Purgert, R.; Eisengart, J. Gonioscopy-Assisted Transluminal Trabeculotomy and Goniotomy, with or without Concomitant Cataract Extraction, inSteroid-Induced and Uveitic Glaucoma: 24-Month Outcomes. *J. Glaucoma* 2023, *32*, 501–510. [CrossRef]
79. Tanev, I.; Kirkova, R. "Ab Interno" Surgery of the Schlemm's Canal in Postuveitic Glaucoma Patients. *J. Pers. Med.* 2023, *13*, 456. [CrossRef]
80. Sachdev, A.; Khalili, A.; Choi, J.; Stead, R.E.; Sung, V.C.T. Gonioscopy-assisted Transluminal Trabeculotomy in Uveitic Glaucoma Secondary to Juvenile Idiopathic Arthritis. *J. Glaucoma* 2020, *29*, e116–e119. [CrossRef]
81. Gunay, M.; Uzlu, D.; Akyol, N. Outcomes of Gonioscopy-Assisted Transluminal Trabeculotomy as a Primary Surgical Treatment for Glaucoma Secondary to Juvenile Idiopathic Arthritis-Associated Uveitis. *Ocul. Immunol. Inflamm.* 2023, *31*, 2060–2064. [CrossRef]
82. Parikh, D.A.; Mellen, P.L.; Kang, T.; Shalaby, W.S.; Moster, M.R.; Dunn, J.P. Gonioscopy-Assisted Transluminal Trabeculotomy for the Treatment of Glaucoma in Uveitic Eyes. *Ocul. Immunol. Inflamm.* 2023, *31*, 1608–1614. [CrossRef]
83. Belkin, A.; Chaban, Y.V.; Waldner, D.; Samet, S.; Ahmed, K., II; Gooi, P.; Schlenker, M.B. Gonioscopy-assisted transluminal trabeculotomy is an effective surgical treatment for uveitic glaucoma. *Br. J. Ophthalmol.* 2023, *107*, 690–697. [CrossRef]
84. Sotani, N.; Kusuhara, S.; Matsumiya, W.; Okuda, M.; Mori, S.; Sotani, R.; Kim, K.W.; Nishisho, R.; Nakamura, M. Outcomes of Microhook ab Interno Trabeculotomy in Consecutive 36 Eyes with Uveitic Glaucoma. *J. Clin. Med.* 2022, *11*, 3768. [CrossRef]
85. Seow, W.H.; Lim, C.H.L.; Lim, B.X.H.; Lim, D.K. Uveitis and glaucoma: A look at present day surgical options. *Curr. Opin. Ophthalmol.* 2023, *34*, 152–161. [CrossRef]
86. Traverso, C.E.; Carassa, R.G.; Fea, A.M.; Figus, M.; Astarita, C.; Piergentili, B.; Vera, V.; Gandolfi, S. Effectiveness and Safety of Xen Gel Stent in Glaucoma Surgery: A Systematic Review of the Literature. *J. Clin. Med.* 2023, *12*, 5339. [CrossRef]
87. Sng, C.C.; Wang, J.; Hau, S.; Htoon, H.M.; Barton, K. XEN-45 collagen implant for the treatment of uveitic glaucoma. *Clin. Exp. Ophthalmol.* 2018, *46*, 339–345. [CrossRef]
88. Qureshi, A.; Jones, N.P.; Au, L. Urgent Management of Secondary Glaucoma in Uveitis Using the Xen-45 Gel Stent. *J. Glaucoma* 2019, *28*, 1061–1066. [CrossRef]

89. Evers, C.; Anton, A.; Böhringer, D.; Kallee, S.; Keye, P.; Neß, T.; Philippin, H.; Reinhar, T.; Lübke, J. XEN®-45 implantation for refractory uveitic glaucoma. *Graefe's Arch. Clin. Exp. Ophthalmol.* **2023**. [CrossRef]
90. Serrar, Y.; Rezkallah, A.; Kodjikian, L.; Poli, M.; Mathis, T.; Denis, P. XEN-63 gel stent to treat a refractory uveitic glaucoma: A case report. *Eur. J. Ophthalmol.* **2023**, *33*, NP32–NP36. [CrossRef]
91. Gambini, G.; Carlà, M.M.; Giannuzzi, F.; Caporossi, T.; De Vico, U.; Savastano, A.; Baldascino, A.; Rizzo, C.; Kilian, R.; Caporossi, A.; et al. PreserFlo® MicroShunt: An Overview of This Minimally Invasive Device for Open-AngleGlaucoma. *Vision* **2022**, *6*, 12. [CrossRef]
92. Triolo, G.; Wang, J.; Aguilar-Munoa, S.; Jayaram, H.; Barton, K. Preserflo microshunt implant for the treatment of refractory uveitic glaucoma: 36-month outcomes. *Eye* **2023**, *37*, 2535–2541. [CrossRef]
93. Obeidan, S.A.; Osman, E.A.; Mousa, A.; Al-Muammar, A.M.; Abu El-Asrar, A.M. Long-term evaluation of efficacy and safety of deep sclerectomy in uveitic glaucoma. *Ocul. Immunol. Inflamm.* **2015**, *23*, 82–89. [CrossRef]
94. Mercieca, K.; Steeples, L.; Anand, N. Deep sclerectomy for uveiticlaucoma: Long-term outcomes. *Eye* **2017**, *31*, 1008–1019. [CrossRef]
95. Xiao, J.; Zhao, C.; Zhang, Y.; Liang, A.; Qu, Y.; Cheng, G.; Zhang, M. Surgical Outcomes of Modified CO_2 Laser-assisted Sclerectomy for Uveitic Glaucoma. *Ocul. Immunol. Inflamm.* **2022**, *30*, 1617–1624. [CrossRef]
96. Salloukh, A.E.; Ansari, A.S.; Chiu, A.; Mathews, D. Evaluating the long-term efficacy and effectiveness of Viscocanalostomy and combined phacoemulsification with Viscocanalostomy in the treatment of patients with uveitic glaucoma: 5-year follow up data. *BMC Surg.* **2021**, *21*, 200. [CrossRef]
97. Papadaki, T.G.; Zacharopoulos, I.P.; Pasquale, L.R.; Christen, W.B.; Netland, P.A.; Foster, C.S. Long-term Results of Ahmed Glaucoma Valve Implantation for Uveitic Glaucoma. *Am. J. Ophthalmol.* **2007**, *144*, 62–69. [CrossRef]
98. Law, S.K.; Nguyen, A.; Coleman, A.L.; Caprioli, J. Comparison of safety and efficacy between silicone and polypropylene ahmed glaucoma valves in refractoryglaucoma. *Ophthalmology* **2005**, *112*, 1514–1520. [CrossRef]
99. Özdal, P.Ç.; Vianna, R.N.G.; Deschênes, J. Ahmed valve implantation in glaucoma secondary to chronic uveitis. *Eye* **2006**, *20*, 178–183. [CrossRef]
100. Bettis, D.I.; Morshedi, R.G.; Chaya, C.; Goldsmith, J.; Crandall, A.; Zabriskie, N. Trabeculectomy with mitomycin c or ahmed valve implantation in eyes with uveitic glaucoma. *J. Glaucoma* **2015**, *24*, 591–599. [CrossRef]
101. Sungur, G.; Yakin, M.; Eksioglu, U.; Satana, B.; Ornek, F. Assessment of conditions affecting surgical success of Ahmed glaucoma valve implants in glaucoma secondary to different uveitis etiologies in adults. *Eye* **2017**, *31*, 1435–1442. [CrossRef]
102. Bao, N.; Jiang, Z.-X.; Coh, P.; Tao, L.-M. Long-term outcomes of uveitic glaucoma treated with Ahmed valve implant in a series of Chinese patients. *Int. J. Ophthalmol.* **2018**, *11*, 629–634.
103. Valenzuela, F.; Oportus, M.J.; Pérez, C.I.; Mellado, F.; Cartes, C.; Villarroel, F.; López-Ponce, D.; López-Solís, R.; Traipe, L. Ahmed glaucoma drainage implant surgery in the management of refractory uveitic glaucoma: Long-term follow up. *Arch. Soc. Esp. Oftalmol.* **2018**, *93*, 431–438. [CrossRef] [PubMed]
104. Chow, A.; Burkemper, B.; Varma, R.; Rodger, D.C.; Rao, N.; Richter, G.M. Comparison of surgical outcomes of trabeculectomy, Ahmed shunt, and Baerveldt shunt in uveitic glaucoma. *J. Ophthalmic Inflamm. Infect.* **2018**, *8*, 9. [CrossRef] [PubMed]
105. Hennein, L.; Hou, J.; Stewart, J.M.; Lowry, E.A.; Jiang, Z.; Enanoria, W.T.; Han, Y. Comparison of Surgical Outcome After Ahmed Valve Implantation for Patients with and without Fluocinolone Intravitreal Implant (Retisert). *J. Glaucoma.* **2016**, *25*, 772–776. [CrossRef] [PubMed]
106. Tang, M.; Gill, N.P.; Tanna, A.P. Effect of Early Aqueous Suppression After ValvedTube Shunt Surgery for Uveitic Glaucoma. *Ophthalmol. Glaucoma* **2023**, *7*, 37–46.
107. Gedde, S.J.; Schiffman, J.C.; Feuer, W.J.; Herndon, L.W.; Brandt, J.D.; Budenz, D.L. Tube versus Trabeculectomy Study Group. Treatment outcomes in the Tube Versus Trabeculectomy (TVT) study after five years of follow-up. *Am. J. Ophthalmol.* **2012**, *153*, 789–803. [CrossRef]
108. Gedde, S.J.; Feuer, W.J.; Lim, K.S.; Barton, K.; Goyal, S.; Ahmed, I.I.; Brandt, J.D.; Primary Tube Versus Trabeculectomy Study Group. Treatment Outcomes in the Primary TubeVersus Trabeculectomy Study after 5 Years of Follow-up. *Ophthalmology* **2022**, *129*, 1344–1356. [CrossRef]
109. Tan, A.N.; Cornelissen, M.F.; Webers, C.A.; Erckens, R.J.; Berendschot, T.T.; Beckers, H.J. Outcomes of severe uveitic glaucoma treated with Baerveldt implant: Can blindness be prevented? *Acta Ophthalmol.* **2018**, *96*, 24–30. [CrossRef]
110. Chabra, R.; Tan, S.Z.; Au, L.; Spencer, A.F.; Fenerty, C.H.; Jones, N.P. Long-Term Outcomes and Complications of Baerveldt Glaucoma Drainage Implants in Adults with Glaucoma Secondary to Uveitis. *Ocul. Immunol. Inflamm.* **2019**, *27*, 1322–1329. [CrossRef]
111. Cazana, I.M.; Böhringer, D.; Reinhard, T.; Anton, A.; Ness, T.; Lübke, J. A comparison of long-term results after Baerveldt 250 implantation in advanced uveitic vs. other forms of glaucoma. *Graefes Arch. Clin. Exp. Ophthalmol.* **2022**, *260*, 2991–3000. [CrossRef] [PubMed]
112. Manako, K.; Takahashi, E.; Saruwatari, J.; Matsumura, T.; Kojima, S.; Inoue, T. Risk factors for Baerveldt glaucom drainage implantation for uveitic glaucoma. *Sci. Rep.* **2023**, *13*, 4473. [CrossRef] [PubMed]
113. Budenz, D.L.; Feuer, W.J.; Barton, K.; Schiffman, J.; Costa, V.P.; Godfrey, D.G.; Buys, Y.M.; Ahmed Baerveldt Comparison Study Group. Postoperative Complications in the Ahmed Baerveldt Comparison Study During Five Years of Follow-up. *Am. J. Ophthalmol.* **2016**, *163*, 75–82. [CrossRef]

114. Sinha, S.; Ganjei, A.Y.; McWatters, Z.; Lee, D.; Moster, M.R.; Myers, J.S.; Kolomeyer, N.; Mantravadi, A.V.; Pro, M.J.; Razeghinejad, R. Ahmed Versus Baerveldt Glaucoma Drainage Device in Uveitic Glaucoma: A Retrospective Comparative Study. *J. Glaucoma* **2020**, *29*, 750–755. [CrossRef] [PubMed]
115. Sinha, S.; Ganjei, A.Y.; Ustaoglu, M.; Syed, Z.A.; Lee, D.; Myers, J.S.; Fudemberg, S.J.; Razeghinejad, R. Effect of shunt type on rates of tube-cornea touch and cornealdecompensation after tube shunt surgery in uveitic glaucoma. *Graefes Arch. Clin. Exp. Ophthalmol.* **2021**, *259*, 1587–1595. [CrossRef] [PubMed]
116. Vuori, M.L. Molteno aqueous shunt as a primary surgical intervention foruveitic glaucoma: Long-term results. *Acta Ophthalmol.* **2010**, *88*, 33–36. [CrossRef] [PubMed]
117. Gkaragkani, E.; Jayaram, H.; Papadopoulos, M.; Pavesio, C.; Brookes, J.; Khaw, P.T.; ElSayed, Y.M.; Clarke, J. Glaucoma Drainage Device Surgery Outcomes in Children with Uveitic Glaucoma. *Am. J. Ophthalmol.* **2023**, *251*, 5–11. [CrossRef] [PubMed]
118. Kubaisi, B.; Maleki, A.; Ahmed, A.; Lamba, N.; Sahawneh, H.; Stephenson, A.; Montieth, A.; Topgi, S.; Foster, C.S. Ahmed glaucoma valve in uveitic patients with fluocinoloneacetonide implant-induced glaucoma: 3-year follow-up. *Clin. Ophthalmol.* **2018**, *12*, 799–804. [CrossRef]
119. Voykov, B.; Doycheva, D.; Deuter, C.; Leitritz, M.A.; Dimopoulos, S.; William, A. Outcomes of Ahmed Glaucoma Valve Implantation for Glaucoma Secondary to Fuchs Uveitis Syndrome. *Ocul. Immunol. Inflamm.* **2017**, *25*, 760–766. [CrossRef]
120. Yakin, M.; Eksioglu, U.; Sungur, G.; Satana, B.; Demirok, G.; Ornek, F. Short-term to Long-term Results of Ahmed Glaucoma Valve Implantation for Uveitic GlaucomaSecondary to Behçet Disease. *J. Glaucoma* **2017**, *26*, 20–26. [CrossRef]
121. Lee, S.Y.; Kim, Y.H.; Kim, K.E.; Ahn, J. Comparison of Surgical Outcomes between Trabeculectomy with Mitomycin C and Ahmed Valve Implantation with Mitomycin C in Eyes with Uveitic Glaucoma. *J. Clin. Med.* **2022**, *11*, 1368. [CrossRef] [PubMed]
122. Iverson, S.M.; Bhardwaj, N.; Shi, W.; Sehi, M.; Greenfield, D.S.; Budenz, D.L.; Kishor, K. Surgical outcomes of inflammatory glaucoma: A comparison of trabeculectomy and glaucoma-drainage-device implantation. *Jpn. J. Ophthalmol.* **2015**, *59*, 179–186. [CrossRef] [PubMed]
123. El-Saied, H.M.A.; Abdelhakim, M.A.S.E. Different surgical modalities for management of uveitic glaucoma: 2 year comparative study. *Acta Ophthalmol.* **2022**, *100*, e246–e252. [CrossRef] [PubMed]
124. Ventura-Abreu, N.; Mendes-Pereira, J.; Pazos, M.; Muniesa-Royo, M.J.; Gonzalez-Ventosa, A.; Romero-Nuñez, B.; Milla, E. Surgical Approach and Outcomes of Uveitic Glaucoma in a Tertiary Hospital. *J. Curr. Glaucoma Pract.* **2021**, *15*, 52–57. [CrossRef]

Disclaimer/Publisher's Note: The statements, opinions and data contained in all publications are solely those of the individual author(s) and contributor(s) and not of MDPI and/or the editor(s). MDPI and/or the editor(s) disclaim responsibility for any injury to people or property resulting from any ideas, methods, instructions or products referred to in the content.

Article

Goniotomy for Non-Infectious Uveitic Glaucoma in Children

Charlotte L. L. I. van Meerwijk [1,*], Astrid B. Edema [1], Laurentius J. van Rijn [2], Leonoor I. Los [1] and Nomdo M. Jansonius [1]

[1] Department of Ophthalmology, University Medical Center Groningen, P.O. Box 30.001, 9700 RB Groningen, The Netherlands; a.b.edema@umcg.nl (A.B.E.); l.i.los@umcg.nl (L.I.L.); n.m.jansonius@umcg.nl (N.M.J.)
[2] Department of Ophthalmology, Amsterdam University Medical Center, location VU University Medical Center, P.O. Box 7057, 1007 MB Amsterdam, The Netherlands; vanrijn@amsterdamumc.nl
* Correspondence: c.l.l.i.van.meerwijk@umcg.nl

Abstract: Secondary glaucoma is still a blinding complication in childhood uveitis, for which most commonly used surgical interventions (trabeculectomy or glaucoma drainage implant) involve multiple re-interventions and/or complications postoperatively. The goniotomy procedure has never been investigated in the current era, in which patients with pediatric uveitis receive biologics as immunosuppressive therapy for a prolonged period, with potential implications for the outcome. The purpose of the study is to evaluate the efficacy and safety of a goniotomy procedure in pediatric non-infectious uveitis in a retrospective, multicenter case series. The primary outcomes were the postoperative intraocular pressure (IOP), number of IOP-lowering medications, and success rate. Postoperative success was defined as $6 \leq IOP \leq 21$ mmHg, without major complications or re-interventions. Fifteen eyes of ten children were included. Median age of the included patients at goniotomy was 7 years; median follow-up was 59 months. Median (interquartile range) IOP before surgery was 30 (26–34) mmHg with 4 (3–4) IOP-lowering medications. At 1, 2, and 5 years after goniotomy, median IOP was 15, 14, and 15 mmHg with 2 (0–2), 1 (0–2), and 0 (0–2) medications, respectively ($p < 0.001$ postoperatively versus preoperatively for all timepoints). Success rate was 100%, 93%, and 80% after 1, 2, and 5 years, respectively. There were no significant changes in visual acuity and uveitis activity or its treatment, and there were no major complications. Our results show that the goniotomy is an effective and safe surgery for children with uveitic glaucoma.

Keywords: glaucoma; surgery; uveitis; childhood

1. Introduction

Children ≤16 years of age constitute 5–10% of the uveitis population [1]. The incidence of uveitis in children is 4–6 per 100,000 person-years [2,3], of which a non-infectious etiology is the most common. Non-infectious pediatric uveitis is a challenge to treat, because of its often-asymptomatic presentation, ocular evaluation difficulties, the high impact of treatment, the chronic course, and the risk of serious complications.

Secondary glaucoma is one of the most common complications, together with cataract, optic disc edema, and cystoid macular edema [4]. Moreover, glaucoma is nonreversible and thereby potentially blinding [5]. Based on a retrospective analysis in a tertiary care referral center, secondary glaucoma developed in 26% of the children with uveitis. In 58% of these children, the required intraocular pressure (IOP) reduction was not achieved with IOP-lowering medication only, and additional surgical interventions were needed in order to prevent or limit optic nerve damage [6].

The pathophysiology of uveitic glaucoma is multifactorial [7]. Typically, there is mechanical obstruction or dysfunction of the trabecular meshwork, which can be blocked by inflammatory cells, proteins, and debris liberated from a disrupted blood-aqueous barrier. In addition, alterations in the trabecular meshwork due to a reaction to steroids may occur. All these factors may result in an obstruction of the aqueous outflow facility [8]. In chronic uveitis, obstruction of aqueous outflow may result from scarring and obliteration of trabecular meshwork beams or Schlemm's canal or from overgrowth of a fibrovascular membrane in the chamber angle [8].

In order to achieve an IOP decrease in this type of secondary glaucoma, various surgical interventions are possible. The most frequently used techniques are trabeculectomy (TE) and implantation of a glaucoma drainage device. Another option is goniotomy. Previous research and a recent review showed no preference for a particular intervention [9,10]. Advantages of goniotomy over the other two types of intervention are a quick surgical procedure and a relatively rapid postoperative recovery.

The goal of goniotomy is to facilitate the entrance of aqueous humor into Schlemm's canal. Incising the trabecular meshwork is presumed to lower aqueous outflow resistance, leading to improved IOP control [11]. Histopathological studies showed a superficial, non-healing incision, with entrance to Schlemm's canal [12]. During goniotomy, the anterior trabecular meshwork is incised just below Schwalbe's line by using a knife or needle under direct visualization of the chamber angle with a gonioscopy lens. Goniotomy is usually performed initially over 4 to 6 clock hours in the nasal, temporal or inferior angle. The procedure can be repeated (extended to more clock hours) in case of an inadequate IOP-lowering effect [13].

Three studies have been published on goniotomy procedures in pediatric uveitis [14–16]. They all showed a significant decrease in IOP and number of IOP-lowering medications, although multiple interventions were often needed. Since these studies were published, however, uveitis treatment has undergone a tremendous development, with stricter control of uveitis activity, early use of systemic disease-modifying antirheumatic drugs (DMARDs), and strict monitoring and early treatment when the IOP rises. Nevertheless, despite these developments, pediatric uveitic glaucoma has not found a gold standard treatment yet.

The aim of the current study was to evaluate the efficacy and safety of goniotomy in pediatric uveitis in an era with a paradigm shift regarding uveitis treatment. For this purpose, we performed a retrospective, multicenter case series study involving all patients from tertiary centers in The Netherlands, where goniotomy is the current approach to treat glaucoma in children with uveitis.

2. Materials & Methods

2.1. Study Population

Patients with non-infectious pediatric uveitis, who underwent a goniotomy procedure from December 2011 until March 2020, were retrospectively included from the departments of Ophthalmology of the University Medical Center (UMC) Groningen (Center 1) and the Amsterdam UMC (Center 2), both in The Netherlands. The diagnosis and classification of uveitis was done by ophthalmologists specialized in pediatric uveitis and according to the Standardization of Uveitis Nomenclature (SUN) criteria [16]. Children were evaluated for the presence of an underlying systemic disease by pediatric rheumatologists. The indication for glaucoma surgery was made by glaucoma specialists and was mostly based on an IOP > 21 mmHg with maximum tolerated IOP-lowering medication and individual patient characteristics. The included goniotomy procedures were done as the first surgical intervention for glaucoma, with a minimal follow-up after the intervention of 1 year. If bilateral goniotomy was performed, both eyes of the patient were included (see Section 2.5 'Statistical analysis'). The study adhered to the tenets of the Declaration of Helsinki. Because the study concerns a retrospective analysis of data that have been collected during regular patient care, no formal approval of a Medical Ethical Committee was required (waiver obtained from the Medical Ethical Committee of both participating centers).

2.2. Technique

A standard goniotomy procedure as described by Worst was used with very little modifications [17]. During the procedure, the anterior trabecular meshwork was incised just below Schwalbe's line by using a knife/needle under direct visualization of the chamber angle with a gonioscopy lens. Usually, 4 to 5 clock hours were treated. After the procedure, a soluble suture was placed at the corneal incision. After surgery, the number of topical steroid administrations per day was increased temporarily. In addition, in Center 1, methylprednisolone 15 mg/kg was given during surgery. The DMARD use remained unchanged in both centers.

2.3. Data Collection

Preoperative data extracted from the patient's electronic medical records included: age at surgery, sex, type of uveitis, etiology of uveitis, antinuclear antibody (ANA) seropositivity, anterior complications at first presentation (peripheral anterior synechiae (PAS), cataract, band keratopathy), posterior complications at first presentation (cystoid macular edema, vasculitis, papillitis), lens status at last visit before surgery, interval between onset of uveitis and surgery, and interval between start of IOP-lowering medication and surgery. Onset of uveitis was defined as the first time uveitis was diagnosed, either in the included centers or elsewhere as specified in the referral letter.

The following information was recorded at the last visit before surgery and every year (±3 months) after surgery up to 5 years of follow-up: IOP, number of different classes of IOP-lowering medication used, use of DMARDs, best-corrected visual acuity, anterior chamber inflammation activity according to the SUN grading system for anterior chamber cells [18], and use of topical steroid medication. End of follow-up was defined as the date of either the last visit in 2022 or failure (as defined below). Complications and additional interventions during follow-up were recorded. The diagnosis of cystoid macular edema was made, when any accumulation of fluid in the macular area was seen by spectral domain optical coherence tomography. Papillitis was defined as blurring of the optic disc margins visible by fundoscopy and/or the presence of optic disc hyperfluorescence on fluorescein angiography. The IOP was measured by Goldmann Applanation Tonometry when possible. Icare rebound tonometer readings were used if the child was unable to cooperate with Goldmann Applanation Tonometry. As systemic anti-inflammatory medication, we scored systemic steroids (excluding short-term perioperative steroid treatment), conventional synthetic (cs)DMARDs such as methotrexate and mycophenolate mofetil, and biologic (b)DMARDs such as adalimumab and infliximab (anti-TNF-alpha).

2.4. Study Outcomes

Primary outcomes were IOP, number of IOP-lowering medication classes after surgery, and success or failure after surgery. Success was defined as no failure regardless of the use of IOP-lowering medication. Failure was defined as any of the following: (1) an IOP > 21 or <6 mmHg on at least 3 consecutive occasions from 3 months after the goniotomy onwards; (2) an IOP <10 mmHg together with a hypotonic maculopathy, optic disc edema, vision loss or choroidal detachment; (3) the need for additional glaucoma-related surgical interventions; (4) loss of light perception. We defined vision loss as a visual acuity loss of more than 2 Snellen chart lines. Secondary outcomes included complications, uveitis activity, and visual acuity.

2.5. Statistical Analysis

For descriptive statistics, we used median and interquartile range (IQR), because of the non-normal distribution of the data. Medians were compared using the Wilcoxon signed rank test (for paired samples) and the Wilcoxon rank sum test (for independent samples). For nominal data, we used the McNemar's test for paired samples and the Pearson chi-square test for independent samples. The effect of goniotomy on IOP and on the number of IOP-lowering medication classes was studied with (generalized) linear mixed-effects models, in order to be able to account for the inclusion of both eyes in some patients and for the assessment of IOP and the number of medication classes at multiple timepoints. Dependent variable was either IOP or the number of medication classes; timepoint was entered in the models as a fixed effect and factorized (with 6 levels: preoperatively and 1, 2, 3, 4, and 5 years postoperatively), with the preoperative time point as reference. Center, patient, and eye were entered as nested random effects. As a secondary analysis, we entered 'center' as a fixed effect, to study if there were any differences in the effect of goniotomy on IOP between the centers. A Kaplan–Meier curve was used to illustrate at which time points during the follow-up failures occurred.

Data were statistically analyzed with SPSS 28.0.0 (SPSS Inc., Chicago, IL, USA). For the (generalized) linear mixed-effects models, we used package 'lme4' in R (version 4.2.2; R Foundation for Statistical Computing, Vienna, Austria) with 'lmer' for IOP and 'glmer' with family = poisson for the number of IOP-lowering medication classes. A p-value of 0.05 or less was considered statistically significant.

3. Results

A total of 15 eyes of 10 patients were included; 8 eyes in Center 1 and 7 eyes in Center 2. Table 1 gives an overview of the demographics. Median age at goniotomy was 7 (IQR 6–11) years and median follow-up after surgery was 59 (37–83) months. The included eyes were most often of female patients, and the uveitis was mainly JIA-related and anteriorly located. In 47% of eyes, pre-existing anterior complications were seen at the first visit in the expert center. Three eyes had had cataract surgery with IOL implantation before their goniotomy procedure, and one eye had PAS in a limited number of clock hours, without clear progress and not involving the goniotomy site. None of the patients were lost to follow-up.

Table 1. Demographics per eye.

Demographics	
Number of patients	10
Number of eyes	15
Sex—Female	13 (87%)
Age at goniotomy (yrs) [a]	7 (6–11)
Localization—anterior uveitis	13 (87%)
Etiology—JIA [b]	9 (64%)
ANA positivity [c]	9 (64%)
Pre-existing complications at first visit UMC	
Anterior complications—yes	7 (47%)
Peripheral anterior synechiae—yes	1 (7%)
Posterior synechiae—yes	6 (40%)
Band keratopathy—yes	3 (20%)
Cataract—yes	0 (0%)
Posterior complications [d]—yes	4 (27%)
Lens status before goniotomy [e]	
Phakic eyes—no cataract	9 (60%)
Phakic eyes—cataract	3 (20%)
Pseudophakic eyes	3 (20%)
Interval (months) [a] between	
Onset of uveitis and goniotomy	22 (9–56)
Start glaucoma medication and goniotomy	9 (6–19)
Postoperative follow-up (months) [a]	59 (37–83)

[a] Median (interquartile range), [b] Juvenile Idiopathic Arthritis, [c] Antinuclear Antibodies, [d] Cystoid macular edema, vasculitis and/or papillitis, [e] No cataract surgery was performed in the period between the first presentation and goniotomy.

Figure 1 and Table 2 show the results for IOP and the number of IOP-lowering medication classes. During follow-up, a significant decrease in IOP and the number of IOP-lowering medication classes was seen at every postoperative time point as compared to the preoperative time point ($p < 0.001$ for both IOP and the number of IOP-lowering medication classes at all timepoints). The greatest reduction of IOP-lowering medication was 1 year after goniotomy, with 7 eyes of 4 patients not receiving any IOP-lowering medication from this moment onwards. In one patient with two eyes, the amount of IOP-lowering medication was slowly tempered over time, ending without IOP-lowering medication from year 4 onwards. Three patients with three eyes included use of two or three types of IOP-lowering medication throughout the postoperative period without tempering medication over time. There was a small difference between the centers regarding the effect of goniotomy on IOP ($p = 0.047$), mainly related to a somewhat higher preoperative IOP in Center 1 (median preoperative IOP 33 versus 26 mmHg for Center 1 versus Center 2, respectively). With regard to visual acuity, uveitis activity, the frequency of topical steroid medication, and use of DMARDs, no clear differences were found between the preoperative and postoperative time points (Table 2).

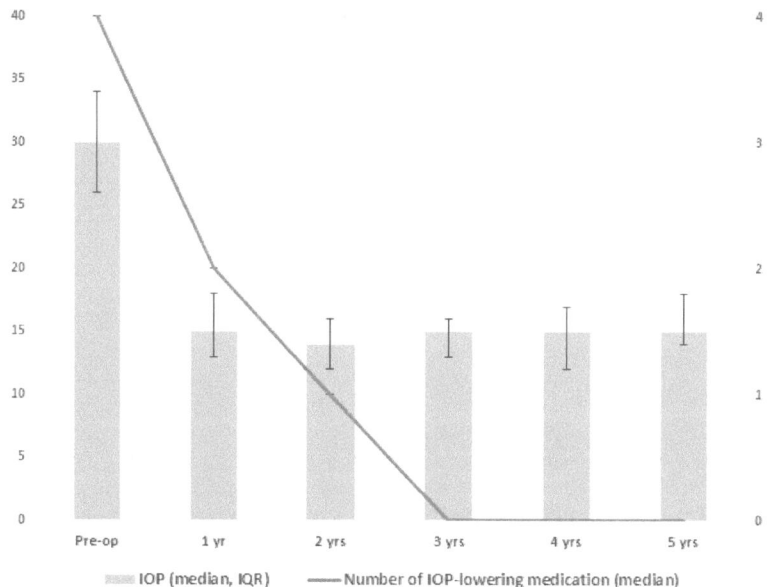

Figure 1. Median intraocular pressure (IOP; gray bars) and median number of IOP-lowering medications (line) after one goniotomy procedure based on 15 eyes in 10 patients. Error bars depict interquartile range of the IOP.

Table 2. Primary and secondary outcomes during the follow-up.

Characteristics	Pre-Operatively	1 Year	2 Years	3 Years	4 Years	5 Years
N (patients/eyes)	10/15	10/15	9/14	7/12	6/10	5/8
IOP (mmHg) [a,b]	30 (26–34)	15 (13–18)	14 (12–16)	15 (13–16)	15 (12–17)	15 (14–18)
IOP lowering medication [a,b,c]	4 (3–4)	2 (0–2)	1 (0–2)	0 (0–2)	0 (0–1)	0 (0–2)
AC inflammation [b,d]	0 (0–1)	0 (0–1)	0 (0–1)	0 (0–0)	0 (0–1)	0 (0–0)
Topical steroid medication [b,e]	2 (1–3)	1 (1–3)	1 (1–3)	1 (1–2)	2 (1–2)	1 (1–2)
Visual acuity (logMAR) [b]	0.05 (−0.03–0.30)	0.10 (0.00–0.13)	0.00 (−0.03–0.03)	−0.05 (−0.10–0.18)	0.00 (−0.10–0.20)	0.00 (−0.10–0.18)
csDMARDS (N pt/eyes) [f]	9/14	9/14	8/13	6/10	3/6	2/4
bDMARDS (N pt/eyes) [g]	5/8	6/10	6/10	4/8	3/6	3/6

[a] Intraocular pressure, [b] Median (interquartile range) per eye, [c] Number of different classes of IOP-lowering medication, [d] Anterior chamber inflammation, graded according to the Standardization of Uveitis Nomenclature (SUN) guidelines (Jabs et al.), [e] In units; prednisolone drops and ointment and dexamethasone drops were scored as 1 unit per drop. Rimexolone (Vexol, Alcon bv) and fluorometholone (FML liquifilm, Abbvie bv) were scored as 0.5 units per drop. No subconjunctival triamcinolone was used, [f] Conventional synthetic disease-modifying antirheumatic drugs, [g] Biologic disease-modifying antirheumatic drugs.

Figure 2 presents a Kaplan–Meier curve. The success rates were 100% ($n = 15/15$), 93% ($n = 14/15$), and 80% ($n = 8/10$), after 1, 2, and 5 years, respectively. The two failures concerned eyes from different patients who underwent additional glaucoma surgery; one eye received a Baerveldt drainage implant 16 months after the goniotomy procedure, because of periods of IOP increase due to low compliance with a glaucomatous excavation of the optic disc; one eye received a TE after 28 months, because of a high IOP with the maximum IOP-lowering medication.

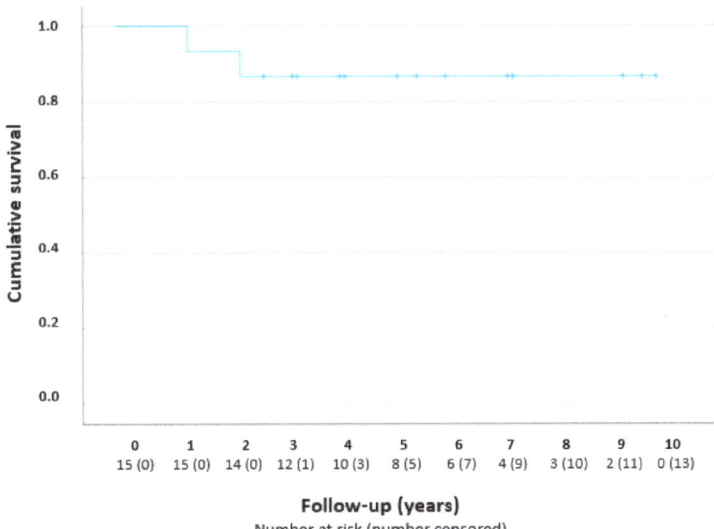

Figure 2. Kaplan–Meier curve—cumulative survival after one goniotomy procedure in years. The number at risk is reported per year during the follow-up.

None of the eyes had major adverse events postoperatively. In one eye a macroscopic hyphema occurred after goniotomy with spontaneous resolution in one week. Three eyes had a mild uveitic reaction after goniotomy that endured for 3 and 8 months, respectively, and persisted in one eye (in a patient without DMARDs). Three eyes had a transient high IOP post-operatively. Two eyes underwent cataract surgery after goniotomy (after 2 and 16 months, respectively); both of them were already diagnosed with cataract before the glaucoma intervention.

4. Discussion

Goniotomy reveals a significant decrease in IOP and the number of IOP-lowering medication classes in non-infectious uveitic glaucoma in children; in our data, the decrease remained stable during a 5-year follow-up. No differences between pre- and postoperative data were found with regard to visual acuity, uveitis activity, frequency of topical steroid medication, and use of different systemic medications, suggesting a safe procedure and a stable uveitis over time.

Previous studies showed similar significant decreases in IOP and number of IOP-lowering medication classes after surgery, but showed a lower success rate after one goniotomy; 72–76% [14,15] after 1 year, 54–61% [14,16] after 2 years, and 47–54% [14,16] after ≥5 years of follow-up. While in earlier studies PAS, aphakia, and multiple previous ocular surgeries were described as predictors of surgical failure, in our study we had only one eye with limited PAS, no aphakic eyes, and no eyes with multiple previous ocular surgeries. It is probable that the more fortunate baseline and preoperative findings in our cohort contributed to a better outcome post-operatively. In the eye with PAS, the areas with synechiae were avoided during the goniotomy procedure and this eye had a successful outcome with no IOP-lowering medication at the end of follow-up.

We did not perform additional analyses to determine potential risk factors for risk of failure because we had just two failures in our cohort. However, the risk factors for failure published by previous studies correspond with the characteristics of our failures.

For example, Ho and Walton [19] found a higher risk of failure in cases with a longer interval between glaucoma diagnosis and surgery (mean 1.1 ± 1.0 years in their success versus 5.1 ± 3.3 years in the failure group, $p = 0.001$). In our cohort, the failures had a longer interval between the start of IOP-lowering medication and surgery as well (16 and 28 months in the failures versus 9 (6–19) months (median (IQR)) in the success group). Additionally, Ho and Walton [19] published a significantly higher age at surgery in the failure group (mean 9.2 ± 3.7 years in their success versus 12.6 ± 4.7 years in their failure group, $p = 0.04$). A difference in age at surgery was also present in our cohort (11 and 13 years in the failures versus 7 (6–10) years (median (IQR)) in the success group). These observations support the advice to perform prompt glaucoma surgery when it is indicated.

Adequate uveitis control in non-infectious pediatric uveitis is of great importance, and an inactive uveitis for at least 3 months before surgery is recommended [7,20]. In order to reach an inactive uveitis, DMARDs were often used preoperatively; csDMARDs in nine patients (90%) and bDMARDs in five patients (50%). None of the patients used systemic steroids for a prolonged period of time. Previous studies also describe the use of csDMARDs and systemic steroids [14,16]. Bohnsack et al. [15]. was the only study that reported more details: 69% of the patients used DMARDs (with no differentiation between csDMARDs and bDMARDs) and 14% of the patients used systemic steroids.

The working mechanism of the goniotomy in uveitic glaucoma is not completely understood. Most likely, incising the damaged trabecular meshwork results in a better aqueous humor outflow, leading to improved IOP control [11]. In a histopathological study after a trabeculodialysis in uveitic glaucoma, the treated meshwork was scarred, with adjacent collagen cores cemented together with loss of endothelial covering and absence of intertrabecular spaces and thereby collapsed structures. However, it is not only the connection with or entrance to Schlemm's canal that seems to influence the outflow of the aqueous humor via the trabecular meshwork pathway. The pulsation mechanism to flush aqueous efficiently to Schlemm's canal and into the draining venous system, activated by stretching of the trabecular meshwork, secondary to IOP rise, is also important for IOP regulation [21]. It is plausible that the fibrosing process, due to chronic inflammation, decreases the ability to pulsate. In addition, pro-inflammatory factors are produced during an IOP increase [22]. Thus, early control of uveitis activity and early surgical treatment of medically uncontrolled elevated IOP could both have a protective effect on the structure of the trabecular meshwork and contribute to the more favorable outcomes of goniotomy surgery now as compared to the past. A major advantage of the goniotomy is the ability to continue DMARD, as the survival of filtering blebs and the occurrence of fibrosis, such as after a glaucoma drainage implant, is not a factor [23–25].

In our study and in the three previous studies about the goniotomy procedure in pediatric uveitis [14–16], exacerbation of uveitis did not occur and no major complications such as infection, iatrogenic damage of intraocular structures or hypotony occurred. A small, transient hyphema, macroscopic but without the need of any intervention, occurred in our cohort. Blood visible in the anterior chamber angle is considered a normal phenomenon after goniotomy, presumed to be caused by reflux and considered a sign of success. Two out of twelve phakic eyes (17%) underwent cataract surgery after goniotomy; both of them were already diagnosed with cataract before the glaucoma intervention. In previous research [14–16], 10–44% of the phakic eyes, which had some lens opacity before glaucoma surgery, needed cataract surgery after a goniotomy procedure. Cataract progressed in only a few cases after goniotomy. The complication profile of the goniotomy procedure is mild when compared to that of TE and glaucoma drainage implants, which have a risk of hypotony and bleb or implant-based complications [10].

In spite of its retrospective design, our study does not suffer from selection bias, due to the fact that goniotomy was the first step in the surgical protocol during the inclusion period (except in one patient, where the first treated eye had failed). In all patients, visualization and accessibility of the chamber angle were sufficient to perform a goniotomy. Goniotomy procedures were performed by two surgeons (one surgeon per center). The relatively long follow-up period and the reporting of data at fixed time points are other strengths of our study. Potential weaknesses of our study include its limited sample size and a lack of predefined standardization in measurements and time points. Success was predominantly based on IOP outcomes. Ideally, visual field outcomes should have been added, but obtaining reliable visual field outcomes in young children is challenging. In addition, the two eyes in which goniotomy failed were treated directly with other forms of glaucoma surgery; therefore, it is unclear whether additional goniotomy would have had an added benefit.

Further research regarding goniotomy in pediatric uveitic glaucoma is warranted, preferably using prospective randomized controlled studies with a larger sample size that compare different types of glaucoma surgery, especially as a function of age.

5. Conclusions

This study indicates that goniotomy might be considered as a primary surgical treatment in children with non-infectious uveitic glaucoma. Goniotomy is a safe and straightforward procedure, and it appears to be effective over a relatively long follow-up period. It might be a definite treatment in the majority of eyes, and it can be supplemented by more extensive glaucoma surgery at a later time point if necessary.

Author Contributions: Conceptualization, N.M.J. and L.J.v.R.; methodology, C.L.L.I.v.M., A.B.E. and L.I.L.; software, C.L.L.I.v.M. and A.B.E.; validation, L.I.L. and N.M.J.; formal analysis, A.B.E., C.L.L.I.v.M. and N.M.J.; investigation, C.L.L.I.v.M., A.B.E. and L.J.v.R.; resources, C.L.L.I.v.M., A.B.E. and L.I.L.; data curation, A.B.E.; writing—original draft preparation, C.L.L.I.v.M. and A.B.E.; writing—review and editing, L.I.L., N.M.J. and L.J.v.R.; visualization, C.L.L.I.v.M. and A.B.E.; supervision, L.I.L., N.M.J. and L.J.v.R.; project administration, C.L.L.I.v.M. and A.B.E.; funding acquisition, C.L.L.I.v.M. All authors have read and agreed to the published version of the manuscript.

Funding: This research received no external funding.

Institutional Review Board Statement: The study adhered to the tenets of the Declaration of Helsinki. Because the study concerns a retrospective analysis of data that have been collected during regular patient care, no formal approval of a Medical Ethical Committee was required (waiver obtained from the Medical Ethical Committee of both participating centers (Amsterdam and Groningen).

Informed Consent Statement: Not applicable.

Data Availability Statement: Not applicable.

Conflicts of Interest: The authors declare no conflict of interest.

References

1. Heinz, C.; Pleyer, U.; Ruokonnen, P.; Heiligenhaus, A. Sekundärglaukom bei kindern mit uveitis. *Ophthalmologe* **2008**, *105*, 438–444. [CrossRef]
2. Päivönsalo-Hietanen, T.; Tuominen, J.; Saari, K.M. Uveitis in children: Population-based study in Finland. *Acta Ophthalmol. Scand.* **2000**, *78*, 84–88. [CrossRef] [PubMed]
3. Chia, A.; Lee, V.; Graham, E.M.; Edelsten, C. Factors related to severe uveitis at diagnosis in children with juvenile idiopathic arthritis in a screening program. *Am. J. Ophthalmol.* **2003**, *135*, 757–762. [CrossRef]
4. de Boer, J.; Wulffraat, N.; Rothova, A.J. Visual loss in uveitis of childhood. *Br. J. Ophthalmol.* **2003**, *87*, 879–884. [CrossRef] [PubMed]
5. Sijssens, K.M.; Rothova, A.; Berendschot, T.T.J.M.; de Boer, J.H. Ocular Hypertension and Secondary Glaucoma in Children with Uveitis. *Ophthalmology* **2006**, *113*, 853–859.e2. [CrossRef]
6. Seth, N.G.; Yangzes, S.; Thattaruthody, F.; Singh, R.; Bansal, R.; Raj, S.; Kaushik, S.; Gupta, V.; Pandav, S.S.; Ram, J.; et al. Glaucoma Secondary to Uveitis in Children in a Tertiary Care Referral Center. *Ocul. Immunol. Inflamm.* **2018**, *27*, 456–464. [CrossRef]
7. Murthy, S.I.; Pappuru, R.; Latha, K.M.; Kamat, S.; Sangwan, V.S. Surgical management in patient with uveitis. *Indian J. Ophthalmol.* **2013**, *61*, 284–290. [CrossRef]
8. Boyle, J.W.; Netland, P.A.; Salim, S. *Uveitic Glaucoma: Pathophysiology and Management*; American Academy of Ophthalmology: San Francisco, CA, USA, 2008.
9. Chen, T.C.; Chen, P.P.; Francis, B.A.; Junk, A.K.; Smith, S.D.; Singh, K.; Lin, S.C. Pediatric glaucoma surgery: A report by the American Academy of Ophthalmology. *Ophthalmology* **2014**, *121*, 2107–2115. [CrossRef]

10. van Meerwijk, C.L.L.I.; Jansonius, N.M.; Los, L.I. Uveitic glaucoma in children: A systematic review on surgical outcomes. *J. Ophthalmic Inflamm. Infect.* **2022**, *12*, 35. [CrossRef]
11. Greenwood, M.D.; Seibold, L.K.; Radcliffe, N.M.; Dorairaj, S.K.; Aref, A.A.; Román, J.J.; Lazcano-Gomez, G.S.; Darlington, J.K.; Abdullah, S.; Jasek, M.C.; et al. Goniotomy with a single-use dual blade: Short-term results. *J. Cataract. Refract. Surg.* **2017**, *43*, 1197–1201. [CrossRef]
12. Worst, J.G. Goniotomy; An improved method for chamber-angle surgery in congenital glaucoma. *Am. J. Ophthalmol.* **1964**, *57*, 185–200. [CrossRef]
13. Walton, D.S.; Hodapp, E. Angle Surgery: Goniotomy. In *Surgical Management of Childhood Glaucoma*; Springer International Publishing: Berlin/Heidelberg, Germany, 2018; pp. 49–55. [CrossRef]
14. Freedman, S.F.; Rodriguez-Rosa, R.E.; Rojas, M.C.; Enyedi, L.B. Goniotomy for Glaucoma Secondary to Chronic Childhood Uveitis. *Am. J. Ophthalmol.* **2002**, *133*, 617–621. [CrossRef]
15. Bohnsack, B.L.; Freedman, S.F. Surgical Outcomes in Childhood Uveitic Glaucoma. *Am. J. Ophthalmol.* **2013**, *155*, 134–142. [CrossRef]
16. Ho, C.L.; Wong, E.Y.M.; Walton, D.S. Goniosurgery for glaucoma complicating chronic childhood uveitis. *Arch. Ophthalmol.* **2004**, *122*, 838–844. [CrossRef]
17. Worst, J.G.F. *The Pathogenesis of Congenital Glaucoma: An Embryological, Gonioscopical, Gonio-Surgical and Clinical Study*; Van Gorcum & Comp. N.V.: Assen, The Netherlands, 1966.
18. Jabs, D.A.; Nussenblatt, R.B.; Rosenbaum, J.T. Standardization of uveitis nomenclature for reporting clinical data. Results of the first international workshop. *Am. J. Ophthalmol.* **2005**, *140*, 509–516. [CrossRef]
19. Ho, C.L.; Walton, D.S. Goniosurgery for glaucoma secondary to chronic anterior uveitis: Prognostic factors and surgical technique. *J. Glaucoma* **2004**, *13*, 445–449. [CrossRef]
20. Rohl, A.; Patnaik, J.L.; Claire Miller, D.; Lynch, A.M.; Palestine, A.G. Timing of Quiescence and Uveitis Recurrences After Cataract Surgery in Patients with a History of Uveitis. *Ophthalmol. Ther.* **2021**, *10*, 619–628. [CrossRef]
21. Johnstone, M.; Martin, E.; Jamil, A. Pulsatile flow into the aqueous veins: Manifestations in normal and glaucomatous eyes. *Exp. Eye Res.* **2011**, *92*, 318–327. [CrossRef]
22. WuDunn, D. Mechanobiology of trabecular meshwork cells. *Exp. Eye Res.* **2009**, *88*, 718–723. [CrossRef]
23. Cunliffe, I.A.; Richardson, P.S.; Rees, R.C.; Rennie, I.G. Effect of TNF, IL-1, and IL-6 on the proliferation of human Tenon's capsule fibroblasts in tissue culture. *Br. J. Ophthalmol.* **1995**, *79*, 590–595. [CrossRef]
24. Ramdas, W.D.; Pals, J.; Rothova, A.; Wolfs, R.C.W. Efficacy of glaucoma drainage devices in uveitic glaucoma and a meta-analysis of the literature. *Graefes Arch. Clin. Exp. Ophthalmol.* **2019**, *257*, 143–151. [CrossRef]
25. Garg, A.; Alió, J.L. *Surgical Techniques in Ophthalmology (Pediatric Ophthalmic Surgery)*, 1st ed.; Jaypee Brothers Medical Publishers (P) Ltd.: New Delhi, India, 2011. [CrossRef]

Disclaimer/Publisher's Note: The statements, opinions and data contained in all publications are solely those of the individual author(s) and contributor(s) and not of MDPI and/or the editor(s). MDPI and/or the editor(s) disclaim responsibility for any injury to people or property resulting from any ideas, methods, instructions or products referred to in the content.

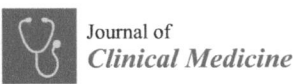

Article

Factors Associated with Visual Acuity in Advanced Glaucoma

Hyun Jee Kim, Mi Sun Sung * and Sang Woo Park *

Department of Ophthalmology, Research Institute of Medical Sciences, Chonnam National University Medical School and Hospital, Gwangju 61469, Republic of Korea
* Correspondence: sms84831@hanmail.net (M.S.S.); exo70@naver.com (S.W.P.); Tel.: +82-62-220-6575 (M.S.S.); +82-62-220-6742 (S.W.P.)

Abstract: This study aimed to comprehensively analyze various parameters in advanced glaucoma patients to identify the factors that can affect best-corrected visual acuity (BCVA) in advanced glaucoma. This cross-sectional retrospective study included 113 patients (mean age, 61.66 ± 13.26 years; males, 67) who had advanced glaucomatous damage (113 eyes; mean BCVA, 0.18 ± 0.38 logMAR; mean deviation of 30-2 visual field [VF], −19.08 ± 6.23 dB). Peripapillary retinal nerve fiber layer (RNFL) and total and segmented macular thickness (RNFL, ganglion cell layer (GCL), and inner plexiform layer (GCL)) were measured using Spectralis optical coherence tomography (OCT). Correlations between BCVA and OCT parameters or 30-2 VF parameters were assessed using Pearson correlation analysis. Multivariate regression analysis was performed to determine the factors associated with BCVA in advanced glaucoma patients. Peripapillary RNFL thickness, subfoveal choroidal thickness, and global macular RNFL, GCL, IPL, and total thickness were found to be significantly correlated with BCVA and central visual function. Multivariate analysis showed a significant correlation between subfoveal choroidal thickness and BCVA. In addition, central VF mean sensitivity, especially inferior hemifield, showed a significant relationship with BCVA. In conclusion, subfoveal choroidal thickness and central VF sensitivity, especially the inferior hemifield area, are factors that affect BCVA in advanced glaucoma.

Keywords: visual acuity; advanced glaucoma; subfoveal choroidal thickness; central visual field

Citation: Kim, H.J.; Sung, M.S.; Park, S.W. Factors Associated with Visual Acuity in Advanced Glaucoma. *J. Clin. Med.* **2023**, *12*, 3076. https://doi.org/10.3390/jcm12093076

Academic Editor: Kevin Gillmann

Received: 28 March 2023
Revised: 19 April 2023
Accepted: 22 April 2023
Published: 24 April 2023

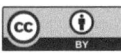

Copyright: © 2023 by the authors. Licensee MDPI, Basel, Switzerland. This article is an open access article distributed under the terms and conditions of the Creative Commons Attribution (CC BY) license (https://creativecommons.org/licenses/by/4.0/).

1. Introduction

Glaucoma is the leading cause of visual dysfunction and blindness worldwide. The disease is associated with various genetic mechanisms and alterations in biochemical pathways that affect the visual system [1]. Therefore, the ultimate purpose of glaucoma treatment is to maintain visual function and vision-related QOL through the early detection and prevention of disease progression [2]. Because of the distinct features of the disease, i.e., it is "chronic and irreversible", it can significantly affect the quality of life (QOL) of glaucoma patients [3,4].

Several parameters are known to be associated with vision-related QOL in glaucoma patients [5–8]. Chun et al. [5] previously showed that visual acuity is the most important factor in severe glaucoma. Similarly, a previous study performed on the Early Manifest Glaucoma Trial (EMGT) cohort demonstrated that visual acuity is significantly correlated with vision-related QOL, independent of visual field (VF) parameters [6]. The central VF remains relatively intact until the severely advanced stage of the disease due to the surplus of retinal ganglion cells in the macular area [9]. However, as the disease progresses, a reduction in best-corrected visual acuity (BCVA) can occur, and this decline can significantly affect the daily life of glaucoma patients. Hence, treatment strategies for preventing BCVA aggravation are clinically important.

A decrease in BCVA is associated with a decrease in VF parameters [10]. However, in clinical practice, some patients experience a rapid decrease in BCVA even when not in the advanced stage, contrary to our expectations [11]. Meanwhile, some patients maintain relatively good visual acuity despite being in the severely advanced stage [9,10]. This suggests that factors other than the extent of VF defects may contribute to BCVA. Takahashi et al. [9] showed that damage to the papillomacular bundle, a specific area of the retina, was strongly associated with BCVA in glaucoma. It has recently been demonstrated that macular vascular density of the deep layer is independently associated with central visual function in glaucoma patients [12–14]. However, information regarding the potential factors influencing visual acuity in advanced glaucoma patients is still limited. Therefore, this study aimed to comprehensively analyze various parameters in glaucoma patients to identify the factors that can affect visual acuity in advanced glaucoma.

2. Materials and Methods

2.1. Participants

We retrospectively reviewed the medical records of 113 patients (113 eyes) who visited the glaucoma clinic and were diagnosed with advanced glaucoma at the Chonnam National University Hospital between February 2019 and May 2022. The Institutional Review Board of the Chonnam National University Hospital approved this retrospective study and waived the need for informed consent due to the use of de-identified patient data. The present study was conducted in accordance with the Declaration of Helsinki.

Each patient received a detailed consultation and underwent a complete ophthalmic examination at the first outpatient visit, which included slit-lamp examination, manifest refraction, BCVA using the logarithm of the minimum angle resolution (logMAR) units, intraocular pressure (IOP) using Goldmann applanation tonometry, optic nerve head (ONH) and peripapillary retinal nerve fiber layer (RNFL) examinations using both color disc photography and red-free RNFL fundus photography, and VF measurements using the Humphrey Field Analyzer (Carl Zeiss Meditec, Dublin, CA, USA) with the Swedish interactive threshold algorithm standard 30-2 program. The axial length and central corneal thickness were measured using optical low-coherence reflectometry (Lenstar; Haag-Streit AG, Koeniz, Switzerland).

The inclusion criteria for the study were age > 18 years; patients with advanced glaucomatous damage with global mean deviation (MD) below -12 dB on the 30-2 VF test according to the simplified modification of the Hodapp–Anderson–Parrish criteria [15]; BCVA of 20/200 or better; and spherical equivalent refractive error within $\pm$ 6.0 D and cylinder refraction within $\pm$ 5.0. The exclusion criteria were any history of ocular surgery other than uncomplicated cataract or glaucoma surgery; presence of any media opacities that could affect the BCVA or VF results; presence of retinal disease, including fine epiretinal membrane, diabetic retinopathy, and drusen; or presence of neurological disease or intracranial lesion. We strictly excluded eyes with cataracts or posterior capsular opacity after mydriasis to prevent the potential influence of their effects on BCVA.

2.2. Visual Field Examination

All patients underwent the 30-2 VF test twice within 2 months of the initial visit. Our protocols for the first VF results were highly variable and inaccurate. The accuracy of the VF results improved across the repetitions. This is called the "learning effect". To exclude the learning effect, we used a second VF test for analysis. The same test-spot size (Goldmann size III stimulus) and standard perimetric conditions (background luminance, 31.5 apostilbs) were used for all VF examinations. Near-refractive correction was performed as necessary. The VF measurements were considered reliable if the fixation losses were <20% and the false-positive response rates were <15%. False-negative responses were not included in the exclusion criteria because the presence of several false-negative responses was associated more with the patient's status than reliability [16]. MD, pattern standard deviation (PSD), VF index (VFI), and foveal sensitivity data were extracted from the VF results. In addition, central VF sensitivity, defined as the central 12 points correlating topographically to the macular area, was analyzed. Each visual sensitivity value of the central 12 test points was converted to a linear scale (1/Lambert value) using the following formula, $1/\text{Lambert} = (10)^{0.1 \times dB}$, and the converted linear scale values were subsequently averaged to obtain the central mean sensitivity values. The central 12 points were further divided topographically into two hemispheres, superior and inferior, based on the Garway–Heath map. Detailed protocols for the analysis of the VF results are described in our previous study [17].

2.3. Spectral-Domain Optical Coherence Tomography

All patients underwent OCT imaging using SD-OCT (Heidelberg Spectralis SD-OCT; Spectralis software version 6.9.4; Heidelberg Engineering GmbH, Heidelberg, Germany) at the initial visit. All OCT scans were performed by an experienced operator (M.Y.H.). The Bruch membrane opening (BMO) area and peripapillary RNFL thickness (along a 3.5 mm diameter-circle scan) were measured using Glaucoma Module Premium Edition software. The global value and six Garway–Heath regional peripapillary RNFL thickness values relative to the FoBMO axis (the line connecting the center of the fovea and the BMO center) were calculated (nasal-superior, 85–125 degrees; nasal, 125–235 degrees; nasal-inferior, 235–275 degrees; temporal-inferior, 275–315 degrees; temporal, 315–45 degrees; and temporal-superior, 45–85 degrees).

Macular scans were performed using the Posterior Pole algorithm and 30-25-degree volume scans centered on the fovea were acquired. The segmentation of individual retinal layers was performed using the Glaucoma Module Premium Edition software. In addition to the total retinal thickness, the macular RNFL, macular ganglion cell layer (GCL), and macular inner plexiform layer (IPL) were measured. All images from the B-scans were reviewed thoroughly for segmentation errors, and any obvious errors were corrected manually.

2.4. Optic Nerve Head Measurements

The Heidelberg Spectralis OCT's enhanced depth-imaging mode was used for the other ONH measurements. The ONH was scanned by centering a 15×10 degree rectangular scan on the ONH. Each OCT volume consisted of 49 serial horizontal B-scans with a length of 4.5 mm in length and 50 images averaged, spaced at approximately 63 µm intervals. Among the B-scans, three sections that passed through the center of the ONH, midsuperior, and midinferior regions were selected for ONH analysis.

The temporal β-parapapillary atrophy margin (β-PPA), BMO, and disc margin were defined using infrared fundus images. The β-PPA width was defined as the distance between the beginning of the retinal pigment epithelium (RPE) (i.e., temporal β-PPA margin) and temporal disc margin on each horizontal B-scan image. Based on the location of the Bruch's membrane (BM) termination, the β-PPA was further divided into PPA_{+BM} and PPA_{-BM}. The PPA_{+BM} width was defined as the distance from the beginning of the RPE to the BM, and the PPA_{-BM} was defined as the distance from the temporal disc margin to the beginning of the BM.

The lamina cribrosa (LC) depth was defined as the vertical distance between the reference line and the anterior LC surface at the center of the ONH from selected horizontal B-scan images. The LC thickness was defined as the perpendicular distance between the anterior and posterior margins of the highly reflective region at the ONH vertical center. In this study, the sclerochoroid junction reference plane was used for the LC depth measurements to overcome the effect of choroidal thickness. The measurement was performed using a built-in caliper tool in the intrinsic OCT viewer, and the average data of three horizontal B-scan images (center, midsuperior, and midinferior) were calculated and used for the analysis. The ONH measurements were performed by two independent examiners (H.J.K. and M.S.S.) blinded to the patients' information, and the means of the values obtained by the two examiners were used in the final analysis. Details regarding the ONH measurements have been described in previous studies [18–21].

2.5. Choroidal Thickness Measurements

Peripapillary choroidal thickness was measured manually using the embedded software [22]. We delineated the upper and lower segmentation lines of the 360-degree circular peripapillary RNFL scan (3.5 mm), centered on the BMO. The lines were adjusted to align with the inner scleral wall and posterior border of the RPE to define the outer and inner boundaries of the choroid, respectively. The software automatically computed the peripapillary choroidal thickness using the RNFL thickness sector algorithms. Subfoveal choroidal thickness was measured manually from a single EDI scan running through the fovea with the caliper function embedded in the Spectralis instrument. Subfoveal choroidal thickness is defined as the vertical distance from the hyperscattering outer border of the RPE to the inner border of the sclera at the fovea. The average measurements from the two independent examiners (H.J.K. and M.S.S.) were used in this study.

2.6. Statistical Analysis

All statistical analyses were performed using SPSS version 23.0 (SPSS, Chicago, IL, USA). Partial correlation analyses were conducted to determine the relationships between the OCT structural parameters and functional parameters such as BCVA and central visual function while adjusting for age. Relationships between the BCVA and several VF parameters were examined using Pearson correlation analyses. The differences in the strength of the correlations between BCVA and the mean sensitivity of the central six points in the superior and inferior hemifields were compared using Steiger's test [23]. Univariate and multivariate regression analyses were performed to determine the significant factors affecting BCVA in advanced glaucoma patients. The statistical significance was set at $p < 0.05$.

3. Results

A total of 113 eyes of 113 patients with advanced glaucoma were included in this cross-sectional retrospective study. The mean age of the patients was 61.66 ± 13.26 years and 57.29% (67 patients) were men. The mean BCVA was 0.18 ± 0.38 logMAR and the mean IOP was 24.96 ± 10.40 mmHg. The MD and PSD values for the 30-2 VF were -19.52 ± 5.51 dB and 12.07 ± 3.43 dB, respectively. The demographic features of the patients with advanced glaucoma are presented in Table 1.

Table 1. Demographic data of patients with advanced glaucoma.

Variable	N = 113
Age (years)	61.66 ± 13.26
Sex (male/female)	67/46
Laterality (right/left)	62/51
BCVA (logMAR)	0.18 ± 0.38
Axial length (mm)	24.49 ± 1.47
Central corneal thickness (μm)	529.28 ± 50.43
Baseline IOP (mmHg)	24.96 ± 10.40
OCT parameters	
BMO area (mm^2)	2.40 ± 0.54
LC thickness (μm)	201.69 ± 36.46
LC depth (μm)	516.93 ± 150.25
PPA$_{+BM}$ width (μm)	251.91 ± 180.14
PPA$_{-BM}$ width (μm)	112.22 ± 192.54
Subfoveal choroidal thickness (μm)	207.69 ± 71.70
Global peripapillary RNFL thickness (μm)	52.16 ± 12.43
Global peripapillary choroidal thickness (μm)	114.18 ± 45.61
Global macular RNFL thickness (μm)	19.81 ± 2.67
Global macular GCL thickness (μm)	30.83 ± 7.32
Global macular IPL thickness (μm)	29.27 ± 4.52

Table 1. Cont.

Variable	N = 113
Global macular thickness (μm)	306.99 ± 18.40
30-2 VF parameters	
MD (dB)	−19.52 ± 5.51
PSD (dB)	12.07 ± 3.43
VFI (%)	40.79 ± 19.91
Foveal sensitivity (dB)	27.24 ± 9.77
Mean sensitivity of the central 12 points (dB)	−19.08 ± 6.23

BCVA = best-corrected visual acuity; logMAR = logarithm of the minimum angle of resolution; IOP = intraocular pressure; OCT = optical coherence tomography; BMO = Bruch's membrane opening; LC = lamina cribrosa; PPA_{+BM} = β-parapapillary atrophy with Bruch's membrane; PPA_{-BM} = β-parapapillary atrophy without Bruch's membrane; RNFL = retinal nerve fiber layer; GCL = ganglion cell layer; IPL = inner plexiform layer; VF = visual field; MD = mean deviation; PSD = pattern standard deviation; VFI = visual field index.

Table 2 shows the results of the partial correlation analysis between the clinical and structural variables and BCVA or central VF sensitivity after adjusting for age in advanced glaucoma patients. Overall, peripapillary RNFL thickness and global macular RNFL, GCL, IPL, and total thickness showed significant correlations with both BCVA and central VF sensitivity (all $p < 0.05$). Furthermore, subfoveal choroidal thickness and the temporal sector of peripapillary choroidal thickness showed significant correlations with the BCVA and VF sensitivity of the central 12 points ($p = 0.001$ and $p = 0.006$, respectively, for BCVA; $p = 0.045$ and $p = 0.048$, respectively, for central VF sensitivity).

Table 2. Correlations between clinical and structural variables and best-corrected visual acuity or central visual function in advanced glaucoma patients.

Variable	BCVA		Central VF Sensitivity on 30-2 VF	
	r	p-Value *	r	p-Value *
Axial length	0.130	0.211	0.158	0.126
Central corneal thickness	0.002	0.987	0.154	0.131
Baseline IOP	0.126	0.184	−0.065	0.495
BMO area	0.032	0.735	0.021	0.826
LC thickness	0.015	0.874	−0.018	0.852
LC depth	−0.166	0.079	0.062	0.511
PPA_{+BM} width	0.003	0.976	−0.072	0.452
PPA_{-BM} width	0.234	**0.013**	0.078	0.414
Subfoveal choroidal thickness	−0.316	**0.001**	0.202	**0.045**
Peripapillary RNFL thickness				
Global	−0.345	**<0.001**	0.387	**<0.001**
Temporal-superior	−0.177	0.060	0.363	**<0.001**
Temporal	−0.393	**<0.001**	0.424	**<0.001**
Temporal-inferior	−0.064	0.499	0.042	0.660
Nasal-inferior	−0.176	0.061	0.086	0.366
Nasal	−0.235	**0.012**	0.234	**0.013**
Nasal-superior	−0.227	**0.015**	0.279	**0.003**
Peripapillary choroidal thickness				
Global	−0.248	**0.008**	0.125	0.189
Temporal-superior	−0.214	**0.023**	0.075	0.430
Temporal	−0.258	**0.006**	0.194	**0.048**
Temporal-inferior	−0.257	**0.006**	0.122	0.199
Nasal-inferior	−0.223	**0.018**	0.108	0.256
Nasal	−0.228	**0.015**	0.096	0.311
Nasal-superior	−0.186	**0.049**	0.158	0.095
Global macular RNFL thickness	−0.376	**<0.001**	0.264	**0.006**
Global macular GCL thickness	−0.473	**<0.001**	0.478	**<0.001**
Global macular IPL thickness	−0.475	**<0.001**	0.413	**<0.001**
Global macular thickness	−0.400	**<0.001**	0.215	**0.026**

BCVA = best-corrected visual acuity; IOP = intraocular pressure; BMO = Bruch's membrane opening; LC = lamina cribrosa; PPA_{+BM} = β-parapapillary atrophy with Bruch's membrane; PPA_{-BM} = β-parapapillary atrophy without Bruch's membrane; RNFL = retinal nerve fiber layer; GCL = ganglion cell layer; IPL = inner plexiform layer; VF = visual field; MD = mean deviation; PSD = pattern standard deviation; VFI = visual field index. * p values from partial correlation analysis adjusted by age. Factors with statistical significance are shown in bold.

Furthermore, we evaluated the association between the 30-2 VF parameters and BCVA in advanced glaucoma patients (Table 3). As expected, as the severity of functional damage increased, patients had worse BCVA. We found a statistically significant correlation in advanced glaucoma patients between the BCVA and functional parameters such as the MD (r = −0.374, $p < 0.001$), PSD (r = −0.397, $p < 0.001$), VFI (r = −0.424, $p < 0.001$), foveal sensitivity (r = −0.549, $p < 0.001$), and mean sensitivity of the central 12 points (r = −0.493, $p < 0.001$). When the central 12 points were further divided into superior and inferior hemifields, both demonstrated significant relationships with BCVA (r = −0.202, $p = 0.015$ for the superior hemifield, and r = −0.445, $p < 0.001$ for the inferior hemifield). However, there was a difference in the strength of the correlations between them; the mean sensitivity of the central six points of the inferior hemifield tended to have a better relationship with BCVA than that of the superior hemifield ($p = 0.044$).

Table 3. Association between BCVA and 30-2 VF parameters in advanced glaucoma patients.

Variable	BCVA	
	r	*p*-Value *
MD	−0.374	**<0.001**
PSD	−0.397	**<0.001**
VFI	−0.424	**<0.001**
Foveal sensitivity	−0.549	**<0.001**
Mean sensitivity of central 12 points	−0.493	**<0.001**
Mean sensitivity of central 6 points in superior hemifield	−0.202	**0.015**
Mean sensitivity of central 6 points in inferior hemifield	−0.445	**<0.001**

BCVA = best-corrected visual acuity; VF = visual field; MD = mean deviation; PSD = pattern standard deviation; VFI = visual field index. * *p* values from Pearson correlation analysis. Factors with statistical significance are shown in bold.

To determine the ocular and structural factors that have a close relationship with BCVA in advanced glaucoma patients, univariate and multivariate regression analyses were performed. We eliminated the factors that were not statistically meaningful in the univariate model before analysis. Because the peripapillary RNFL thickness and global macular RNFL, GCL, IPL, and total thickness showed significant multicollinearity, we only used the global macular GCL thickness out of the macular parameters, and the peripapillary RNFL thickness and global macular GCL thickness were used in a different multivariate regression model. The macular GCL thickness was chosen as it showed the strongest correlation with BCVA in the univariate regression analysis. As summarized in Table 4, the PPA$_{-BM}$ width ($p = 0.001$), subfoveal choroidal thickness ($p = 0.001$), peripapillary RNFL thickness ($p < 0.001$), and global macular GCL thickness ($p < 0.001$) showed significant associations with BCVA in the univariate analysis. Through multivariate regression analysis, the subfoveal choroidal thickness ($p = 0.020$ in model 1 and $p = 0.043$ in model 2), peripapillary RNFL thickness ($p = 0.001$), and global macular GCL thickness ($p < 0.001$) were identified as statistically meaningful factors associated with BCVA in advanced glaucoma patients. Figure 1 illustrates the relationship between the subfoveal choroidal thickness and BCVA. It can be seen that as the subfoveal choroidal thickness decreased, the patients' BCVA became significantly worse ($r^2 = 0.100$, r = 0.316, $p = 0.001$).

Table 4. Multivariate analysis of the associations between BCVA and ocular and structural parameters.

Variable	Univariate			Multivariate (Model 1)			Multivariate (Model 2)		
	Coefficient	95% CI	*p*-Value *	Coefficient	95% CI	*p*-Value *	Coefficient	95% CI	*p*-Value *
PPA$_{-BM}$ width	0.001	0.000–0.001	**0.001**	0.00038	0.000–0.001	0.056	0.00025	0.000–0.001	0.120
Subfoveal choroidal thickness	−0.002	−0.003–−0.001	**0.001**	−0.001	−0.002–0.000	**0.020**	−0.001	−0.002–0.000	**0.043**
Peripapillary RNFL thickness	−0.010	−0.016–−0.005	**<0001**	−0.009	−0.014–−0.004	**0.001**			
Global macular GCL thickness	−0.023	−0.031–−0.015	**<0.001**				−0.020	−0.029–−0.012	**<0.001**

BCVA = best-corrected visual acuity; CI = confidence interval; PPA$_{-BM}$ = β-parapapillary atrophy without Bruch's membrane; RNFL = retinal nerve fiber layer; GCL = ganglion cell layer. * *p* values from multivariate regression analysis. Factors with statistical significance are shown in bold.

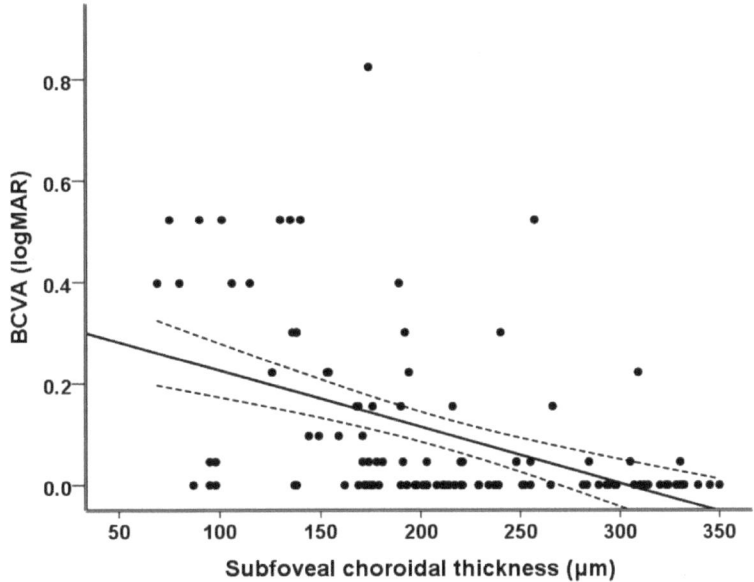

Figure 1. Scatter plots showing the relationship between BCVA and subfoveal choroidal thickness. The dashed lines represent the 95% confidence intervals for the solid trend lines.

4. Discussion

Central visual function is closely related to patients' QOL [7]. Thus, maintaining BCVA and central VF is important in glaucoma patients [9]. Either a loss of the central VF or a decrease in the BCVA can significantly affect vision-related QOL [11]. Generally, it is known that central VF is relatively well-preserved until the late stage of glaucoma [24]. However, as the severity of glaucoma increases, a deterioration of central vision inevitably occurs. In clinical situations, the degree of central VF damage and BCVA is highly variable among patients, even in those with similar severity of disease. Specifically, some patients maintain a good BCVA and reserved central VF until the terminal stage of glaucoma, whereas other patients exhibit BCVA deterioration even before advanced glaucomatous damage. In the present study, we focused on the factors affecting BCVA in eyes with advanced glaucomatous damage. Although BCVA is an important factor in determining the visual function and vision-related QOL in glaucoma patients, information regarding BCVA is scarce compared to information regarding VF parameters. Hence, in this study, we focused on BCVA in advanced glaucoma patients and comprehensively investigated the various factors affecting BCVA.

In this study, the peripapillary RNFL thickness and global macular RNFL, GCL, IPL, and total thickness showed significant correlations with BCVA and central visual function. Our findings indicate that as the degree of structural damage increases, a significant decrease in BCVA occurs in patients with advanced glaucoma. These findings are consistent with those of previous studies [9,25,26]. Kim et al. [25] observed significant correlations between the logMAR BCVA and peripapillary RNFL thickness in glaucoma eyes with severe disease status. Among the sectors of the peripapillary RNFL area, Takahashi et al. [9] demonstrated that the temporal sector, which corresponds to the location of the papillomacular bundle, had a strong relationship with BCVA in glaucoma patients. The papillomacular bundle is an axonal fiber bundle emanating from the macula and fovea that carries information from the macula [27,28]. Since visual acuity is dependent on the spatial resolution capacity of the visual system, it is, in turn, influenced by the RGC density at the foveal lesion. Thus, the papillomacular bundle, which is responsible for central visual function, is considered a predictive marker for poor vision [27]. We also found that peripapillary RNFL thickness, especially the temporal sector, and the global macular thickness parameters showed significant associations with BCVA in advanced glaucoma patients.

Of note, the subfoveal choroidal thickness showed a significant correlation with BCVA and central VF sensitivity on 30-2 VF in advanced glaucoma patients. The effect of subfoveal choroidal thickness on BCVA remained statistically significant, even after controlling for the severity of structural damage by multivariate regression analysis. Previously, a report from the Beijing Eye Study, a population-based study of a large Chinese cohort, demonstrated an association between BCVA and subfoveal choroidal thickness [29]. In that study, eyes with thinner subfoveal thickness tended to have lower BCVA, whereas eyes with thicker subfoveal choroidal thickness were associated with better BCVA [29]. In another study, Nishida et al. [30] demonstrated that the only significant predictor of visual acuity in myopic eyes without other retinal pathology was subfoveal choroidal thickness. Although our results cannot be directly compared to those of prior studies because of differences in the study populations, our findings are consistent with those of prior studies.

The outer retinal segment of the fovea, especially the photoreceptor layer, is the most important area for determining BCVA. Moreover, the fovea is mainly nourished by choroidal circulation. Although the role of the choroid in the pathogenesis of glaucoma remains unclear, we suggest that a thin subfoveal choroid may be associated with decreased blood flow in the fovea region, which can lead to photoreceptor dysfunction that subsequently affects the functional status of the overlying outer retina. Recently, associations between macular microvasculature and central visual function or BCVA have been reported by several studies using OCT angiography [12–14], which found that macular microvascular density, especially from the deep layer, was an important independent predictor of BCVA [12–14]. Additionally, Song et al. [14] demonstrated that the severity of central VF impairment can vary significantly according to the status of deep macular microvasculature, despite similar VF MD and macular structural damage. Since the parafoveal region can support central visual function, impairment of the blood flow at the parafoveal retina can affect central visual function. In terms of highlighting the role of blood flow in the functional status of glaucoma, the findings of Song et al. are consistent with our results. However, the thinning of the choroid may not necessarily indicate the impairment of the blood flow. Meanwhile, Egawa et al. [31] reported a thinning of subfoveal choroid in eyes with retinitis pigmentosa (RP) and found that central visual function was significantly correlated with the ratio of the luminal/total choroidal area representing the inner subfoveal choroidal structure rather than the subfoveal choroidal thickness. Further research is needed to clarify the role of the subfoveal choroid in central visual function in glaucoma patients.

We observed significant relationships between the BCVA and 30-2 VF parameters. Among them, parameters representing the central visual function, such as the VFI, foveal sensitivity, and mean sensitivity of the central 12 points, showed strong correlations with BCVA. Our findings indicate that BCVA can also be used as an important indicator for the progression of glaucoma in patients with advanced disease. When the central 12 points were further divided into superior and inferior hemispheres, the strength of the correlations varied significantly. Interestingly, we found that the mean sensitivity of the central six points in the inferior hemifield tended to have a better relationship with BCVA than that in the superior hemifield in advanced glaucoma patients. Previously, Sawada et al. [8] explored the correlations between vision-specific QOL and clustered VF in glaucoma patients, using the Japanese version of the 25-item National Eye Institute Visual Function Questionnaire (NEI VFQ-25), which comprises 12 subscales related to the status of vision-related activities, social functioning, and emotional well-being. The study found that the VF in the better eye, particularly the lower hemifield, had a stronger correlation with QOL than that in the worse eye. Similarly, Cheng et al. [32] reported that glaucoma patients with superior hemifield VF defects had difficulty in near activities that required close-up vision, whereas patients with inferior hemifield VF defects reported more difficulties with general and peripheral vision and were more likely to report vision-related role difficulties. In our study, BCVA was measured at a distance of 5 m, which is closer to far vision than near vision. Accordingly, the mean sensitivity of the central six points in the inferior hemifield may have a stronger relationship with BCVA. Our findings are clinically significant as they highlight the importance of the inferior central VF for maintaining BCVA in advanced glaucoma patients.

This study has several limitations. First, the sample size was relatively small. Second, some bias may exist because of the study's retrospective nature. Third, only Korean patients were included in this study and our findings may not be applicable to other ethnicities. Thus, studies including larger and more diverse populations are needed. Fourth, because this study was conducted on patients from tertiary glaucoma clinics, our findings may not reflect the experience of glaucoma patients treated in other clinical settings. Fifth, although we excluded patients with cataracts or retinol lesions that could affect BCVA, several confounding factors may have affected our findings. However, we applied strict inclusion and exclusion criteria to minimize the impact of these factors. Finally, we did not consider systemic conditions, such as blood pressure and diabetes mellitus, or the use of systemic drugs that may affect the visual function of glaucoma patients. Future studies should take into account various systemic factors to further clarify the factors affecting BCVA in glaucoma patients.

In conclusion, the severity of the structural glaucomatous damage, such as peripapillary RNFL thickness and macular RNFL, GCL, IPL, and total thickness, was associated with BCVA in patients with advanced glaucomatous damage. Moreover, the subfoveal choroidal thickness and central VF sensitivity, especially in the inferior hemifield area, are factors that affect BCVA. Clinicians should carefully consider these findings when treating advanced glaucoma patients.

Author Contributions: Conceptualization, M.S.S. and S.W.P.; methodology, H.J.K., M.S.S. and S.W.P.; validation, H.J.K., M.S.S. and S.W.P.; formal analysis, H.J.K. and M.S.S.; investigation, H.J.K. and M.S.S.; resources, H.J.K. and M.S.S.; data curation, H.J.K. and M.S.S.; writing—original draft preparation, H.J.K. and M.S.S.; writing—review and editing, M.S.S. and S.W.P.; visualization, H.J.K., M.S.S. and S.W.P.; supervision, M.S.S. and S.W.P.; funding acquisition, M.S.S. and S.W.P. All authors have read and agreed to the published version of the manuscript.

Funding: This research was supported by a Patient-Centered Clinical Research Coordinating Center grant funded by the Ministry of Health and Welfare, Republic of Korea (HI19C0481, HC19C0276), and a Chonnam National University Hospital Biomedical Research Institute grant (BCRI23078). The funding organizations had no role in the design of this research.

Institutional Review Board Statement: This study was conducted in accordance with the Declaration of Helsinki and approved by the Institutional Review Board of Chonnam National University Hospital (CNUH-2022-441).

Informed Consent Statement: The Institutional Review Board of the Chonnam National University Hospital waived the need for informed consent, considering the use of de-identified patient data.

Data Availability Statement: The datasets used and/or analyzed during the current study are available from the corresponding author on reasonable request.

Conflicts of Interest: The authors declare no conflict of interest.

References

1. Surgucheva, I.; Park, B.-C.; Yue, B.Y.J.T.; Tomarev, S.; Surguchov, A. Interaction of myocilin with gamma-synuclein affects its secretion and aggregation. *Cell Mol. Neurobiol.* **2005**, *25*, 1009–1033. [CrossRef]
2. Quigley, H.A. Glaucoma. *Lancet Lond. Engl.* **2011**, *377*, 1367–1377. [CrossRef] [PubMed]
3. Pascolini, D.; Mariotti, S.P. Global estimates of visual impairment: 2010. *Br. J. Ophthalmol.* **2012**, *96*, 614–618. [CrossRef] [PubMed]
4. Guedes, R.A.P.; Guedes, V.M.P.; Freitas, S.M.; Chaoubah, A. Quality of Life of Medically Versus Surgically Treated Glaucoma Patients. *Eur. J. Gastroenterol. Hepatol.* **2013**, *22*, 369–373.
5. Chun, Y.S.; Sung, K.R.; Park, C.K.; Kim, H.K.; Yoo, C.; Kim, Y.Y.; Park, K.H.; Kim, C.Y.; Choi, K.; Lee, K.W.; et al. Factors influencing vision-related quality of life according to glaucoma severity. *Acta Ophthalmol.* **2019**, *97*, e216–e224. [CrossRef] [PubMed]

6. Peters, D.; Heijl, A.; Brenner, L.; Bengtsson, B. Visual impairment and vision-related quality of life in the Early Manifest Glaucoma Trial after 20 years of follow-up. *Acta Ophthalmol.* **2015**, *93*, 745–752. [CrossRef] [PubMed]
7. Murata, H.; Hirasawa, H.; Aoyama, Y.; Sugisaki, K.; Araie, M.; Mayama, C.; Aihara, M.; Asaoka, R. Identifying areas of the visual field important for quality of life in patients with glaucoma. *PLoS ONE* **2013**, *8*, e58695. [CrossRef] [PubMed]
8. Sawada, H.; Yoshino, T.; Fukuchi, T.; Abe, H. Assessment of the Vision-specific Quality of Life Using Clustered Visual Field in Glaucoma Patients. *Eur. J. Gastroenterol. Hepatol.* **2014**, *23*, 81–87. [CrossRef]
9. Takahashi, N.; Omodaka, K.; Kikawa, T.; Akiba, M.; Nakazawa, T. Association between Topographic Features of the Retinal Nerve Fiber Bundle and Good Visual Acuity in Patients with Glaucoma. *Curr. Eye Res.* **2021**, *46*, 1724–1731. [CrossRef]
10. Asaoka, R. The relationship between visual acuity and central visual field sensitivity in advanced glaucoma. *Br. J. Ophthalmol.* **2013**, *97*, 1355–1356. [CrossRef]
11. Sugisaki, K.; Inoue, T.; Yoshikawa, K.; Kanamori, A.; Yamazaki, Y.; Ishikawa, S.; Uchida, K.; Iwase, A.; Araie, M. Factors Threatening Central Visual Function of Patients with Advanced Glaucoma: A Prospective Longitudinal Observational Study. *Ophthalmology* **2022**, *129*, 488–497. [CrossRef] [PubMed]
12. Jeon, S.J.; Park, H.-Y.L.; Park, C.K. Effect of Macular Vascular Density on Central Visual Function and Macular Structure in Glaucoma Patients. *Sci. Rep.* **2018**, *8*, 16009. [CrossRef] [PubMed]
13. Hsia, Y.; Wang, T.-H.; Huang, J.-Y.; Su, C.-C. Relationship Between Macular Microvasculature and Visual Acuity in Advanced and Severe Glaucoma. *Am. J. Ophthalmol.* **2021**, *236*, 154–163. [CrossRef]
14. Song, W.K.; Kim, K.E.; Yoon, J.Y.; Lee, A.; Kook, M.S. Association of macular structure, function, and vessel density with foveal threshold in advanced glaucoma. *Sci. Rep.* **2022**, *12*, 19771. [CrossRef] [PubMed]
15. Hodapp, E.; Parrish, R.; Anderson, D.R. *Clinical Decisions in Glaucoma*, 1st ed.; C.V. Mosby: St Louis, MO, USA, 1993.
16. Bengtsson, B.; Heijl, A. False-negative responses in glaucoma perimetry: Indicators of patient performance or test reliability? *Invest. Ophthalmol. Vis. Sci.* **2000**, *41*, 2201–2204. [CrossRef]
17. Sung, M.S.M.; Ji, Y.S.M.; Heo, H.M.; Park, S.W.M. Comparison of the Structure-Function Relationship between Advanced Primary Open Angle Glaucoma and Normal Tension Glaucoma. *Eur. J. Gastroenterol. Hepatol.* **2022**, *31*, 574–583. [CrossRef]
18. Sung, M.S.; Heo, H.; Piao, H.; Guo, Y.; Park, S.W. Parapapillary atrophy and changes in the optic nerve head and posterior pole in high myopia. *Sci. Rep.* **2020**, *10*, 4607. [CrossRef]
19. Kim, Y.W.; Lee, E.J.; Kim, T.-W.; Kim, M.; Kim, H. Microstructure of β-Zone Parapapillary Atrophy and Rate of Retinal Nerve Fiber Layer Thinning in Primary Open-Angle Glaucoma. *Ophthalmology* **2014**, *121*, 1341–1349. [CrossRef]
20. Yamada, H.; Akagi, T.; Nakanishi, H.; Ikeda, H.O.; Kimura, Y.; Suda, K.; Hasegawa, T.; Yoshikawa, M.; Iida, Y.; Yoshimura, N. Microstructure of Peripapillary Atrophy and Subsequent Visual Field Progression in Treated Primary Open-Angle Glaucoma. *Ophthalmology* **2016**, *123*, 542–551. [CrossRef]
21. Lee, S.H.; Lee, E.J.; Kim, T.-W. Topographic Correlation Between Juxtapapillary Choroidal Thickness and Microstructure of Parapapillary Atrophy. *Ophthalmology* **2016**, *123*, 1965–1973. [CrossRef]
22. Sung, M.S.; Jin, H.N.; Park, S.W. Clinical Features of Advanced Glaucoma With Optic Nerve Head Prelaminar Schisis. *Am. J. Ophthalmol.* **2021**, *232*, 17–29. [CrossRef]
23. Steiger, J.H. Tests for comparing elements of a correlation matrix. *Psychol. Bull.* **1980**, *87*, 245–251. [CrossRef]
24. Weber, J.; Schultze, T.; Ulrich, H. The visual field in advanced glaucoma. *Int. Ophthalmol.* **1989**, *13*, 47–50. [CrossRef] [PubMed]
25. Kim, J.H.; Lee, H.S.; Kim, N.R.; Seong, G.J.; Kim, C.Y. Relationship Between Visual Acuity and Retinal Structures Measured by Spectral Domain Optical Coherence Tomography in Patients with Open-Angle Glaucoma. *Investig. Opthalmol. Vis. Sci.* **2014**, *55*, 4801–4810. [CrossRef] [PubMed]
26. Suzuki, Y.; Kiyosawa, M. Visual Acuity in Glaucomatous Eyes Correlates Better with Visual Field Parameters than with OCT Parameters. *Curr. Eye Res.* **2021**, *46*, 1717–1723. [CrossRef] [PubMed]
27. Baek, S.U.; Lee, W.J.; Park, K.H.; Choi, H.J. Health screening program revealed risk factors associated with development and progression of papillomacular bundle defect. *EPMA J.* **2021**, *12*, 41–55. [CrossRef]
28. Leung, C.K.S.; Guo, P.Y.; Lam, A.K.N. Retinal Nerve Fiber Layer Optical Texture Analysis: Involvement of the Papillomacular Bundle and Papillofoveal Bundle in Early Glaucoma. *Ophthalmology* **2022**, *129*, 1043–1055. [CrossRef]
29. Shao, L.; Xu, L.; Bin Wei, W.; Chen, C.X.; Du, K.F.; Li, X.P.; Yang, M.; Wang, Y.X.; You, Q.S.; Jonas, J.B. Visual Acuity and Subfoveal Choroidal Thickness: The Beijing Eye Study. *Am. J. Ophthalmol.* **2014**, *158*, 702–709.e1. [CrossRef]
30. Nishida, Y.; Fujiwara, T.; Imamura, Y.; Lima, L.H.; Kurosaka, D.; Spaide, R.F. Choroidal thickness and visual acuity in highly myopic eyes. *Retina* **2012**, *32*, 1229–1236. [CrossRef]
31. Egawa, M.; Mitamura, Y.; Niki, M.; Sano, H.; Miura, G.; Chiba, A.; Yamamoto, S.; Sonoda, S.; Sakamoto, T. Correlations between choroidal structures and visual functions in eyes with retinitis pigmentosa. *Retina* **2019**, *39*, 2399–2409. [CrossRef]
32. Cheng, H.-C.; Guo, C.-Y.; Chen, M.-J.; Ko, Y.-C.; Huang, N.; Liu, C.J.-L. Patient-Reported Vision-Related Quality of Life Differences Between Superior and Inferior Hemifield Visual Field Defects in Primary Open-Angle Glaucoma. *JAMA Ophthalmol.* **2015**, *133*, 269–275. [CrossRef] [PubMed]

Disclaimer/Publisher's Note: The statements, opinions and data contained in all publications are solely those of the individual author(s) and contributor(s) and not of MDPI and/or the editor(s). MDPI and/or the editor(s) disclaim responsibility for any injury to people or property resulting from any ideas, methods, instructions or products referred to in the content.

MDPI AG
Grosspeteranlage 5
4052 Basel
Switzerland
Tel.: +41 61 683 77 34

Journal of Clinical Medicine Editorial Office
E-mail: jcm@mdpi.com
www.mdpi.com/journal/jcm

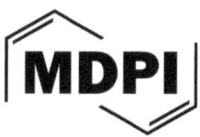

Disclaimer/Publisher's Note: The title and front matter of this reprint are at the discretion of the Guest Editor. The publisher is not responsible for their content or any associated concerns. The statements, opinions and data contained in all individual articles are solely those of the individual Editor and contributors and not of MDPI. MDPI disclaims responsibility for any injury to people or property resulting from any ideas, methods, instructions or products referred to in the content.

www.ingramcontent.com/pod-product-compliance
Lightning Source LLC
LaVergne TN
LVHW072352090526
838202LV00019B/2527